Congenital toxoplasmosis

Scientific Background, Clinical Management and Control

W0049913

Springer-Verlag France S.A.R.L

Pierre Ambroise-Thomas
Eskild Petersen (Eds)

Congenital toxoplasmosis

Scientific Background, Clinical Management
and Control

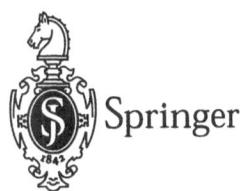
Springer

Pierre Ambroise-Thomas
Faculté de Médecine de Grenoble
Université Joseph Fourier
Grenoble - France

Peter Eskild Petersen
Statenserum Institut
Copenhagen, Denmark

Cover photo © Peter Eskild Petersen, Copenhagen, Denmark

ISBN 978-2-287-59664-3   ISBN 978-2-8178-0847-5 (eBook)
DOI 10.1007/978-2-8178-0847-5

© Springer-Verlag France 2000
Originally published by Springer-Verlag,France, Berlin, Heidelberg in 2000

Spin: 10706585

Cip requested

List of Contributors

ALEXANDER J.
Department of Immunology
University of Strathclyde
Glasgow, UK

Department of Pathobiology
School of Veterinary Medicine
University of Pennsylvania
Philadelphia, USA

AMBROISE-THOMAS P.
Department of Medical and Molecular Parasitology-Mycology
CNRS UPRES A 5082
Faculty of Medicine - Joseph Fourier University
Laboratory of Parasitic Diseases at the University Hospital
Grenoble, France

ASPÖCK H.
Abteilung für Medizinische Parasitologie
Klinisches Institut für Hygiene der Universität
Wien, Austria

BRÉZIN A.P.
Service d'ophthalmologie
Hôpital Cochin
Paris, France

BOYER K.
Rush Presbyterian St. Luke's Medical Center
Chicago, USA

BUXTON D.
Moredun Research Institute
Edinburgh, UK

CANDOLFI E.
Faculté de Médecine
Institut de Parasitologie et de Pathologie tropicale
Strasbourg, France

DEROUIN F.
Laboratory of Parasitology-Mycology
Saint-Louis Hospital
Paris, France

DOWELL M.
Departments of Medicine and Pediatrics
The University of Chicago
Chicago, USA

DUBEY J.P.
US Department of Agriculture
Livestock and Poultry Sciences Institute
Parasite Biology and Epidemiology Laboratory
BARC-East, Beltsville, USA

EATON R.
New England Newborn Screening Programme
Boston, USA

EBBESEN P.
Danish Cancer Research Foundation
Copenhagen, Denmark

FOULON W.
Department of Gynecology and Obstetrics
Academisch Ziekenhuis
Free University of Brussels, Belgium

FRENKEL J.K.
Department of Biology
University of New Mexico
Santa Fe, USA

GILBERT R.
Department of Epidemiology and Public Health
Institute of Child Health
University College London Medical School
London, UK

GROSS U.
Department of Bacteriology
University of Göttingen
Göttingen, Germany

HAYDE M.
Department of Neonatalogy & Intensive Care Medicine
University Children's Hospital of Vienna
Wien, Austria

HUNTER C.A.
Department of Pathobiology
School of Veterinary Medicine
University of Pennsylvania
Philadelphia, USA

INNES E.A.
Moredun Research Institute
Edinburgh, UK

JACQUEMARD F.
Institut de Puériculture de Paris
Service de Diagnostic Prénatal et de Médecine Foetale
Paris, France

KIJLSTRA A.
Department of Ophtalmo-Immunology
Netherlands Ophtalmic Research Institute
Amsterdam, Netherlands

LIND P.
Department of Biochemistryand Immunology
National Veterinary Laboratory
Copenhagen, Denmark

MC LEOD R.
Division of Infectious Diseases
Michael Reese Hospital and Medical Centre
Chicago, USA

NIELSEN H.V.
Laboratory of Parasitology
Statens Serum Institut
Copenhagen, Denmark

PELLOUX H.
Department of Medical and Molecular Parasitology-Mycology
Faculty of Medicine
Laboratory of Parasitic Diseases
University Hospital
Grenoble, France

PETERSEN E.
Laboratory of Parasitology
Statens Serum Institut
Copenhagen, Denmark

POLLAK A.
Department of Pediatrics
University Children's Hospital of Vienna
Wien, Austria

REICHMANN G.
Department of Pathobiology
School of Veterinary Medicine
University of Pennsylvania
Philadelphia, USA

Institute for Medical Microbiology & Virology
Heinrich-Heine University
Düsseldorf, Germany

ROBERTS C.W.
Department of Immunology
University of Strathclyde
Glasgow, UK

ROMAND S.
Institut de Puériculture
Paris, France

ROTHOVA A.
Department of Ophtalmo-Immunology
Netherlands Ophtalmic Research Institute
Amsterdam, Netherlands

STANFORD M.
The Rayne Institute St Thomas' Hospital
London, UK

STRAY-PEDERSEN B.
Department of Obstetrics and Gynecology
Rikshospitalet
Oslo, Norway

THULLIEZ P.
Laboratory of Toxoplasmosis
Institut de Puériculture
Paris, France

WALKER W.
Department of Pathobiology
School of Veterinary Medicine
University of Pennsylvania
Philadelphia, USA

Contents

1.1. Congenital toxoplasmosis: past, present and future

P. Ambroise-Thomas, E. Petersen

Toxoplasmosis is the first infection of the TORCH complex (Toxoplasmosis, Rubella, Cytomegalovirus and Herpes simplex) and one of the most important congenital diseases. Consideration is too often limited to the cases of very severe toxoplasmosis with numerous and spectacular symptoms at birth, such as hydrocephalus, neurological disorders and ocular involvement, which lead to major handicaps. However, the frequency of attenuated, asymptomatic or poorly symptomatic congenital toxoplasmosis is often disregarded. The asymptomatic infections may give rise to very late reactivation, which sometimes occurs in puberty or even adulthood. The reactivation of unrecognised congenital toxoplasmosis is sometimes accompanied with neurological disorders, and is a common cause of retinochoroiditis. The retinochoroiditis can be very disabling and the majority cases of retinochoroiditis in young adults are thought to be secondary to untreated congenital toxoplasmosis. This is the most severe medical and socio-economical consequence of congenital toxoplasmosis and is the reason behind the pre- and neonatal screening programmes.

The screening and prevention of congenital toxoplasmosis is difficult despite advances over the last decades in our understanding of the disease and in the diagnostic tools available.

This book presents our present knowledge on congenital *Toxoplasma* infection and highlights current problems in managing the disease from both the clinical and public health point of view.

Congenital toxoplasmosis is a relatively rare disease and advances can mainly be obtained through multicentre studies, with a careful interpretation of data corresponding to different epidemiological situations, to avoid erroneous conclusion from a too general overview . One attempt to obtain new insight into the disease has been a European Union funded research programme " The European Research Network on Congenital Toxoplasmosis ", which includes forty specialised centres in fourteen different European countries and was created in 1993 [1], and some of its major results are presented in this book.

Previous fundamental research

The complete life cycle of *Toxoplasma gondii* was finally found in the early seventies. It established the cat as the final host and the importance of oocysts shed by infected cats as a major reservoir for transmission of the infection to humans.

The source of infection by herbivores, unexplained so far, could then be accounted for. At the same time, it became possible for physicians to supplement the prophylactic precautions and recommendations given in order to avoid primary infection during pregnancy [2, 3].

In the following years, the level of our knowledge mainly increased in cellular biology, immunology and molecular biology. It should be noted that most advances have been made possible when cases of *Toxoplasma*-encephalitis occurred in patients with AIDS, in the early eighties [4]. Because they are frequent and extremely severe, these forms of toxoplasmosis in HIV-infected patients have been studied in vast research programmes. It has thus been possible to learn more about both the biology of *Toxoplasma* in the host cell and the different intra- and extracellular messengers, more particularly cytokines, which control these interrelations and are involved in the tachyzoite-bradyzoite interconversions.

Some of the discoveries gave rise to expectations for future new therapies, like the use of interferon-γ (IFNγ) to prevent the reactivation of quiescent chronic toxoplasmosis which unfortunately did not not prove valuable in the clinical situation.

The genotype of some *Toxoplasma gondii* strains has been characterized allowing a typing of isolates in virulent and avirulent isolates [5]. It was expected that this would be an important element of prognosis in human disease, in the assessment, for example, of the risk of mother-to-foetus transmission or late recurrence or reactivation of latent congenital toxoplasmosis. Unfortunately, these hopes have not been confirmed because the experimental results obtained on mice cannot be transposed to humans [6].

The evolution of diagnostic methods

Until the early sixties, the only really precise method was the Sabin-Feldman dye test which was first developed in 1948. Since live Toxoplasma was required, it was difficult to perform, and was only used in a small number of laboratories, probably not more than ten or twelve all over Europe. *Toxoplasma*-serology was therefore concentrated in a few highly-specialised laboratories, and each of them performed a limited number of tests.

The introduction of indirect immunofluorescence (IF) in the sixties was a real breakthrough. Detection of Toxoplasma-specific antibodies became within all hospitals and most private laboratories reach. Programmes of routine serologic screening became possible and were launched in some European countries, as in France and Austria [7-11]. In addition, both IF and the dye test make use of somatic antigens, preferably surface antigens, composed of whole organisms. This is one of the reasons why IF results can almost be superimposed on those of the dye test, so that result interpretation was easier right from the start. After *Toxoplasma* infection by both techniques remain positive for life and are therefore used to verify the acquired immunity of patients already infected at some time in their lives.

The serological assays were further refined with the establishment of the first international serum reference by the WHO, which defined an international unit of total antibody reactivity against *Toxoplasma gondii* in International Units [12].

In the past twenty years the development of diagnostic tools has concentrated on the Enzyme-Linked Immuno-Sorbent-Assay (EIA, ELISA) and direct EIA of specific IgG-antibodies and immunocapture tests of specific IgM-antibodies have become ever more refined.

Other procedures, such as Enzyme-Linked Immuno-Filtration Assay (ELIFA) or Western-blot, have allowed the comparison of the mother and child serologic profiles, with the detection of newly synthesised antibodies in case of congenital toxoplasmosis. More recently, the IgG avidity test, used to determine the time of infection, has been another contribution to the arsenal of diagnostic assays [13].

The use of well defined recombinant antigens in diagnosis has just begun, and the first antigen to be used was the dominant surface antigen the SAG1 (P30), but the place in clinical use of such assays has not yet been defined.

In addition to the improvement of both techniques and reagents, new biological samples became available with the advances in ultrasonography which made cordocentesis possible and analysis of foetal blood samples for *Toxoplasma*-specific antibodies. The procedure implied a too high rate of foetal losses and has now been replaced by direct detection of *Toxoplasma*-specific DNA in amniotic fluid [14].

The Polymerase Chain Reaction (PCR) which amplifies a small amount of specific DNA was also applied in the early nineties to the diagnosis of acute infection with *Toxoplasma gondii* [15-17] and found its place in diagnosis of foetal infection, where the presence of *Toxoplasma*-DNA in amniotic fluid is taken as a certain sign of maternal-foetal transmission.

However, progress made in the medical field has not been restricted to biology. Over the last decades, medical imaging has also seen spectacular advances, which have undeniably been beneficial to the diagnosis of congenital toxoplasmosis. The classical cranial X-rays examination used to diagnose intracerebral calcifications has been replaced by CT-scan and ultrasonography which give much more informative results. In particular, the contribution of ultrasonography should be emphasised, mainly in the prenatal diagnosis of severe foetal malformations that may lead to the decision of induced abortion.

Epidemiology and public health

Although no firm data are available, the severe forms of congenital toxoplasmosis seem to be considerably rarer than they used to be years ago, at least in some countries. It is not known to what extent it is a result of prenatal screening and prevention efforts. On the whole, there is no doubt that our knowledge remains limited.

In the field of epidemiology, the age-specific seroprevalence is not known in detail in most countries. It is known to be variable and sometimes very different from one country to another, or even from one region to another, although the reasons for these differences are barely known [18, 19]. No data exists either on the importance of the different sources of transmission: sporulated oocysts from cat faeces or by ingestion of undercooked infected meat.

The exact prevalence of congenital toxoplasmosis is not known in most countries, and no precise figures are available on the frequency of not only symptomatic toxoplasmosis but mainly of asymptomatic congenital toxoplasmosis which is revealed only by serology and which may result in delayed complications. The frequency, the time delay and the circumstances under which such complications occur are also unknown. It is true that these epidemiological data are probably the most difficult to collect since they require a very strict and very long (for over 15 years, sometimes) follow-up of the offsprings in whom asymptomatic congenital toxoplasmosis has been detected at birth.

Problems for the future

In a pregnant woman, it is possible to precisely detect acquired immunity, resulting from primary *Toxoplasma* infection. Recently-acquired toxoplasmosis can also be diagnosed with a high degree of accuracy, even though this requires the simultaneous use of several serologic tests, each of them providing different, yet complementary data.

On the contrary, determination of the time of maternal toxoplasmic infection in relation to the beginning of pregnancy remains quite inaccurate and speculative in many cases. Yet, this element is essential to evaluate the risk of toxoplasmic transmission from mother to foetus.The factors enhancing or, on the contrary, limiting transplacental transmission are still poorly known, as whether the origin of these factors is in the placenta, the immunity system or the parasite, with perhaps specific transmissibility for some toxoplasmic strains.

It is indisputable that prenatal diagnosis performed on the foetus has been much improved thanks to PCR on amniotic fluid. However, it cannot be performed during the first twelve weeks of pregnancy for practical reasons, and even after the third month, it is often uncertain. The same is true, but much less frequently, for the serologic diagnosis at birth, despite progress made thanks to the use of procedures such as Western-blot or detection of newly-synthesised antibodies. For this reason in many cases, the diagnosis of congenital toxoplasmosis can only be confirmed by a serologic follow-up at regular intervals during the first twelve months of life [20].

Treatment

Therapeutic tools have not improved as much as our diagnostic tools, and remain quite limited. If some therapeutic problems are almost solved, others are only partly solved. These concern mainly the best therapeutic regimen to be initiated in order to : 1) avoid mother-to-foetus transmission ; 2) treat a foetus already infected ; 3) complete the results of the first parasiticidal therapy by an appropriate maintenance therapy (nature and mainly duration ?), and 4) treat asymptomatic clinical toxoplasmosis immediately after birth to prevent the risks of recurrences or late complications, such as retinochoroiditis or central nervous system involvement. Thus, no drugs active against *Toxoplasma* cysts, and therefore able to prevent reactivation of quiescent toxoplasmosis are available. But above all, due to the shortcomings of our diagnostic tools, it is often not possible to precisely determine the cases where the prescription of antiparasitic drugs would be justified, even though these drugs are not devoid of serious adverse side effects [21].

The situation is difficult because physicians avoid therapy potentially dangerous for the foetus because they are concerned about side effects of the drugs prescribed during pregnancy. With no drugs available which are both effective and safe, and with often no possibility to evaluate the potential benefits of treatment, the decision to treat is often empirical and primarily guided by the concern for " *primum non nocere* ". In concrete terms, this is what happens when serology findings reveal that maternal infection has occurred probably or certainly during pregnancy. Transplacental transmission is not systematic and the frequency of transmission varying with the gestational age at the time of maternal infection. The consequences on the foetus also vary widely. In such circumstances, which is often encountered in daily practice, there is no mainstay for the prescription of a very active but potentially toxic drug. Doing nothing when a potential risk exists is, of course, not acceptable. Under such conditions, the solution frequently used in some countries consists of prescribing spiramycin, which is known to concentrate in placenta, to have no toxicity for the foetus, but to have only a moderate anti-toxoplasmic action. It is very difficult to assess to what extent this treatment of the mother reduces the transmission to the foetus ; however it is active in the foetus and alleviates the consequences of transmission to the same.

Priorities for the future

It is always risky to speculate on the future. Ten years ago nobody would have imagined what molecular biology could bring to toxoplasmosis. Conversely, five years ago, most authors would greatly have overevaluated the progress that molecular biology could permit. Yet, in the years to come, several major advances will probably be achieved, their seeds being already present in today's results.

After that of *Plasmodium falciparum*, the genomic structure of *Toxoplasma gondii* will probably be known in the next few years. The advances resulting from this knowledge will certainly be important, although they remain difficult to assess. The genotyping of *Toxoplasma gondii* strains and better knowledge of the cellular and molecular biology of the parasite should explain several aspects of the epidemiology and pathophysiology of congenital toxoplasmosis: the factors involved in mother-to-foetus transmission, as well as the mechanisms involved in tachyzoite-bradyzoite interconversion and in reactivation of quiescent toxoplasmosis. In parallel, these scientific gains will undoubtedly give more chances to targeted pharmacological researches.

The serologic procedures will certainly become more accurate, primarily thanks to more specific reagents, particularly antigens. However, serology gives only indirect evidence and results, which obviously vary from one individual to another. Whatever the extent of progress, these techniques will then probably come close to the limits of their possibilities.

Molecular biology, using PCR or other techniques which are still experimental, will presumably allow major advances in diagnosis, but these cannot be evaluated yet.

In fact, the main problem with congenital toxoplasmosis today is that prevention is not satisfactory for different reasons. Prevention is limited to the serologic screening for evidence of past infection, to recommendations given to seronegative pregnant women, and to pre- and perinatal diagnoses and treatments, their efficacy being often uncertain [22-30]. The only really effective measures would be the disappearance of the sources of infection, or protection against infection. The vaccines currently under study or already used in veterinary medicine should bring this contribution to human medicine.

References

1. Petersen E, Ambroise-Thomas P, Foulon W et al (1994) Congenital toxoplasmosis. The European Research Network on Congenital Toxoplasmosis. A concerted action under the EU research programm Biomed. J Obst Gynecol 14 (Suppl 2):112-117
2. Frenkel JK (1990) Diagnosis, incidence and prevention of congenital toxoplasmosis. Am J Dis Child 144:956-958
3. Newton LH, Hall SM (1995) A survey of health education material for the primary prevention of congenital toxoplasmosis. Commun Dis Rep CDR Rev 5:R21-R27
4. Ambroise-Thomas P, Pelloux H (1993) Toxoplasmosis congenital and in immuno-compromised patients. A parallel. Parasitol Today 9:61-63
5. Cristina N, Darde ML, Boudin C et al (1995) A DNA finger-printing method for individual characterization of *Toxoplasma gondii* strains: combination with isoenzymatic characters for determination of linkage groups. Parasitol Res 81:32-37
6. Frenkel JK, Ambroise-Thomas P (1997) Genomic drift of *Toxoplasma gondii*. Parasitol Res 23:1249-1254
7. Ancelle T, Goulet V, Tirard-Fleury V et al (1996) La toxoplasmose chez la femme enceinte en France en 1995. BEH 51:227-229
8. Aspock H, Pollak A (1992) Prevention of prenatal toxoplasmosis by serological screening of pregnant women in Austria. Scand J Infect Dis (Suppl) 84:32-37
9. Bourget P, Lesne-Hulin A, Forestier F et al (1996) Prévention de la Toxoplasmose congénitale par la spiramycine: valeur et limites des concentrations dans le liquide amniotique. Therapie 51:685-687
10. Daffos F, Forestier F, Capella-Pavlovski M et al (1988) Prenatal management of 746 pregnancies at risk for congenital toxoplasmosis. N Engl J Med 318:271-275
11. Desmonts G, Daffos F, Forestier F et al (1985) Prenatal diagnosis of congenital toxoplamosis. Lancet 1:500-504
12. Petithory JC, Ambroise-Thomas P, de Loye J et al (1996) Sero-diagnostic de la toxoplasmose. Etude comparative multicentrique d'une gamme étalon par les différents tests actuels et avec expression des résultats en Unités Internationales. Bull OMS 74:291-298

13. Pelloux H, Brun E, Vernet G et al (1998) Determination of anti-*Toxoplasma gondii* immuno-globulin G avidity: application to the Vidas system. Diagn Microbiol Infect Dis 32:69-73
14. Fricker-Hidalgo H, Pelloux H, Muet F et al (1997) Prenatal diagnosis of congenital toxoplas-mosis: comparative value of fetal blood and amniotic fluid using serological technics. Pren Diagn 17:831-885
15. Guy EC, Pelloux H, Lappalainen M et al (1996) Interlaboratory comparison of Polymerase Chain Reaction for the detection of *Toxoplasma gondii* DNA added to samples of amniotic fluids. Eur J Clin Microbiol Infect Dis 15:36-839
16. Pelloux H, Weiss J, Simon J et al (1996) A new set of primers for the detection of *Toxoplasma gondii* in amniotic fluid using polymerase chain reaction. FEMS Microbiol Lett 138:1-15
17. Pelloux H, Guy E, Angelici MC et al (1998) A second european collaborative study on polyme-rase chain reaction for *Toxoplasma gondii*, involving 15 teams. FEMS Microbiol Lett 165:231-237
18. Contreras M, Schenone H, Salinas P et al (1996) Seroepidemiology of human toxoplasmosis in Chile. Rev Inst Med Trop Sao Paulo 38:431-435
19. Jenum PA, Stray-Pedersen B, Melby KK et al (1998) Incidence of *Toxoplasma gondii* infection in 35,940 pregnant women in Norway and pregnancy outcome for infected women. J Clin Microbiol 36:2900-2906
20. Fricker-Hidalgo H, Pelloux H, Bost M et al (1996) Toxoplasmose congénitale : apport du suivi biologique post-natal. Presse Méd 25:1868-1872
21. McAuley J, Boyer KM, Patel D et al (1994) Early and longitudinal evaluation of treated infants and children and untreated historical patients with congenital toxoplamosis:the Chicago col-laborative treatment trial. Clin Infect Dis 18:38-72
22. Foulon W, Naessens A, Lauwers S et al (1988) Impact of primary prevention on the incidence of toxoplasmosis during pregnancy. Obst Gynecol 72:363-366
23. Foulon W (1992) Congenital toxoplasmosis: is screening desirable? Scand J Infect Dis (Suppl) 84:11-17
24. Foulon W, Naessens A, Derde MP (1994) Evaluation of the possibilities for preventing conge-nital toxoplasmosis. Am J Perinatol 11:57-62
25. Guerina NG, Hsy HW, Meissner C et al (1994) Neonatal serologic screening and early treat-ment for congenital *Toxoplasma gondii* infection. N Engl J Med 330:1858-1863
26. Hohlfeld P, Biedermann K, Extermann P et al (1995) Toxoplasmose pendant la grossesse : pré-vention, diagnostic prénatal et traitement. Schweiz Med Wochenschr (Suppl), 65:62S-69S
27. Holliman RE (1995) Congenital toxoplasmosis: prevention, screening and treatment. J Hosp Infect 30:179-190
28. Lappalainen M, Sintonen H, Koskiniemi M et al (1995) Cost-benefit analysis of screening for toxoplasmosis during pregnancy. Scand J Infect Dis 27:265-272
29. Szenasi Z, Ozsvar Z, Nagy E et al (1997) Prevention of congenital toxoplasmosis in Szeged, Hungary. Int J Epidemiol 26:428-435
30. Wallon M, Mallaret MR, Mojon M et al (1994) Toxoplasmose congénitale, évaluation de la pré-vention. Presse Méd 23:1467-1470

1.2. Biology of *Toxoplasma gondii*

J.K. FRENKEL

Life cycle of *Toxoplasma*

Toxoplasma is a protozoan of the phylum Apicomplexa [1], the term referring to the apical complex of the cytoskeleton of this organism, also present, for example, in the Coccidia and the sporozoites of the malaria organisms. There are 2 stages of *Toxoplasma* which are encountered in human patients, other mammalian and avian hosts: tachyzoites and bradyzoites (Fig. 1) [2]. I will describe a variety of features of *Toxoplasma* that may confront clinicians in relation to *Toxoplasma* and the infection and disease it produces, and refer to scientific sources and more detailed information in the references. Because *Toxoplasma gondii* is the only species in the genus, I will refer to it simply by genus rather than using the binomial.

Tachyzoites are the rapidly multiplying forms of *Toxoplasma*, which account for most cytopathology, and tissue destruction. Tachyzoites grow only intracellularly (Fig. 1), in many types, of nucleated cells, dividing by a sequential division in two (endodyogeny) within a parasitophorous vacuole [3], which ultimately harbors 8-32 tachyzoites by the time the cell bursts. Different cells of different hosts vary in their capacity to support tachyzoite multiplication and in supporting different division times, often every 4-6 hours. Tachyzoites measure about 2-3 x 6-7µm, with the size of intracellular groups of tachyzoites depending largely on the capacity of the host cell cytoplasm to support them. Penetration of the host cell [4] and the formation of the parasitophorous vacuole [3] have been the subject of several studies. When tachyzoites are set free after death of the host cell, they enter other cells and resume rapid multiplication. With the development of antibodies and cellular immunity, tachyzoite multiplication decreases and another stage, bradyzoites, become progressively more numerous.

Bradyzoites are slowly multiplying organisms, of slightly smaller size, which characteristically continue to live with their host cells for months or years. Cysts with infectious bradyzoites can be regarded as essential resting stages, waiting to be ingested by another host. Bradyzoites are usually acid-pepsin resistant, although this is being re-investigated [5]; the occasional finding of survival of tachyzoites in acid pepsin could be due to a technical error, such as occasional autodigestion of pepsin or overloading the system.

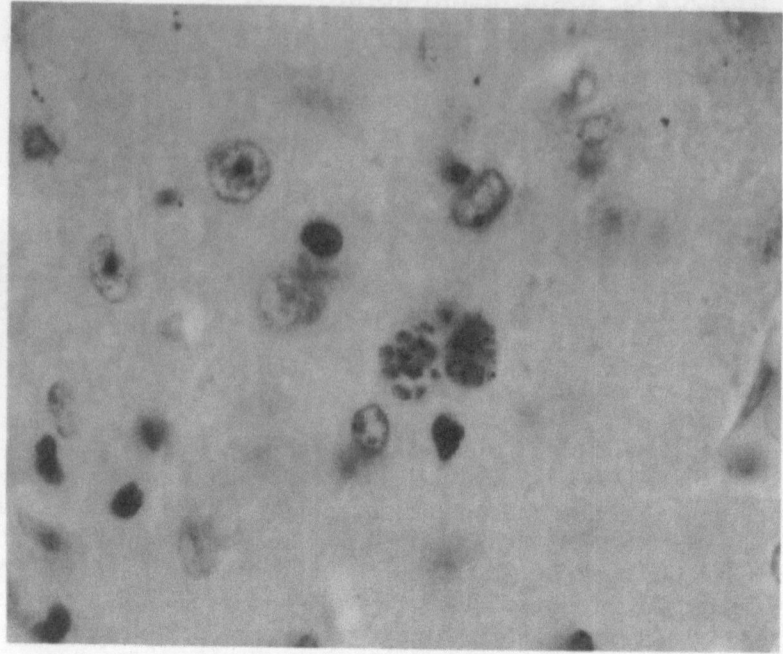

Fig. 1. Comparison of loosely-grouped tachyzoites (*left*) and a young tissue cyst (*right*) with densely packed bradyzoites of *Toxoplasma gondii* in brain of mouse after 2 weeks infection. The glycogen-like amylopectin in bradyzoites, stained with PASH, adds a dense hue to the cyst contents. Periodic acid Schiff (PASH), hematoxylin and eosin, x 1000

Bradyzoites accumulate amylopectin, a variety of glycogen, in their cytoplasm staining red with leukofuchsin after oxidation in periodic acid (PAS positive), which serves as energy source for the invasion of cells [6]. Cysts are surrounded by a thickened parasitophorous membrane, the cyst wall, which has been shown to resist pressure, tearing with jagged edges [7], is weakly PAS-positive and impregnates with several silver methods (Fig. 1).

Bradyzoites in cysts are generally the only stage found late during infection when some immunity is present in the host. However, cysts also form in cultured cells [8, 9]. When cysts disintegrate in the immune host, the bradyzoites are generally killed [10]; nevertheless they may give rise to focal necrosis, interpreted as resulting from delayed type of hypersensitivity. Conversely, in humans with AIDS, or in patients treated with corticosteroids, or in other immunodepressed states, bradyzoites transform into tachyzoites resuming active multiplication [11, 7].

Limited role of bradyzoites in transmission by carnivorism

Bradyzoites in cyst are transmissible by carnivorism, probably explaining how carnivores and omnivores become infected. Tachyzoites account for infection of the human placenta and for transmission to the fetus. However, after the development of serologic tests it became apparent from serologic surveys of animals, verified by subinoculation of their tissues, that many herbivores and humans who were strict vegetarians were *Toxoplasma*-infected, and it remained a mystery for many years how these become infected.

How to explain infection in herbivores?

The many mammalian and avian species studied harbored tissue cysts with bradyzoites in their tissues, whereas immediately after subinoculation into mice, hamsters or other experimental animals, showed proliferative tachyzoites. These tachyzoites are disseminated in the blood stream and via lymphatics. Attempts to transmit tachyzoites by hematophagous arthropods were negative [12, 13]. Animals with early infections, harboring only or mainly tachyzoites, were not regularly infectious by feeding their tissue, however animals with chronic infections, with bradyzoites in their brain and muscles regularly transmitted *Toxoplasma* to animals to whom they were fed.

Against this background, William Hutchison about 1965, fed some chronically infected mice to 2 cats and found that cat feces transmitted *Toxoplasma* [14-16]. This started the search for the morphology of *Toxoplasma* in cat feces. At first, eggs of the common cat nematode, *Toxocara cati*, were suspected to contain *Toxoplasma* [13] which was seemingly confirmed by a number of investigations. These eggs were indeed prominently present in cat feces that were purified by flotation in density gradients. However, more detailed coproscopic analysis revealed smaller 10 x 12μm cystic structures which divided and developed 8 elongate bodies which turned out to be the carrier of *Toxoplasma* infectivity [17-19] (Fig. 2).

Sporozoites in oocysts from cats

Sporozoites in oocysts from cats are shed containing a single cytoplasmic mass, the sporont, which at ambient temperature and under aerobic conditions divides into 2 sporoblasts, each of which becomes enclosed by a sporocyst wall, and subsequently develops 4 slender sporozoites in each sporocyst, or 8 sporozoites per oocyst. These sporozoites become infectious about 3-5 days after they are shed (Fig. 3).

Verification that infectivity resides in oocysts/sporozoites

Infectivity was titrated in laboratory mice, and correlated with oocyst numbers in sucrose density gradient and electrophoresis gradient fractions, and in filtrates through graded-size filters. Infectivity could also be recovered from cats that had been de-wormed, excluding a role of cat nematodes in transmission, as had been previously postulated [17, 18, 20].

Behavior of *Toxoplasma* in its hosts

Toxoplasmosis in cats

Cats will shed 10^6-10^8 of oocysts after first infection, mainly from eating chronically infected birds and rodents [21, 22]. Re-infection is rarely followed by re-shedding of oocysts because of developing immunity and this observation was the conceptual prerequisite for the development of a vaccine [23, 24].

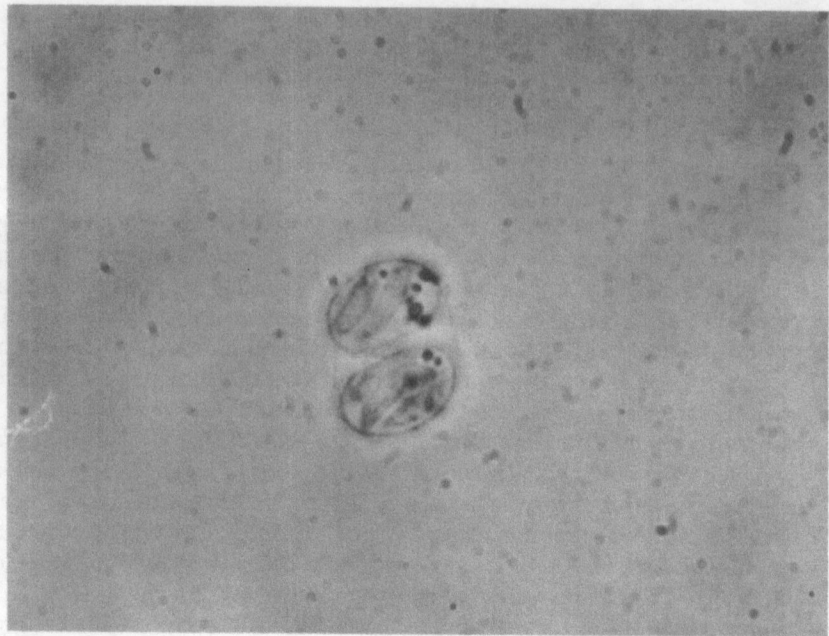

Fig. 2. Sporulated oocyst of *Toxoplasma gondii*, slightly flattened to show individual sporo-zoites in the 2 sporocysts. The oocyst wall is very delicate after exposure to 6% sodium hypo-chlorite, and encloses the 2 sporocysts. There are 4 elongate sporozoites in each sporocyst but only 2 or 3 are shown in the optical section. Several refractive granules are also present in sporocysts. Following density gradient washing, a few fecal bacteria are still floating in the surrounding water. Unstained, X 1600. [20]

However, passively transferred maternal antibody in newborn kittens does not inhibit infection by bradyzoites, followed by oocysts shedding, because such kittens usually give rise to millions of oocyst, starting 3-5 days and continuing for 10-20 days [21].

Not only domestic cats, but various members of the family of Felidae will shed oocysts as shown by experimental infections [25, 26], and from serologic tests [27]. At least 17 species of wild cats that been reported to shed oocysts of *Toxoplasma* [28].

Adult cats usually survive primary *Toxoplasma* infection, generally with minimal symptoms, or even cellular responses [29]; however, kittens often succumb to infection, and newborn kittens have been used to study the deve-lopmental stages in the intestine preceding oocyst formation [30].

Definitive and intermediate hosts of Toxoplasma

Felidae which harbor tachyzoites and bradyzoites and that produce *Toxoplasma* oocyst, after sexual conjugation, are called *complete, definitive,* or *primary hosts.* Humans, other non-feline mammalian hosts, and birds develop only tachyzoites and bradyzoites, and are called *incomplete, intermediate,* or *secondary hosts*. Figure 3 shows the *Toxoplasma* life cycle in relation to the host and the infectious function of the stages and Figure 4 the direct, indirect and transplacental means of transmission.

LIFE CYCLE OF TOXOPLASMA

Fig. 3. Life cycle of *Toxoplasma gondii*. The 3 cats, above, are the definitive hosts in which the enteroepithelial cycle takes place, culminating in the shedding of oocysts. The sporulation time to the oocysts becoming infectious is shown as 3-4 days under aerobic conditions, but may be delayed under microaerophilic circumstances. The pre-patent periods from ingestion of infected tissue from an intermediate host, symbolized by the mice, to shedding of oocysts varies according to the stage of *Toxoplasma* ingested. Minimal pre-patent periods are 3-6 days after ingestion of many bradyzoites (in tissue cysts), 4-10 days after ingestion of a few bradyzoites, and 21-40 days after the ingestion of either sporozoites (in oocysts) or tachyzoites. During the first 3-6 weeks of infection, tachyzoites give rise to a generalized infection in the cat leading eventually to formation of bradyzoites in tissue cysts, which in turn initiate the enteroepithelial cycle in the same cat.

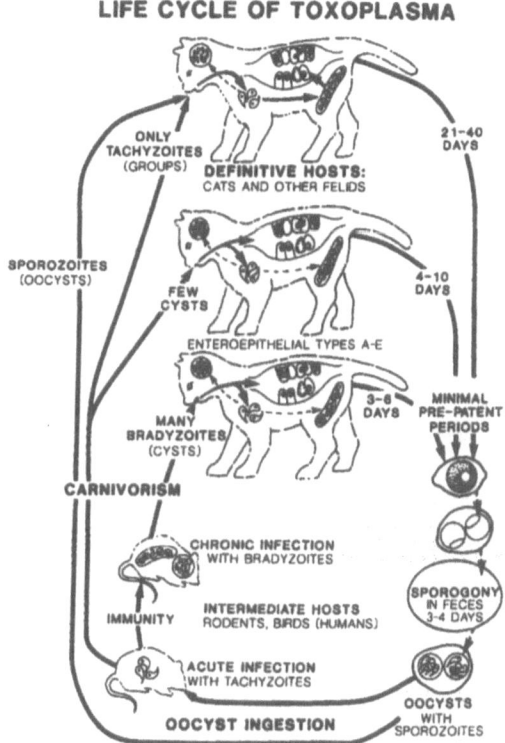

Infectivity of oocysts and disinfection

Oocyst infectivity

Oocyst infectivity starts after sporulation and, based on experience in Kansas, USA, with hot summers and freezing winters, and in Costa Rica with a more equitable climate, infectious titers persist for months to over a year; 548 days was the longest survival time we recorded in slightly moist soil or sand, in which cats deposit their feces, or cover their feces with [31, 32]. In an area where cats, and especially non-immune kittens are prevalent, all soil should be considered contaminated, because of the frequency of new litters, the millions of oocysts shed [21] and chances for repeated contamination during the period of oocyst viability [33].

Disinfection of oocysts

Infectivity of oocyst is impaired after heating and storage at 30C [34] and is abolished by heating to 60° C-70° C for 1-2 min, or by boiling which would be necessary to inactivate accompanying fecal organisms. Because of the high degree of impermeability of the oocysts, they are routinely maintained either in 2% sulfuric acid or in 2% potassium dichromate [30, 35]. Chemical disinfection is difficult. Liquid ammonia, 35%, was better than 7% tincture of iodine; household ammonia, containing 4.6-5.5% ammonia killed oocysts in 3 hours [22]. Sodium hypochloride (bleach) is ineffective after several hours, and proprietary disinfectants used in the hospital are likely to be ineffective [36]. Bradyzoites in tissue cysts are killed safely by 70° C.

Transmission mechanisms of Toxoplasma

Oral transmission by meat and contamination with cat feces

Ingestion appears to accounts for practically all infections (Fig. 4). Tissue cysts from meat and of oocysts from cat fecally-contaminated soil statistically account for all population infections, such as of women who are or may be pregnant. In Europe and the USA, infection by meat are probably more important, and in Latin America, oocyst-related transmission, except for where churrasco is eaten.

Blood-borne, placental transmission

Blood-borne, placental transmission of tachyzoites gives rise to placental and fetal infection (Fig. 4), even though the maternal infection may have been asymptomatic. Because of the short duration of hematogenous dissemination, transmission by blood transfusion is very unlikely. This, and the following are rare events of clinical, but not epidemiological, importance.

Transplantation transmission

Transplantation transmission has occurred mainly after heart transplants, but also transplants of kidneys and other tissues. The frequency of these events is dependent on the prevalence of chronic latent Toxoplasma infection in the donor population, and the inverse, the prevalence of susceptible, non-immune individuals in the recipient population, modified by the likelihood of infectedness of the donor organ with bradyzoites (heart > kidney). Although primary infection in immunocompetent humans is usually subclinical, because organ transplant recipients are immunosuppressed they are more often subject to illness and even death [37-42].

These are occurrences preventable by serologic screening of donor and recipient, and in case of failure, early diagnosis in the recipient by PCR and mitigation by chemotherapy [43].

Pathogenicity of Toxoplasma

Toxoplasma "virulence"

Virulence refers to a pathogenic microbial quality, often known to be the expression of a gene, which is observed relatively consistently against all hosts or cells. An example could be the virulence of toxigenic

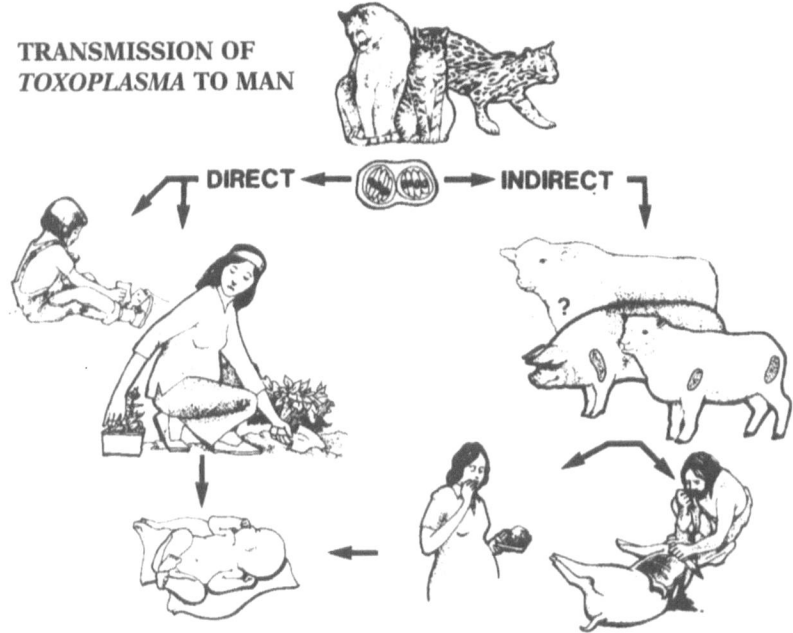

Fig. 4. Transmission of *Toxoplasma gondii* to humans. Domestic, feral and 17+ species of wild cats shed the oocysts after ingestion of any stage of *Toxoplasma*, as shown in Fig. 7. Humans can become infected *directly* by ingesting oocysts from cat feces-contaminated soil, fur of dogs, or food contaminated directly or by flies or cockroaches. Humans can also become infected *indirectly* from the raw or incompletely cooked meat of herbivores, that at times ingest oocyst-contaminated soil when grazing. Transplacental transmission occurs in up to 40% of women, who became infected during their pregnancy, and rarely in immunosuppressed women with chronic, latent *Toxaplasma* infection

Corynebacterium diphtheriae, from which even a soluble toxin can be isolated. The presence of toxicity is sometimes mistakenly inferred by some, from the name *Toxoplasma*, which however, is derived from toxon (Greek), referring to the bowed shape of the organism, not to toxicon (Greek) for toxin.

Firstly, there is no soluble toxin in *Toxoplasma* proper, such reports can be attributed to tissue breakdown products. Secondly, one might ask is there a consistent pathogenic microbial quality? I think not. Some might think from the behavior of *Toxoplasma* in laboratory animals that there was. However, we have a tendency to work with *Toxoplasma* – host combinations in which effects are clearly evident; hence a preponderance of studies where infection leads to disease or is fatal.

Toxoplasma isolates

Toxoplasma isolates from chronically infected wild mice in nature were generally (90%) non-pathogenic on first passage to laboratory mice [44]. Similar observations were made on isolates from wild birds [45]. In order to initiate passages of such isolates in the laboratory, it is often required that mice are immunosuppressed with corticosteroids to provide time for the tachyzoites to become plentiful in the peritoneum. With time, after many passage as tachyzoites, they became more pathogenic, and killed mice after shorter and shorter intervals.

It would appear, therefore, more meaningful to speak of the **pathogenicity**, rather than of virulence. This pathogenicity is not widely applicable to mice or birds from which *Toxoplasma* was isolated, neither to rats, chickens, cats, or to man, considering the prevalent asymptomatic infections.

A well-adapted parasite

To the contrary, *Toxoplasma* is an example of a well-adapted parasite which can survive in most hosts. It is probable that many hosts which normally come in contact with *Toxoplasma* are selected for resistance, if they were not already resistant genetically.

Toxoplasma infection in rats is a good example [46]. Infections in most animals in nature are diagnosed as chronic, latent infections [47-53, 44, 45]. This does not exclude that some animals are killed, and not found; we see only the survivors. Very young animals of many species are killed by infections that older animals can resist by developing a timely immunity. Even very young rats are killed by *Toxoplasma* infection; however, rats started to survive by 23 days of age [54].

A few exceptions

Fatal epidemics of acute toxoplasmosis are known from European hares, *Lepus europeus* [55], more severe in the winter, suggesting that hares ate cat feces more frequently in the winter, when their normal plant diet tends to be covered by snow. It also suggests that they have not been selected for resistance by *Toxoplasma*. A fatal outbreak of toxoplasmosis has been described from carrier pigeons in Panama [56]. However, chickens in general are pretty resistant [57-59]. Other fatal outbreaks occurred in South American chinchillas which were bred in captivity in the USA [60] in Hyrax in several zoos [61], where it can be suspected that these mountain dwellers do not in their normal habitat became in contact with *Toxoplasma*, and have not been selected. Most of these animals were exposed to *Toxoplasma* in an artificial environment. There are a number of sporadic observations as in a manatee [62] normally a herbivore, who may have become infected from contaminated water. Of course, Australian marsupials and Madagascan lemurs are highly susceptible to the pathogenic effects of *Toxoplasma* infection; they are from localities where cats were absent prior to being introduced by British seafarers about the end of the 18th century [63] and marsupials and lemurs have not been selected for resistance in the interval.

Gondis

Gondis are wild rodents from South Tunisia in North Africa; they were used for leishmaniasis and typhus research in the Pasteur Institute of Tunisia and in which *Toxoplasma* was first found by Nicolle and Manceaux [64]. These animals are severely affected by toxoplasmic infection, and even show

Toxoplasma tachyzoites in their bloodstream during primary, fatal infection according to Ambroise-Thomas and Pelloux [65]; probably one of the few mammals in which infection can be diagnosed regularly from a blood smear. Gondis were not infected in nature [66], but were infected in the laboratory probably from cats that used to be kept in animal colonies to catch escaped mice; actually, Nicolle was pictured with his cat in the laboratory.

Mutations in *Toxoplasma* and selection by hosts

Loss of oocyst-formation

When investigating the supposed nematode transmission of *Toxoplasma* [14], we found that 3 lines of *Toxoplasma*, RH, Beverley and AJH did not produce fecal infectivity in cats but a fourth one, M-7741, did [67]. The first 3 lines of *Toxoplasma* had been passaged as tachyzoites in mice twice a week, but the latter was maintained as chronic infection in tissue cysts. Hence, we set out to study how stable oocyst formation was when M-7741 was passaged in the tachyzoite stage.

Tachyzoites were passaged intraperitoneally in mice and after every 5 passages also into sulfadiazine-treated mice, to permit the development of tissue cysts. Such chronically infected mice were fed to seronegative cats which were then checked for oocyst shedding [67]. Tissue cysts derived from the 10-30 tachyzoite mouse passages, when fed to cats, gave rise to oocyst shedding. However, tissue cysts in mice obtained after 35-61 tachyzoite passages in mice, when fed to cats, failed to give rise to oocysts [67]. This was repeated several times with permutations yielding similar results. We do not know why the oocyst stage gets lost after atypical passage, used routinely for maintenance of lines in many laboratories.

Tissue cysts, contrary to oocysts, are not easily lost by simple passage, but there are some RH strains which form few or no cysts [46]. For creation of the ts-4 vaccine, which does not form tissue cysts, the strain was mutagenized, selected for temperature-sensitivity and clones were chosen and tested for pathogenicity and persistence [68].

Genomic drift

The *Toxoplasma* genome is remarkably stable, compared to the related genus *Sarcocystis*, which has a similar oocyst configuration but includes a multitude of species. However, the oocyst-loss phenomenon suggests a slow genomic drift. Several allelic configurations have been found in isolates grown in the same environment, which do not appear to be affected by selection pressures. However, the gametocyte-forming-ability is under selection pressure of the host and depends on the availability of sufficient time to develop bradyzoites in tissue cysts, rather than tachyzoites [69]. This may not only be a laboratory phenomenon. Thirty-five passages in mice require about 122 days. If *Toxoplasma* persisted exclusively in the tachyzoite stage in some humans with AIDS, gametocyte-forming capacity may also be lost.

Clonal structure of Toxoplasma

Toxoplasma gondii comprises 3 clonal lineages [70]. Each clonal type was isolated from a variety of hosts. Clonal type one was more common in human
congenital toxoplasmosis and it has also been associated with "mouse virulence" associated with markers at chromosome VIII [71, 72]. Type 2 was identified more commonly in humans, especially in AIDS and congenital cases.
Type 3 was most commonly isolated from animals. Two recombinants were
observed. When analyzing several laboratory stocks of the RH strain, genetic
heterogeneity was also found [73], suggesting either genomic drift or laboratory mix-ups. When describing these clones in 1992-1996 [70, 71, 72], the
authors list the persons from whom the strains were obtained. However, they
failed to indicate the year of isolation, or the number of passages in mice or
cell cultures, which would provide an indication of the mutations and selection pressure these strains had been under, and to possibly shed light on the
genesis of "mouse virulence".

Development of increasing pathogenicity to laboratory hosts by frequent passage

This process can be observed regularly when new isolates are passaged as
tachyzoites, either intraperitoneally in mice, in cell cultures, or chick
embryos. This process is generally progressive, although there is evidence
that by changing hosts, it can be modified [74]. However, by maintaining new
isolates as chronic infections in the cyst stage, and subinoculating brain tissue, by feeding or injection, the isolates tend to retain longer their level of
pathogenicity and maintain an important attribute, gametocyte formation.
Nevertheless, the mice die eventually after progressively shorter periods of
chronicity. One can then maintain these strains on sulfamerazine-sodium
15mg% in the drinking water for 3 weeks, while mice develop immunity.
However, after several months progressively higher doses are often necessary.
We must conclude, that by continuous passage, isolates are selected for being
able to multiply fast in the particular host environment; this section is probably different from the genetic pathogenicity markers associated with the
type one clone. Organisms are stabilized in respect to gametocyte-forming
ability by passing through the bradyzoite state. To have a standard strain
"stand still" it must be kept in the frozen state.

Tissue effect of Toxoplasma in mother and child

With the increasingly sensitive diagnosis and the spectacular effect of chemotherapy in neonatal toxoplasmosis [75, 76, 77], pathologic lesions from
Toxoplasma are rarely seen at present. Therefore it appears well to outline the
processes that patients progressed through without treatment, to provide a
rational base for the imperative of early diagnosis, early treatment and ultimately prevention. The brain and the eyes are the most severely affected organs.

Maternal Toxoplasma infection

This is generally unrecognized and subclinical, because a woman is usually
immunocompetent and develops immunity in a timely fashion. Occasionally

fatigue, fever and organ-related lesions have been recalled, however lympha-denopathy is the most frequent clinical manifestation noted [78]. The process is one of lymphoreticular cell hyperplasia without tachyzoites or cell necrosis and only few cysts, interpreted as an immune reaction [79].

Congenital toxoplasmosis

The infection is first a generalized one, persisting longer in the brain and eyes, which become more severely damaged because of delay in acquiring effective immunity and because of deficient regenerative capacity and other factors.

1. Proliferating tachyzoites destroy parasitized cells giving rise to pneumo-nia, myocarditis, orchitis and hepatitis. Neurons and other neural cells are destroyed giving rise to individual cell necrosis with mononuclear inflamma-tion or glial nodules in the brain (Fig. 5). Glial nodules are the tombstones of destroyed cells. All parts of the brain are involved. Focally, they may be larger, confluent foci of necrosis, probably because of thrombosis of a single vessel, in the basal ganglia or the cortical gray matter, extending to the meninges. Lesions heal by astrocytic gliosis. In the retina, cell necrosis is accompanied by inflammation extending into the choroid and spilling into the vitreous.

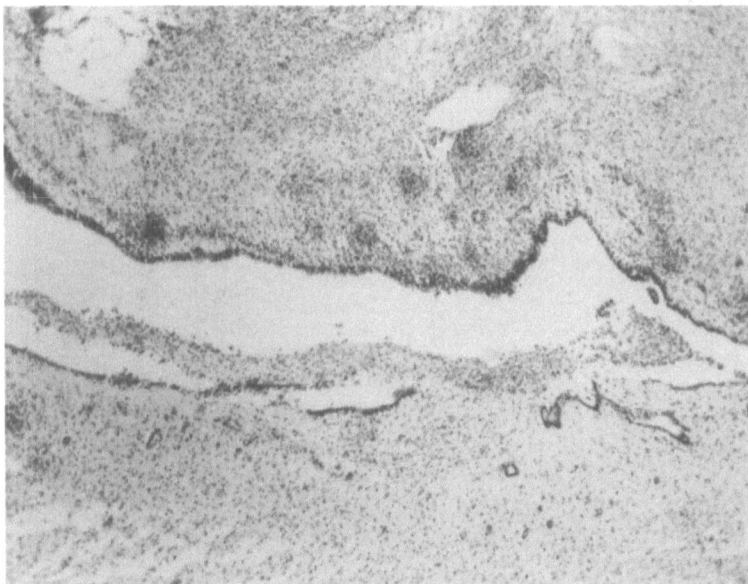

Fig. 5. Fourth ventricle of 4 week-old child with congenital toxoplasmosis. Glial nodules are present in the subependymal areas. There is an ependymal ulcer, below, with glial prolife-ration and inflammation extending into the ventricular lumen. The 4th ventricle was not dila-ted, hence equilibrated with the spinal fluid, with a protein content of 576mg per 100 ml. Nissl stain, x 43. [80]

2. Bradyzoites within intact cysts are scattered throughout the brain, eyes, heart and other tissues but do not produce inflammation. However, a disintegrated cyst is surrounded by tissue necrosis and inflammatory reaction (Fig. 6), even though the free bradyzoites are lysing or have been phagocytized [10]. This cysts rupture necrosis is particularly serious in the retina where function is highly concentrated and regeneration absent [79].

3. Periventricular necrosis (Fig. 7) is a unique lesion and involves the dilated, hydrocephalic, lateral and third ventricles and the obstructed aqueduct. Because most ependyma and choroid plexus epithelium has been destroyed, in part by *Toxoplasma* [79, 80], trapped antigen from the ventricle seeps into the surrounding tissues, reacting with antibody in the arterioles, leading to vasculitis, thrombosis, exudation of fluid and necrosis, sometimes with calcification (Fig. 8). There is often an innermost zone showing granulation tissue extending from the walls of the thrombosed vessels, also indicating that the antigen-excess zone is not toxic to cells (Fig. 8).

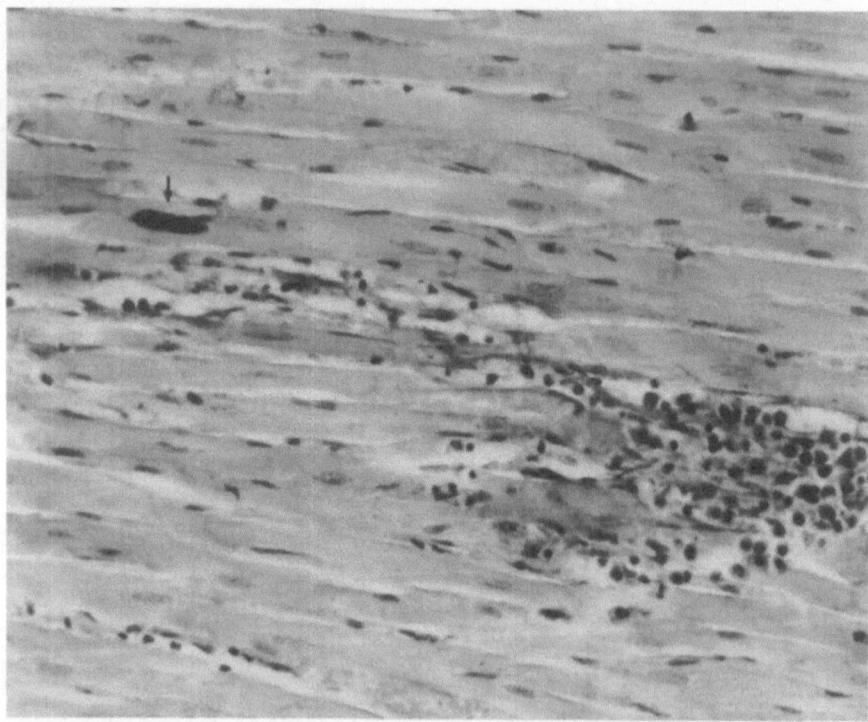

Fig. 6. Intact tissue cyst of *Toxoplasma* (arrow) in myocardium, with focus of myocardial necrosis with inflammatory cells and absence of tachyzoites, typical of a cyst-rupture lesion. PASH & eosin x 300 [From 81]

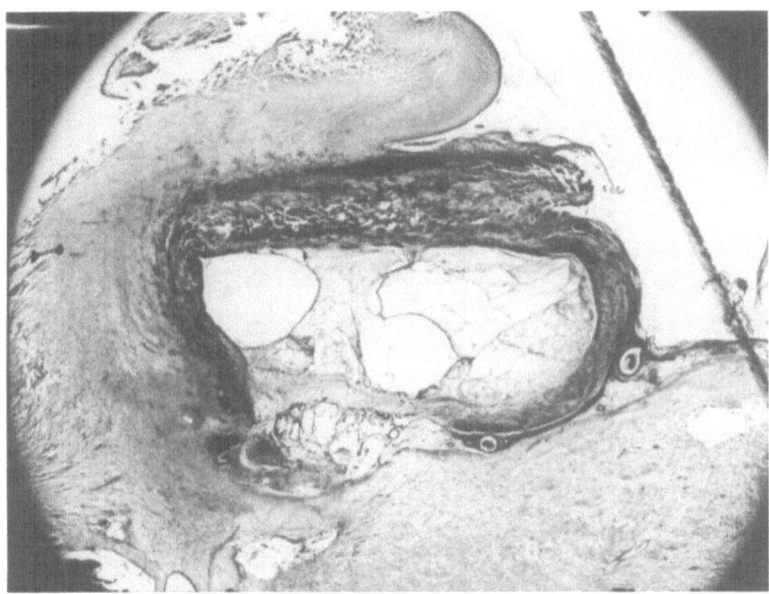

Fig. 7. Dilated lateral ventricle with periventricular necrosis from same child as Fig. 5, from which *Toxoplasma* was isolated. This reaction is absent where the choroid plexus, below, is lined by ependyma. The exudation of fibrin from damaged blood vessels is well shown in this section stained with phosphotungstic acid hematoxylin (PTA). Ventricular fluid from this ventricle elicited a reaction of delayed hypersensitivity in a *Toxoplasma*-infected guinea pig, but not in an uninfected animal. Granulation tissue extends from the choroid plexus into the ventricular lumen, which also contains fibrin strands. Protein concentration of this ventricular fluid was 2600 mg per 100 ml. X 4.5 [From 80]

The periventricular reaction has been interpreted as an antigen-antibody reaction [79, 80] possibly with immune complexes or a precipitin reaction; however, this reaction has not yet been examined by modern histochemical techniques. This ventricular fluid can serve as skin test antigen and is high in protein content, up to grams percent, whereas the fluid of the fourth ventricle has only a slightly increased protein content (Legends to Figs. 5 and 7). Ependymal ulcers in the non-obstructed fourth ventricle are not accompanied by this reaction), apparently because it is adequately drained by the Foramina of Luschka and Magendi, and *Toxoplasma* antigen does not accumulate [79, 80]. This reaction was present in all advanced cases of neonatal toxoplasmic encephalitis in the US, although one may need large cross-sections (Fig. 7) to properly evaluate it. However, I have not seen it in similar Costa Rican cases, where the illness was complicated by marked malnutrition and possibly low antibody levels.

The periventricular necrosis may involve and obliterate the corpus callosum and markedly attenuate especially the inferior and temporal parts of the brain. There may be hemorrhage into the subcortical white matter superiorly, probably due to ischemia secondary to the hydrocephalus. The manner of regeneration of brain tissue in treated cases of encephalitis [75] has not yet been studied.

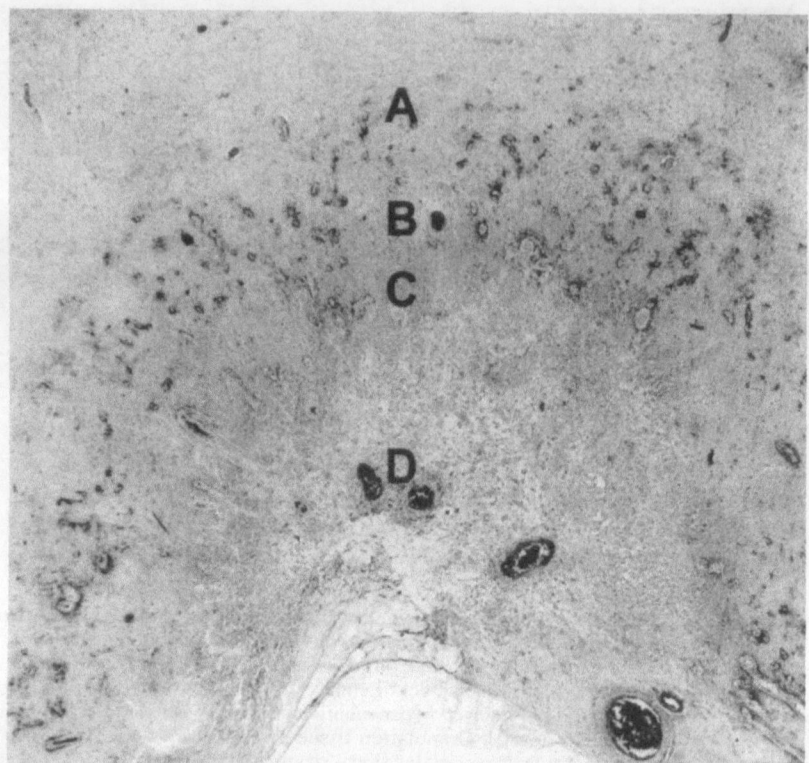

Fig. 8. Lateral ventricle with detail of subzones of periventricular necrosis in a 5 week old child with congenital toxoplasmosis. At level A, in white matter there are glial nodules, many of which are associated with tachyzoites. At level B, blood vessels show protein leakage and inflammatory cells indicated by dark staining, and many vessels are thrombosed; this reaction is considered compatible with an antigen-antibody reaction. Level C shows infarction of white matter. Level D shows viable granulation tissue extending from the walls of a few larger vessel. Vascular spaces are numerous but contain few erythrocytes. Level D is considered a zone of antigen excess; the proliferating fibroblasts indicate that the fluid was not toxic. [From 80]

Lesions in the immunosuppressed patient are more profound in the brain. However, the inflammatory component is deficient or absent, and necrosis predominates.

Infection necrosis is a progressive cell destruction by *Toxoplasma* which leads to ever enlarging foci of necrosis in the brain and occasionally other organs [79, 82].

Infarction necrosis of brain is seen when *Toxoplasma* multiplies in the wall of an artery or arteriole, leading to vascular thrombosis and brain infarction at some distance [82]. The lesions are similar to infection necrosis, but without *Toxoplasma* accompanying the necrosis.

Bibliography

1. Levine ND (1973) Protozoan Parasites of Domestic Animals and Man. 2nd Ed, Burgess, Minneapolis MN
2. Frenkel JK, Hammond DM, Long PL (eds) (1973). The Coccidia. *Eimeria, Isospora, Toxoplasma* and Related Genera. University Park Press, Baltimore, p 9; Toxoplasmosis: parasite life cycle, pathology and immunology. pp. 343-410
3. Lingelbach K, Joiner KA (1998) The parasitophorous vacuole membrane surrounding *Plasmodium* and *Toxoplasma*: an unusual compartment in infected cells. J Cell Science 111:1467-1475
4. Carruthers VB, Sibley LD (1997) Sequential protein secretion from three distinct organelles of *Toxoplasma gondii* accompanies invasion of human fibroblasts.Europ J Cell Biol 73/114-123
5. Dubey JP (1998) Re-examination of resistance to *Toxoplasma gondii* tachyzoites and bradyzoites to pepsin and trypsin. Parasitol 116:43-50
6. Sasono PMD, Smith JE (1998) *Toxoplasma gondii*: an ultrastuctural study of host cell invasion by the bradyzoite stage. Parasitol Res 84:640-645
7. Frenkel JK (1956a) Pathogenesis of toxoplasmosis and of infections with organisms resembling Toxoplasma. Ann NY Acad Sciences 64:215-251
8. Hoff RL, Dubey JP, Behbehani AM, Frenkel JK (1977) *Toxoplasma gondii* cysts in cell culture: new biologic evidence. J Parasitol 63:1121-1124
9. Lindsay DS, Tovio-Kinnucan MA, Blagburn BL (1993) Ultrastructural determination of cystogenesis by various *Toxoplama gondii* isolates in cell culture. J Parasit 79:289-292
10. Frenkel JK, Escajadillo A (1987) Cyst rupture as a pathogenic mechanism of toxoplasmic encephalitis. Am J Trop Med Hyg 36:517-522
11. Frenkel JK (1956b) Effects of hormones on the adrenal necrosis produced by *Besnoitia jellisoni* in golden hamsters. J Exp Med 103:375-398
12. Woke PA, Jacobs L, Jones FE, Melton ML (1953) Experimental results on possible arthropod transmission of toxoplasmosis. J Parasitol 39:523-532
13. Frenkel JK (1965) Attempted transmission of *Toxoplasma* with arthropods. Progr Protozool, London, Excerpta Med Inter Cong Series 91:190
14. Hutchison WM (1967) The nematode transmission of *Toxoplasma gondii*. Trans R Soc Trop Med Hyg 61:80-89
15. Hutchison WM, Dunachie JF, Work K (1968) Brief report. The faecal transmission of *Toxoplasma gondii*. Acta Path Microbiol Scand 74:462-464
16. Hutchison WM (1965) Experimental transmission of Toxoplasma gondii. Nature 206:961-962
17. Frenkel JK, Dubey JP, Miller NL (1969) *Toxoplasma gondii*: fecal forms separated from eggs of the nematode *Toxocara cati*. Science 164:432-433
18. Frenkel JK, Dubey JP, Miller NL (1970) *Toxoplasma gondii* in cats: fecal stages identified as coccidian oocysts. Science 167:893-896
19. Frenkel JK (1973a) *Toxoplasma* in and around us. BioScience 23:343-352
20. Dubey JP, Miller NL, Frenkel JK (1970) The *Toxoplasma gondii* oocyst from cat feces. J Exp Med 132:636-662
21. Dubey JP, Swan GV, Frenkel JK (1972) A simplified method for isolation of *Toxoplasma gondii* from the feces of cats. J Parasitol 58:1005-1006
22. Frenkel JK, Dubey JP (1972) Toxoplasmosis and its prevention in cats and man. J Infect Dis 126:664-673
23. Frenkel JK, Smith D (1982) Immunization of cats against shedding of *Toxoplasma* oocysts. J Parasitol 85:744-748
24. Frenkel JK, Pfefferkorn ER, Smith DD, Fishback JL (1991) A *Toxoplasma* vaccine for cats using a new mutant. Am J Vet Res 52:759-763
25. Jewell ML, Frenkel JK, Johnson KM, Reed V, Ruiz A (1972) Development of *Toxoplasma* oocysts in neotropical felidae. Am J Trop Med & Hyg 21:512-517
26. Miller NL, Frenkel JK, Dubey JP (1972) Oral infections with *Toxoplasma* cysts and oocysts in felines, other mammals, and in birds. J Parasitol 58:928-937
27. Lappin MR, Jacobson ER, Kollias GV, Powell CC (1991) Comparison of serologic assays for the diagnosis of toxoplasmosis in nondomestic felids. J Zoo Wild 22(2):169-174
28. Lukesova D, Literak I (1998) Shedding of *Toxoplasma gondii* by Felidae in zoos in the Czech Republic. Veterinary Parasitology 74:1-7
29. Lin DS, Bowman DD (1991) Cellular responses of cats with primary toxoplasmosis. J Parasit 77:272-279
30. Dubey JP, Frenkel JK (1972) Cyst-induced toxoplasmosis in cats. J Protozool 19:155-177
31. Frenkel JK, Dubey JP (1973) Effects of freezing on the viability of *Toxoplasma* oocysts. J Parasitol 59:587-588
32. Frenkel JK, Ruiz A, Chinchilla M (1975) Soil survival of *Toxoplasma* oocysts in Kansas and Costa Rica. Am J Trop Med & Hyg 24:439-443

33. Ruiz A, Frenkel JK, Cerdas L (1973) Isolation of *Toxoplasma* from soil. J Parasitol 59:204-206
34. Dubey JP (1998) *Toxoplasma gondii* oocysts survival under defined temperatures. J Parasit 84:862-865
35. Frenkel JK (1974) Toxoplasmosis. In : Kirk RW (ed) Current Veterinary Therapy. WB Saunders, Philadelphia, pp. 775-780
36. Ito S, Tsunoda K, Shimada K, Taki T, Matsui T (1975) Disinfectant effects of several chemicals against *Toxoplasma* oocysts. Jpn J Vet S 37:229-234
37. Slavin MA, Meyers JD, Remington JS, Hackman RC (1994) *Toxoplasma gondii* infection in marrow transplant recipients - a 20 year experience. Bone Mar Tr 13:549-557
38. Chandrasekar P, Momin F, Karanes C, Abella S, Ratanat. V, Sensenbrenner L (1997) Disseminated toxoplasmosis in marrow recipients-a report of 3 cases and a review of the literature. Bone Marrow Tr 19:685-689
39. Orr KE, Gould FK, Short G, Dark JH, Hilton CJ, Corris PA, Freeman R. (1994) Outcome of *Toxoplasma gondii* mismatches in heart transplant recipients over a period of 8 years. J Infection 29:249-253.
40. Singer MA, Hagler WS, Grossnik HE (1993) *Toxoplasma gondii* retinochoroiditis after liver transplantation. Retina 13(1):40-45
41. Wreghitt TG et al (1989) Toxoplasmosis in heart-lung transplant recipients. J Clin Path 42:194-199
42. Michel G, Thuret I, Chambost H, Scheiner C, Mary C, Perrimon H (1994) Lung toxoplasmosis after HLA mismatched bone marrow transplantation. Bone Mar Tr 14(3):455-457
43. Collogno J, Verhulst D, Bigaigno J, Doyen C, Chatelai C, Bosly A (1994) Rapid diagnosis of cerebral *Toxoplasmosis* by PCR in allogeneic BMT leads to early and successful treatment. Blood 84:A489
44. Ruiz A, Frenkel JK (1980) Intermediate and transport hosts of *Toxoplasma gondii* in Costa Rica. Amer J Trop Med & Hyg 29:1161-1166
45. Frenkel JK, Hassanein KM, Hassanein RS, Brown E, Thulliez P, Quintereo-Nuñez R (1995) Transmission of *Toxoplasma* in Panama City, Panama: A five-year prospective cohort study of children, cats, rodents, birds, and soil. Am J Trop Med & Hyg 53:458-468
46. Dubey JP, Frenkel JK (1998) Toxoplasmosis of rats: a review, with consideration of their value as an animal model and their possible role in epidemiology. Veterinary Parasitology 77:1-32
47. Hejlicek K, Literák I, Nezval J (1997) Toxoplasmosis in wild mammals from the Czech republic. J Wildlife Diseases 33:480-485
48. Literak I, Hejlicek K, Nezval J, Folk C (1992) Incidence of *Toxoplasma gondii* in populations of wild birds in the Czech Republic. Avian Path 21(4):659-665
49. Roelke ME, Forrester DJ, Jacobson ER, Kollias GV, Scott FW, Barr MC, Evermann JF, Pirtle EC. (1993) Seroprevalence of infectious-disease agents in free-ranging Florida panthers (*Felis concolor coryi*). Journal of Wildlife Diseases 29(1):36-49
50. Smith DD, Frenkel JK (1995) Prevalence of antibody to *Toxoplasma gondii* in wild mammals of Missouri and east central Kansas: biological and ecologic considerations of transmission. J Wildlife Diseases 31:15-21
51. Frenkel JK, Sousa OE (1983) Antibodies to *Toxoplasma* in panamanian mammals. J Parasitol 69:244-245
52. Frenkel JK, Dubey JP, Miller NL (1970) *Toxoplasma gondii*: a coccidian of cats, with a wide range of mammalian and avian hosts. J Parasitol 56:107-108
53. Dubey JP, Humphreys JG, Thulliez P (1995) Prevalence of viable *Toxoplasma gondii* tissue cysts and antibodies to *T. gondii* by various serologic tests in black bears (*Ursus americanus*) from Pennsylvania. J Parasitol 81:109-112
54. Kulasiri CS (1962) The behaviour of suckling rats to oral and intraperitoneal infection with a virulent strain of *Toxoplasma gondii*. Parasit 52:193-198
55. Christiansen M, Siim JC (1951) Toxoplasmosis in hares in Denmark. Lancet June:1201
56. Johnson CM (1943) Immunological and epidemiological investigation under the direction of C.M. Johnson protozoologist. Ann Report of the Gorgas Memorial Laboratory:15-16
57. Jacobs L, Melton ML (1966) Toxoplasmosis in chickens. J Parasitol 52:1158-1162
58. Beauregard M, Magwood SE, Bannister GL, Robertson A, Boulanger P, Ruckerbauer GM, Appel M (1965) A study of *Toxoplasma* infection in chickens and cats on a family farm. Canadian Journal of Comparative Medicine & Veterinary Science 29:286-291
59. Dubey JP, Ruff MD, Camargo ME, Shen SK, Wilkins GL, Kwok OCH, Thulliez P. (1993) Serologic and parasitological responses of domestic chickens after oral inoculation with *Toxoplasma gondii* oocysts. Am J Vet Res 54(10):1668-1672
60. Keagy HF (1949) *Toxoplasma* in the Chinchilla. JAVMA 114:15
61. Nobel TA, Neuman F, Klopfer U (1965) An outbreak of toxoplasmosis in Hyrax (Procavia capensis syriacus). Refuah Vet 22:56-59
62. Buergelt CD, Bonde RK (1983) Toxoplasmic meningoencephalitis in a West Indian manatee. J Am Vet Med Assoc 183:1294-1296
63. Frenkel JK (1989) Tissue-dwelling intracellular parasites: infection and immune responses in the Mammalian host to *Toxoplasma*, *Sarcocystis* and *Trichinella*. Amer Zool 29:455-467

64. Nicolle MMC, Manceaux L (1908) Sur une infection a corps de Leishman (ou organismes voisins) du gondi. Comptes Rendus Acad Sci (Paris) 147:763-766
65. Ambroise-Thomas P, Pelloux H (1993) Le toxoplasme et sa pathologie. Med Mal Inf 23(NSI):121-128
66. Chatton E, Blanc G (1917) Notes et reflexions sur le Toxoplasme et le Toxoplasmose du Gondi. (*Toxoplasma gondii* Ch. Nicolle et Manceaux 1909). Arch Inst Pasteur Tunis 10:1-41
67. Frenkel JK, Dubey JP, Hoff RL (1976) Loss of stages after continuous passage of *Toxoplasma gondii* and *Besnoitia jellisoni*. J Protozool 23:421-424
68. Waldeland H, Pfefferkorn ER, Frenkel JK (1983) Temperature-sensitive mutants of *Toxoplasma gondii:* pathogenicity and persistence in mice. J Parasitol 69:171-175
69. Frenkel JK, Ambroise-Thomas P (1997) Genetic drift of *Toxoplasma gondii*. Parasitol Rev 83: 1-5
70. Howe DK, Sibley LD (1995) *Toxoplasma gondii* comprises three clonal lineages: Correlations of parasite genotype with human disease. J Inf Dis 172:1561-1566
71. Sibley LD, Boothroyd JC (1992) Virulent strains of *Toxoplasma gondii* comprise a single clonal lineage. Nature 359:82-85
72. Howe DK, Summers BC, Sibley LD (1996) Acute virulence in mice is associated with markers on chromosome VII in *Toxoplasma gondii*. Infec Immun 64:5193-5198
73. Howe DK, Sibley LD (1994) *Toxoplasma gondii* - analysis of different laboratory stocks of the RH strain reveals genetic heterogeneity. Exp Parasitology 78:242-245
74. Lecomte V, Chumpitazi BFF, Pasquier B, Ambroise-Thomas P, Santoro F (1992) Brain cysts in rats infected with the RH strain of *Toxoplasma gondii*. Parasitol Res 78:267-269
75. McAuley JB, Boyer KM, Patel D, Mets MB, Swisher C, Roizen N, Wolters C, Stein L, Stein M, Schey W et al (1994) Early and longitudinal evaluations of treated infants and children and untreated historical patients with congenital toxoplasmosis - the Chicago collaborative treatment trial. Clin Inf Dis 18:38-72
76. Roizen N, Swisher CN, Stein MA, Hopkins J, Boyer KM, Holfels E, Mets MB, Stein L, Patel D, Meier P et al (1995) Neurologic and developmental outcome in treated congenital toxoplasmosis. Pediatrics 95:11-20
77. Mets MB, Holfels E, Boyer KM, Swisher CM, Roizen N, Stein L, Stein M, Hopkins J, Withers S, Mack D et al (1996) Eye manifestations of congenital toxoplasmosis. Am J Ophthalm 122:309-324
78. McCabe RE, Brooks RG, Dorfman RF, Remington JS (1987) Clinical spectrum in 107 cases of toxoplasmic lymphadenopathy. Rev Infect Dis 9:754-774
79. Frenkel JK (1971) Toxoplasmosis. Mechanisms of infection, laboratory diagnosis and management. Curr Topics in Path 54:28-75
80. Frenkel JK, Friedlander S (1951) Toxoplasmosis: Pathology of neonatal disease. Pathogenesis, diagnosis and Treatment. Publ Health Serv Publication 141, US Government Printing Office, Washington, DC
81. Hackel DB et al (1953) Pathologic lesions in captured wild animals. Toxoplasmosis in a kangaroo. Lab Invest 2:154-163
82. Bertoli F, Espino M, Arosemena JR, Fishback JL, Kel JK (1995) A spectrum in the pathology of toxoplasmosis in patients with AIDS. Arch Pathol Lab Med 119:214-224

1.3. Placenta physiology

P. Ebbesen

Placenta physiology primarily deals with the production of hormones needed to keep pregnancy ongoing, foetal invasion into maternal tissue and the resulting dual immune function of avoiding maternal-foetal immune rejection while retaining the capacity for preventing vertical infections, and of course with transit of nutrients, waste, antibodies and microbes.

Embryology

Placenta physiology is most easily understood in relation to the embryology of the organ. The early embryo nidated into the endometrium (decidua) is a fluid-filled sphere which contains smaller fluid-containing sacs in addition to the embryonic disc. It rapidly consolidates into essentially one sphere enveloping the amnion cavity and having a local wall thickening the placenta. Placenta consists of the villous bearing chorion plate, the intervillous space where maternal blood enters, and decidua basalis (Fig. 1).

The outer surface of the nidated blastocyst develops into the single-celled cytotrophoblasts. At day 14, the cytotrophoblasts proliferate and penetrate into the decidua basalis, forming the primary villi with cytotrophoblasts and on the surface of these a continuous layer of syncytiotrophoblasts. Mesoderm enters these villi and also vessels. By their continued proliferation the villi reach through the blood-filled space between maternal and foetal tissue and anchor on the endometrium; spreading laterally they cover this surface, on which in direct contact a layer of fibrin is deposited between foetal and maternal cells. Furthermore, the trophoblasts invade and destruct maternal endometrial artery and venous walls, leading to leaking of maternal blood through clefts in the cytotrophoblastic shell into the intervillous space. The intervillous space becomes lined with multinucleated syncytiotrophoblasts. In the third trimester the underlying cytotrophoblast largely disappears, and the syncytia layer becomes quite thin.

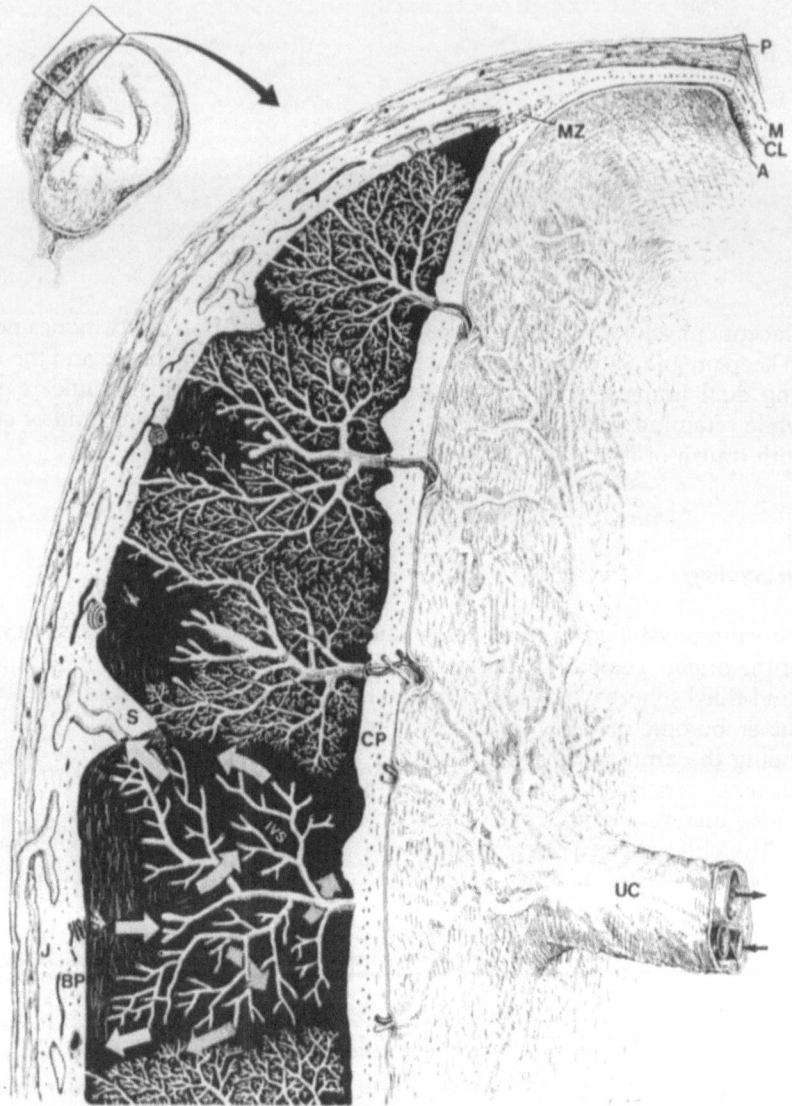

Fig. 1. Mature human placenta *in situ*. It is composed of the chorionic plate (CP) and the basal plate (BP) surrounding the intervillous space (IVS) as cover and as bottom. The fetally vascularized villous trees project from the chorionic plate into the intervillous space and are directly surrounded by the maternal blood that circulates through the intervillous space. The loose centers of villous trees, arranged around the maternal arterial inflow area, are frequent features. P = perimetrium; M = myometrium; CL = chorion leave; A = amnion; MZ = marginal zone between placenta and fetal membranes, with obliterated intervillous space and ghost villi; * = cell island, connected to a villous tree; S = placental septum; J = junctional zone; UC = umbilical cord. ([32], with permission)

Production of signal molecules

Hormones

After the sixth week, placenta produces enough oestrogen and progesterone to take over the function of the corpus luteum. In addition, the placenta syncytiotrophoblasts produce human chorionic gonadotropin (hCG), which is specific to pregnancy. The syncytiotrophoblasts also produce the lactogenic human chorionic somatomammotropin (hCS), also called human placental lactogen (hPL).

Interferons and other cytokines

Many cell types secrete interferons (IFNs) alpha and beta in response to virus or other stimulation, whereas IFNs gamma are produced only by activated T-lymphocytes and NK cells. Alpha and beta interferons share receptors. Trophoblasts have been shown *in vitro* to produce mostly beta interferon, but also considerable amounts of alpha interferon upon stimulation [1]. A key question is whether trophoblasts, in contrast to other tissues, may have a constitutive interferon production, and if so, what is the function. Low levels of interferons have been reported for both foetal and placental tissues during pregnancy and in cord blood in absence of evidence of infections [2, 3].

Prostaglandin E_2 may inhibit interferon effects [4].

Epidermal Growth Factor (EGF) induces differentiation in non-invasive villous trophoblasts [5], whereas it enhances the invasion of extravillous trophoblasts [6]. The observed inhibition of EGF-R by trophoblast-induced interferon may therefore suggest one of the mechanisms involved in the regulation of normal trophoblast differentiation. *In vitro* differentiation of cytotrophoblasts to syncytiotrophoblasts is also linked to increased expression of epidermal growth factor receptor (EGF-R) [7].

C-fos/CSF-1 (colony stimulating factor-1) enhances growth and promotes the secretion of hCG and human placenta lactogen/hPL) in trophoblasts [8] and enhances trophoblast interferon production. Tropho-blast IFNs have antiproliferative effects on trophoblasts *in vitro* [9], and trophoblast interferon downregulates the expression of CSF-IR. Thus, interferons of the placenta may well turn out to have roles in normal placenta physiology in addition to their classical antimicrobial effects.

Invasion control

Invasion *control is a necessity*. Too little invasion is associated with small placentas and preeclampsia, and in case of choriocarcinomas an unrestricted invasion takes place.

The *invasive* function segregates from the absorptive and endocrine functions of trophoblasts by formation of a distinct subset, the extravillous trophoblasts. Invasion requires binding, proteases and migration.

Villous trophoblasts express the integrins alpha 6, beta 4 and alpha 3/beta 1, which anchor them to the basal lamina as they are laminin and collagen4 receptors. In contrast, the extravillous trophoblasts first loose expression of these integrins and then switch to alpha 5/beta 1, a fibronectin receptor. In addition, the extravillous trophoblasts secrete metalloproteases type 4 collagenase (92 kDa) [10].

A number of factors are known to influence the various steps of the controlled invasion, characteristically those stimulating proliferation have no effect on migration and invasion and vice versa.

Stimulants of extravillous trophoblast proliferation are: EGF (paracrine effect), transforming growth factor (TGF, autocrine), colony stimulating growth factor (CSF-1, auto and paracrine), vascular endothelial growth factor (VEGF-1, paracrine (macrophages)) and placenta growth factor PIGF (autocrine effect).

A stimulant of the cells' migration and invasion are insulin-like growth factor (IGF-11) produced by trophoblasts and with receptors on decidua, thus acting as a signal between the two tissues. It has no effect on proteases.

Blockers of extravillous trophoblast proliferation, migration and invasion are TGF beta (auto and paracrine), which act as antiproliferative and anti-invasive by upregulating integrins, downregulating urokinase plasminogen activator (uPA) and promoting fusion into giant cells.

Tissue inhibitor of metalloprotease TIMP is a paracrine, decidua-derived inhibitor of metalloproteinases, but not urokinases.

Some immune function may also be involved in invasion control. Firstly, type one inteferons will in vitro inhibit trophoblast invasion [11], and in vitro work shows invading extravillous trophoblasts to be killed by NK cells [12].

The immunological barrier function

The immune system has two barrier functions. One prevents the active immunological distinction between self and non-self from causing a maternal rejection of the invading foetus. The other is the immunological barrier preventing vertical transmission of microorganisms.

How maternal host-versus-graft responses and foetal graft-versus-host responses are avoided is only partly known. As the foetally-derived cell in closest contact with maternal tissue, the trophoblast has to be directly involved. A thin layer of fibrin is often/always? deposited between invading trophoblasts and invaded endometrium, but this putative physical barrier does not explain why floating maternal T-cells of the intervillous space do not kill the syncytiotrophoblasts.

Human cells derived from the inner cell mass of the blastocyst give rise to the embryonic tissues and gradually express classical class 1 molecules. Cells from the trophextoderm layer of the blastocyst, which give rise to the trophoblast cells constituting the placenta and extraplacental membranes, do not express classical HLA class 1 or class 2 antigens. An antigen masking seems to be at work. However, of these cells, those in close contact with maternal cells, such as extravillous invading cytotrophoblasts and cells of the basal plate, express nonclassical nonpolymorphic HLA-G and C, while chorion laeve exclusively expresses HLA-G [13, 14]. It has been suggested that these non-classical class 1 molecules might have an immune inhibitory function, and indeed transfectants demonstrated that HLA-G is capable of inhibiting *in vitro* natural killer activity. However, neither uninfected, nor HSV-infected mononuclear or syncytial term villous trophoblast cultures which are free of HLA-G expression are susceptible to lysis by maternal NK cells or foetal cord NK cells, but extravillous trophoblasts expressing HLA-G are *in vitro* susceptible to NK killing even in absence of virus. All this speaks against a protective role of HLA-G, leaving the problem unresolved [12].

Interferons can stimulate immune reaction at a low concentration and inhibit at high concentrations, but their role in regulating the placenta immune reactions has not been determined. Another possible factor in prevention of allogeneic foetal rejection is the trophoblast metabolism removing tryptophan needed for T-cell activity [15].

The foetal stroma and endothelial cells of the villi express these transplantation antigens. It has been suggested that the internal cells of the villi serve as an immunological filter, binding maternal antibodies so that they do not reach the foetus.

Although actively avoiding a host-versus-graft response from the mother and a foetal graft-versus-host response, the immune systems of the placenta must be capable of fending off invasion of microorganisms entering from the mother.

The antimicrobial capacity of the placental immune system is little studied. The maternal decidua basalis is rich in leukocytes, including large granular leukocytes (LGL) cells, and the intervillous space is filled with floating maternal blood. Furthermore, placental site giant (trophoblast) cells in the decidua contain the major basic protein, which comprises the core of the eosinophilic granules and is known to be toxic to several parasites [16] and bacteria. The foetal part of the placenta has a flow through of foetal leukocytes which, however, do not reach full *in vitro* reactivity before birth [17]. To this should be added that the syncytiotrophoblasts themselves seem capable of eradicating e.g. virus that has entered these cells [18].

Transport across the placenta

Nutrients and waste

The human placenta is hemochorial in structure, i.e. the trophoblasts directly face the maternal blood, and monochorial in that only one trophoblast layer is present in the term placenta. The blood flow of maternal and foetal blood is neither concurrent (same direction), nor countercurrent, but an intermediate labelled multivillous flow. The syncytiotrophoblasts expression of nitric oxide synthase [19] may indicate that secreted NO takes part in regulation of the blood flow.

The physical barriers to be transversed when moving from maternal intervillous blood to the foetus are: 1) the microvillous plasma membrane of the syncytiotrophoblast, as here there is no lateral intercellular space; 2) the transport then goes through the interior of the trophoblast and the basal or foetal plasma membrane; 3) finally, the amniotic basal lamina and the foetal capillary endothelium where there is a lateral intercellular space (Fig. 2).

The modes of transportation are passive diffusion (gasses, urea, steroids, fatty acids and nutrients); facilitated diffusion (glucose); *active transport* (amino acids, electrolytes and vitamin C and endocytosis (transferri, vitamin B12).

The placenta's own metabolism, which is primarily based on glucose, consumes approximately half the oxygen received from the mother.

Antibodies

A receptor mediated endocytosis is active for IgG. Following binding of ligands to receptors, the receptors aggregate in coated pits containing the protein clatrin. The pits invaginate, are then pinched off and fuse with one another to form endosomes. The IgG is again released on the basal side of the trophoblast. It is the only maternal immunoglobulin that crosses to the foetus, which is of course the rationale for using foetal IgM as a marker of foetal infection.

Passage of maternal cells into the foetal circulation

Anatomy indicates a physical enclosure of the foetus, but maternal cells are demonstrable in the blood of the unborn child [20]. Nevertheless, most acute infections of the mother with virus, bacteria and protozoans rarely result in infection of the foetus [21], demonstrating the paramount importance of other protective mechanisms, including the immune processes.

Infectious agents

With regard to transmission of infectious agents across the trophoblast barrier, the cytomegalovirus, rubella virus and parvovirus B19 are the viruses found to infect the foetus commonly, whereas hepatitis B and C and HIV are transmitted less frequently.

Among the bacteria, syphilis is commonly transmitted, and among the parasites, *Toxoplasma* stands out.

Looking at the various transmittable agents, only a few common rules seem to apply. Primary infection during pregnancy and a high titer of microbes in maternal blood prior to the development of circulating antibodies increases the risk of transmission [21]. Furthermore, the timing of the primary infection of the mother in relation to start of pregnancy can be of importance, but the period of highest risk varies among the infectous agents.

Transmission of microbes is considered possible, both as free entities and as cell-born agents [22]).

For toxoplasmosis there is also firm evidence that vertical infection takes place as a result of primary maternal infection [23], and the transmission rate here seems the highest in the third trimester [24]. Luckily, the risk of lasting severe sequela for the child is inversely related to its intrauterine age at the time of infection. Transmission can take place in presence of maternal antibodies [25], but there is evidence that foetuses of mothers with high avidity of IgG antibodies during the first trimester are at a low risk of getting congenital toxoplasmosis [26].

Histology and cultivation have demonstrated toxoplasma cysts in chorionic tissues [27], endometrium [28], amniotic fluid [29], villi and possibly also within trophoblasts [30]. Furthermore, cysts can be found in foetal blood [31]. Maternal-to-fetal transmission is assumed to be always produced by organisms circulating in the maternal blood. The exact mechanisms involved are, however, unknown.

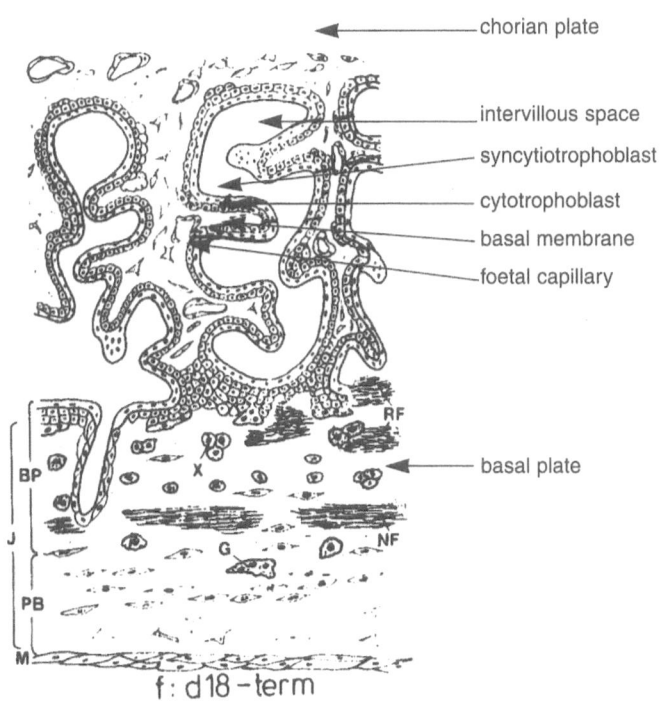

Fig. 2. Tertiary stage of villous development. Anchoring villi connecting chorion plate to basal plate

References

1. Aboagye-Mathiesen G, Tóth FD, Zdravkovic M, Ebbesen P (1999) (in press), Interferon Production at the Feto-Placental Interface
2. Paulesu L, Romagnoli R, Bellizzi E, Cintorino M, Ricci MG, LaRosa R (1991) Immunohistochemical localization of interferons-gamma and interferon-gamma receptors in human placental tissue. Placenta 12:427
3. Ebbesen P, Hager H, Nørskov-Lauritsen N, Aboagye-Mathiesen G, Zdravkovic M, Villadsen J, Liu X, Mosborg Petersen P, Bambra C, Nyongo A, Temmerman M, Zachar V (1995) Concurrence of High Levels of Interferons α and β in Cord and Maternal Blood and Simultaneous Presence of Interferon in Trophoblast in an African Population. J Interferon Cytokine Research 15:123-128
4. Khyatti M, Menezes J (1990) The effect of indomethacin, prostaglandin E2 and interferon on the multiplication of herpes simplex virus type 1 in human lymphoid cells. Antiviral Res 14:161-172
5. Morrish DW, Bhardwaj D, Dabbagh LK, Marusyk H, Siy O (1987) Epidermal growth factor induces differentiation and secretion of human chorionic gonadotropin and placental lactogen in normal human placenta. J Clin Endocrinol Metab 65:1282-1290
6. Bass KE, Morrish D, Roth I, Bhardwaj D, Taylor R, Zhou Y, Fisher SJ (1994) Human cytotrophoblast invasion is upregulated by epidermal growth factor: evidence that paracrine factors modify this process. Dev Biol 164:550-561
7. Muhlhauser J, Crescimanno C, Kaufmann P, Hofler H, Zaccheo D, Castellucci M (1993) Differentiation and proliferation patterns in human trophoblast revealed by c-erbB-2 oncogene product and EGF-R. J Histochem Cytochem 41:165-173
8. Saito S, Fukunaga R, Ichijo M, Nagata S (1994) Expression of granulocyte colony-stimulating factor and its receptor at the fetomaternal interface in murine and human pregnancy. Growth Factors 10:135-143
9. Aboagye-Mathiesen G, Tóth F, Zdravkovic M, Ebbesen P (1995) Human trophoblast interferons: Production and possible roles in early pregnancy. Early Pregnancy: Biology and Medicine 1:1-53
10. St.-Jacques S, Forte M, Lye SJ, Letarte M (1994) Localization of endoglin, a transforming growth factor-beta binding protein, and of CD44 and integrins in placenta during the first trimester of pregnancy. Biol Reprod 51:405-413
11. Horikoshi T, Fukuzawa K, Hanada N, Ezoe K, Eguchi H, Hamaoka S, Tsujiya H, Tsukamoto T (1995) In vitro comparative study of the antitumor effects of human interferon-alpha, beta and gamma on the growth and invasive potential of human melanoma cells. J Dermatol 22:631-636
12. Zdravkovic M, Aboagye-Mathiesen G, Lala PK, Hager H, Ebbesen P Susceptibility of Extravillous Trophoblast Cells to Killing by Natural Killer Cells. (Submitted)
13. Kovats S, Main EK, Librach C, Stubblebine M, Fisher SJ, DeMars R (1990) A class I antigen, HLA-G, expressed in human trophoblasts. Science 248:220-223
14. Johnson PM, Brown PJ (1981) Fc receptors in the human placenta. Placenta 2:355
15. Munn DH, Zhou M, Attwood JT, Bondarev I, Conway SJ, Marshall B, Brown C, Mellor AL (1998) Prevention of allogeneic fetal rejection by tryptophan catabolism. Science 281:1191-1193
16. Maddox DE, Kephart GM, Coulam CB, Butterfield JH, Benirschke K, Gleich GJ (1984) Localization of a molecule immunochemically similar to eosinophil major basic protein in human placenta. J Exp Med 160:29-41
17. Paiva A, Freitas A, Loureiro A, Couceiro A, Martinho A, Simoes O, Santos P, Tomaz J, Pais ML, Breda Coimbra H (1998) Functional aspect of cord blood lymphocytes response to polyclonal and allogeneic activation. Bone Marrow Transplantation 22 (Suppl 1):31-34
18. Zachar V, Nørskov-Lauritsen N, Juhl C, Spire B, Chermann JC, Ebbesen P (1991) Susceptibility of cultured human trophoblasts to infection with human immunodeficiency virus type-1. J Gen Virol 72:1253-1260
19. Lyall F, Jablonka-Shariff A, Johnson RD, Olson LM, Nelson DM (1998) Gene expression of nitric oxide synthase in cultured human term placental trophoblast during in vitro differentiation. Placenta 19:253-260
20. Petit T, Dommergues M, Socie G, Dumez Y, Gluckman E, Brison O (1997) Detection of maternal cells in human fetal blood during the third trimester of pregnancy using allele-specific PCR amplification. Br J Haematol 97:767-771
21. Schwartz DA, Nahmias AJ (1991) Human immunodeficiency virus and the placenta. Current concepts of vertical transmission in relation to other viral agents. Ann Clin Lab Sci 21:264-274
22. Ebbesen P, Tóth F, Aboagye-Mathiesen G, Zachar V, Hager H, Nørskov-Lauritsen N, Mosborg Petersen P, Juhl C, Villadsen J, Zdravkovic M, Dalsgaard AM (1994) Vertical transmission of HIV: Possible mechanisms and placental responses. Trophoblast Research 8:1-17
23. Beazley DM, Egerman RS (1998) Toxoplasmosis. Semin Perinatol 22:332-338

24. Jenum PA, Stray-Pedersen B, Melby KK, Kapperud G, Whitelaw A, Eskild A, Eng J (1998) Incidence of *Toxoplasma gondii* infection in 35,940 pregnant women in Norway and pregnancy outcome for infected women. J Clin Microbiol 36:2900-2906

25. Forther B, Aissi E, Ajana F, Dieusart P, Denis P, de Lasalle EM, Lecomte-Houcke M, Vinatier D (1991) Spontaneous abortion and reinfection by *Toxoplasma gondii*. Lancet 338:444

26. Lappalaninen M, Koskiniemi M, Hiilesmaa V, Ammala P, Teramo K, Koskela P, Lebech M, Raivio KO, Hedman K (1995) Outcome of children after maternal primary *Toxoplasma* infection during pregnancy with emphasis on avidity of specific IgG. The Study Group. Pediatr Infect Dis J 14:354-361

27. Larsen JW (1977) Congenital toxoplasmosis. Teratology 15:213-218

28. Altschuler G (1973) Toxoplasmosis as a cause of hydranencephaly. Am J Dis Child 125:251-252

29. Stray-Pedersen B, Lorentzen-Styr AM (1977) Uterine *Toxoplasma* infections and repeated abortions. Am J Obstet Gynecol 128:716-721

30. Benirschke K, Driscoll SG (1967) The Pathology of the Human Placenta. Springer-Verlag, New York

31. Daffos F, Forester F, Capella-Pavlovsky M, Thulliez P, Aufrant C, Valenti D, Cox WL (1988) Prenatal management of 746 pregnancies at risk for congenital toxoplasmosis. N Engl J Med 318:271-275

32. Kaufmann P, Scheffen I (1992) Placental development in neonatal and fetal medicine. In : Polin R, Fox W (eds) Physiology and Pathophysiology. Saunders, Orlando, pp. 47-55

1.4. Basic immunology: the fetus and the newborn

R. McLeod, M. Dowel[†]

Introduction

Immaturity of the developing immune system in the fetus and neonate renders them susceptible to a variety of pathogens, including *Toxoplasma gondii*. Recent advances in understanding fetal and neonatal immunity, cytokines, and immunogenetics, combined with new knowledge of the biology of *T. gondii* provide important insights relevant to this potentially devastating infection. Cell-mediated immune responses are the major mechanisms of host defense against *T. gondii* infection. Herein, we consider ontogeny of innate and specific cell-mediated immune responses in the human fetus and neonate in conjunction with a discussion of immune mechanisms likely to protect humans against *T. gondii*, studies of immunity of humans with congenital and postnatally acquired toxoplasmosis, and work which demonstrates immune mechanisms important in protection against toxoplasmosis in murine models.

Manifestations of *T. gondii* infection acquired during and after fetal life differ [1]. Recent studies using a murine model of congenital infection [2] are of interest in this regard because the types of central nervous system abnormalities noted in congenitally infected mice were the same as those in congenitally infected humans (e.g. ventriculitis, calcifications) and were different from those in infections acquired by adult humans and mice. It remains to be determined whether differences between outcomes of fetal and postnatally acquired infections are related to immaturity of the fetal immune system, different interactions of *T. gondii* antigens with the fetal versus postnatal immune systems, unique aspects of development of the fetal brain and eye or some combination of these factors. In this context, it is of interest that there was concordance of results of studies on immunogenetics of susceptibility to human congenital toxoplasmosis with those of susceptibility of mice to toxoplasmosis when mice had genes that govern immune specific responses replaced with homologous human transgenes [3]. Such models may be particu-larly useful in mechanistically characterizing the roles that development of the immune system during fetal and newborn life play in susceptibility to congenital toxoplasmosis.

Innate host defenses

NK cells

Natural killer (NK) cells are a subset of lymphocytes able to lyse their target cell using perforins and granzymes and without MHC restriction or presensitization (Table 1) [4-6]. They are important in early defense against intracellular pathogens before specific T cell differentiation and recognize absence of self-MHC expression [7]. The receptors involved in this recognition are not well characterized but are thought to involve the zeta chain of the CD3 molecule and the Fc receptor (CD16) on NK cells [7, 8]. In association with an antigen- IgG complex, CD16 triggers an antibody-dependent cell mediated cytotoxic reaction (ADCC) by the NK cells. In addition, NK cells also bind and destroy their target cells lacking self-MHC without antibody assistance. IL-2 is the primary cytokine involved in NK cell proliferation and with high levels can enhance their cytolytic effects resulting in lymphocyte activated killer cells (LAK) with broad target specificity. IL-15 initiates the proliferation of NK cells and is enhanced by IL-12, IL-7 and TNF-α. The cytolytic effect of NK cells is similarly enhanced by IL-2, IL-12 and IFN-α, β, and γ. More importantly, through synergy of TNF-α and IL-12 in the early phases of an immune response, NK cells produce IFN-γ that can positively influence the development of Th1 subset of CD4+ T cells [9]. NK cells interact with certain MHC class I molecules, which can down-modulate their activity [10]. Killer cell inhibitory receptors bind to parts of MHC Class I molecules on target cells and thus deliver inhibitory signals to the lytic machinery of NK cells [11, 12]. Human NK cells also bind to MHC Class I bearing cells using a cell surface molecule BY55 providing an additional and/or alternative pathway to CD28 costimulation [13].

Development of NK cells in the fetus and neonate

NK cells are detected as early as the 6th week of gestation in human fetal liver (Table 2) [14-16]. These cells are cytotoxic T lymphocyte-like in nature, but lack the usual CD3 phenotype of T lymphocytes and develop without thymic involvement. The percentage of NK cells in the term human neonate is similar to the adult at 15% of total lymphocyte ; however, the total number is nearly double that of the adult [14, 17]. NK cells are identified by surface CD16 (a low affinity FcRγ IIIA receptor) and most express CD56 (neural adhesion molecule, NCAM) and CD57 as well. The CD16+CD56+CD57+NK cells reportedly have the strongest cytolytic potential compared to their CD56⁻or CD57⁻ ounterparts.

NK cytolytic activity at term is estimated to be 50% of that of adults and approaches 100% by late infancy. This diminished cytolytic activity is thought to be associated with the prevalence of the CD56⁻ and CD57⁻ phenotype [18]. This response remains below the adult level even after induction with exogenous IL-12 and IL-15 [19]. In addition to the impaired cytolytic activity, ADCC ability is also diminished by 30-35% [20]. By 1-4 months of age, NK cells

Table 1.

Cell type and function	Cell surface	Stimulated by	Produces and/or secretes	Inhibited by
NK cells Lymphocytes Lyse target cells Produce cytokines Early defense	CD2 (some) CD3 ζ CD16 (FcγRIII) CD56 CD57 CD11b	IL-2 IL-7 IL-12 IFN-γ IFN-α/β	IFN-γ TNF-α GM-VSF Perforins Granzymes	Certains MHC molecules
Monocyte and Macrophage Produce cytokines Present antigen Phagocytose Early defense	CD9 CD11b/CD18 (Mac-1) CD13 CD14 CD16 (FcγRIII) CD23 (FcεRII) CD32 (FcγRII) CD40 CD64 (FcγRI) CD80 (B7.1) CD86 (B7.2)	M-CSF	IL-1 IL-6 IL-10 IL-12 IFN-γ IFN-α TNF-α TGF-β O2- NO	IL-4 (Th2 cell) IL-10 (Th2 cell)
Neutrophil Phagocytose Early defense	CD18 (B2 integrin) CD11a/CD18 (LFA-1) CD11b/CD18 (Mac-1)	IL-3 G-CSF GM-CSF	LTB4 IL-1 IL-8 TNF-α	prostaglandins iron
Eosinophil Early defense Produce cytokines	CD32 (FcγRII)	IFN-γ TNF-α GM-CSF	IL-1 IL-6 IL-8 IL-10 TNF-α G/M-CSF	
T cells Lymphocytes Produce cytokine MHC class recognition Helper and cytolytic role	TCR MHC I or II IL-2R CD1 CD2 (LFA-2) CD3 complex CD4 or CD8 CD5 CD7 CD11a/CD18 (LFA-1) CD28 CD29 CD34 CD38 CD40L CD45RO/A CD54 (ICAM) CTLA-4	IFN-γ IL-2 IL-4 (Th2 cell)	IL-2 (Th1 cell) IL-3 IL-4 (Th2 cell) IL-5 IL-6 IL-9 IL-10 IFN-γ (Th1 cell) TNF-α GM-CSF TGF-β	IL-10
B cells Lymphocytes Produce antibody Present antigen	CD5 (some) CD9 CD10 CD22 CD23 (FcεRII) FcεRI CD40		immuno- globulin	

Table 2.

	Gestation	Birth	6 months	1 year
NK cell	6 weeks, present in liver	15% of total lymphocytes Double absolute number present in adults 50% of adult cytolytic activity Overall increase number but decrease function		Full cytolytic activity reached in late infancy
Monocyte/ Macrophage & Denditric cell	4 weeks, detected in yolk sac then liver and bone marrow	Monocytes number > adults IL-1 equals adult Diminished IL-6 and TNF-α Cord blood DC less effective than adult in T cell support		Chemotaxis < adult for 6-10 years
Neutrophil	Limited storage pool. 14-16 weeks, precursors seen 22-24 weeks, 10% of circulating leukocytes	50-60% of circulating leukocytes 40-45% adhesive capability to endothelium Poor chemotactic ability Normal superoxide anion Decreased hydroxyl radicals		
Eosinophil	18-30 weeks, 10-20% of total granulocytes	Post-natal peak at 3-4 weeks		
T cell	7 weeks, detected in yolk sac and liver 8 weeks, lymphoid colonization and reduced TCR diversity and TdT enzyme activity 10 weeks, lymphoid tissues, liver and bone marrow 14 weeks, all three thymocytes in proper location 16 weeks, improved TCR diversity and TdT activity	Virgin subset T cells Normal IL-2 synthesis and IL-2R expression Reduced TNF-α, IL-3, IL-4, IL-5, IFN-γ and GM-CSF CTL acticity variable Diminished production of IFN-γ No DTH skin reaction to antigens and diminished reaction after stimulation	Peak T cell number	Adult T cell number, age 4 Peak size of thymus, age 10 Decreased skin reaction persists to age 1
B cell	8 weeks, maternal IgG crosses placenta (majority in utero) 15 weeks, IgM secreting plasma cells present 17 weeks, some circulating fetal IgG may first be seen 20-30 weeks, IgG and Iga plasma cells first appear	T1-type 1 antigen response T-dependent response primary	T1-type 2 antigen response to encapsulated organisms Maximum IgM at 2-6 months	Circulating IgG is nearly all from infant (nadir at 3-4 months)
CD type	NK CD16 at 6 weeks gestation T cell thymocytes express CD7 at 7 weeks gestation T cell thymocytes express CD3, CD7, CD4 and CD8 at 12-14 weeks gestation T cell thymocytes express CD4 or CD8 > 14 weeks gestation	NK CD56 50% NK CD57 decreased Most CD4· T cells express CD45RA· marker (naïve)	CD45RA· cells → CD45RO· with age and antigen stimulation	

develop adequate cytotoxicity in addition to their increased numbers [21]. IL-2 and IFN-γ are potent activators of NK cells and IL-2 enhanced cytolytic activity is greater in the neonate than the adult. Cytolytic activity of neonatal cells, however, is less responsive to interferons [18, 22, 23]. Thus, it appears that although NK cell numbers are increased in the neonate, their function is decreased.

NK cells and T. gondii infection

In humans, NK and LAK cells are activated by *T. gondii* (Fig. 1) [24, 25]. In response to IL-12, TNF-γ, IL-15 and IL-1B produced by *T. gondii*-infected macrophages, NK cells produce large amounts of IFN-γ. IFN-γ (in conjunction with TNF-γ) activates murine macrophage and monocyte effect or function by stimulating reactive nitrogen intermediates (RNI) and oxygen free radical killing and tryptophan starvation. In mice, control of both acute and chronic *T. gondii* infection is dependent on IFN-γ as shown by increased susceptibility to infection in mice treated with anti-IFN-γ antibody [26]. Knockout of β2 microglobulin, which makes Class I MHC molecules nonfunctional, in a murine model, resulted in Class I dependent CD8+ deficiency and these mice had a robust expansion of NK cells and were protected against *T. gondii* infection [27]. In severe combined immunodeficiency (SCID) murine models where B and T cells are deficient, IFN-γ production by NK cells is regulated by IL-10, IL-2 and TNF-α [28]. Additional regulation by aco-stimulatory molecule, CD28, is involved in murine NK cell IFN-γ production after *T. gondii* infection [29]. Interestingly, NK cells are able to respond to IL-12 in the absence of IFN-γ by way of constitutive IL-12 receptor expression. This innate immune system mechanism alone, however, is unable to provide resistance to reactivation of toxoplasmic encephalitis in chronic infection of nude and SCID mice [30, 31] (Suzuki, personal communication). The early activation of NK cells with production of IFN-γ contributes to limiting tachyzoite replication prior to recruitment of immune T cell and drives differentiation of Th precursor cells to Th1 effector cells, potentiating specific cell-mediated immunity. Controversy remains, however, as to the role of NK cells in direct lysis of *T. gondii*-infected cells [24, 32].

Antigen presenting cells and phagocytes: monocytes and macrophages and dendritic cells

Mononuclear phagocytes include circulating monocytes and macrophages and are involved in the immune response through cytokine production, antigen processing and presentation, activation of T cells, phagocytosis and killing of pathogens and ADCC (Table 1).

Monocytes circulate in the blood for approximately 1-3 days prior to migrating into the tissues where they differentiate into macrophages. The vast majority of mononuclear phagocytes are macrophages and they persist in the tissues for approximately 4-12 weeks [33]. These cells have some innate microbicidal capacity and can be stimulated by TNF-α and IFN-γ to have enhanced microbicidal activity.

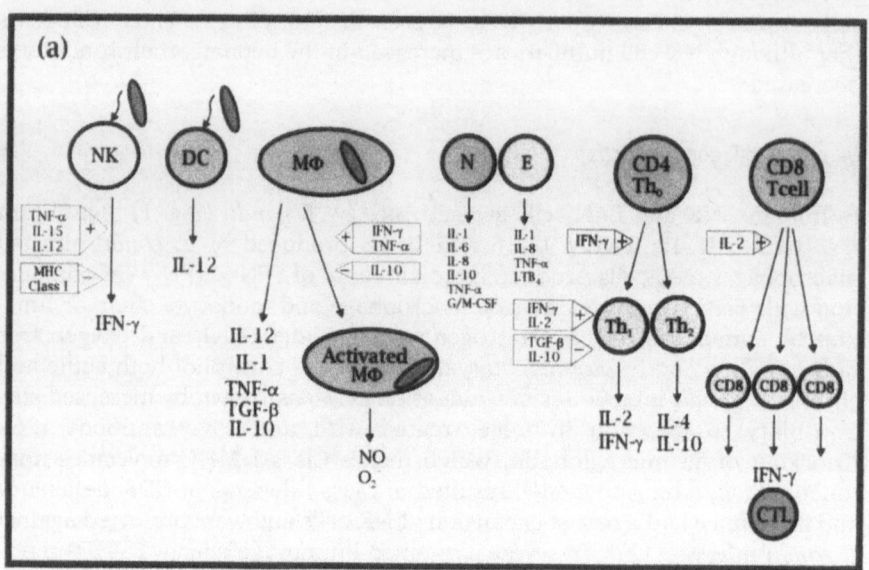

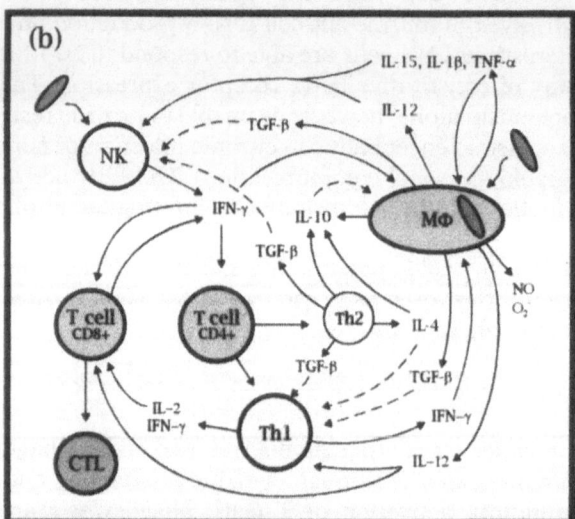

Fig. 1 a, b. Schematic illustration of representative immune cells, cytokines they produce (a) and their interrelationships important in protection and pathogenesis of toxoplasmosis (b). The data which support the importance of these representative interrelationships are largely derived from studies of mice and are only inferred for humans.
Solid line = stimulatory effect; dotted line = inhibitory effect

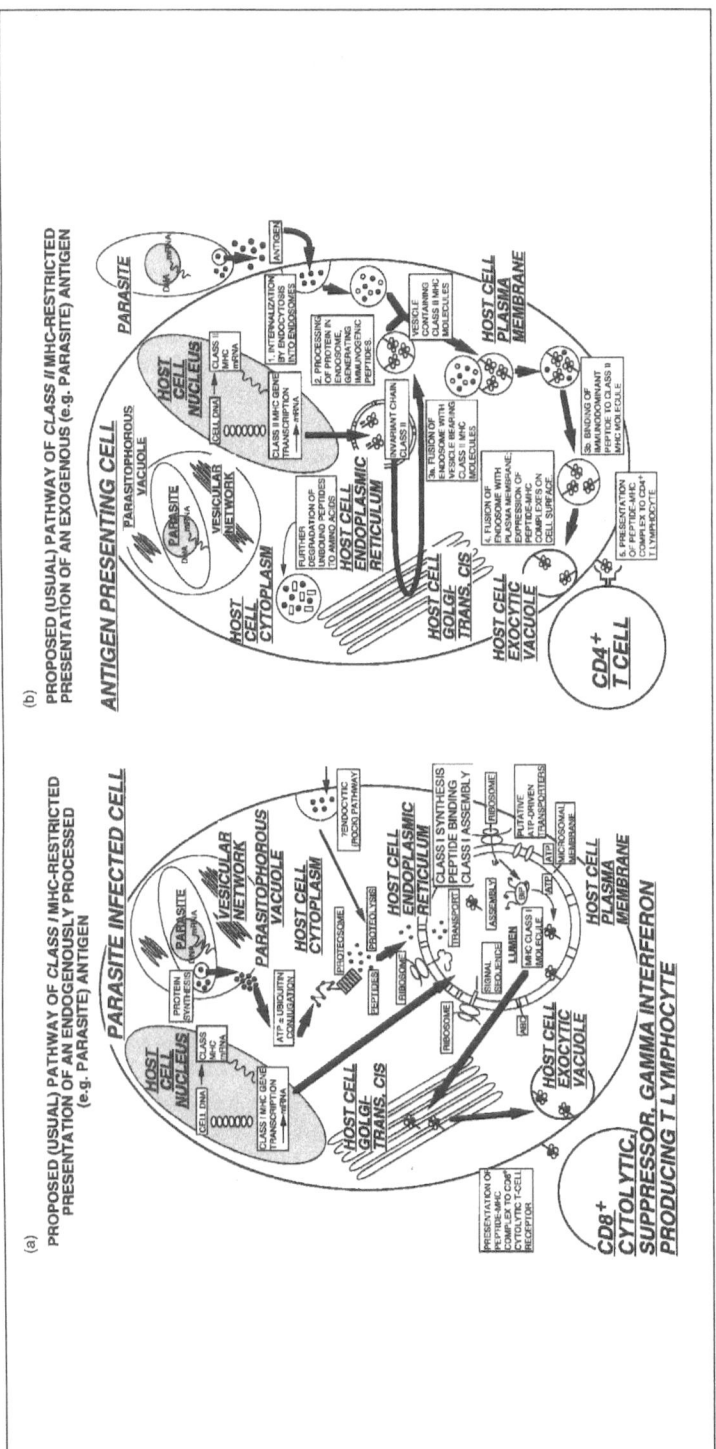

Fig. 2. Usual pathways of MHC Class I and Class II restricted processing and presentation of peptides to CD8- or CD4- T cells. (a) Class I cytoplasmic processing usually results instimulation of CD8- T lymphocytes that are cytolytic and/or produce IFN-γ or are suppressor T lymphocytes (b) Class II processing usually results in stimulation of CD4- T lymphocytes. Development of a Th1 (i.e IFN-γ and IL-2 producing) versus Th2 (i.e, IL-4 IL-5 and IL-10) phenotype depends in part on the interaction with costimulatory molecules such as B7-1 and B7-2 during sensitization. Adapted from Abbas [39] with modifications, and from McLeod et al [40] with permission

Mononuclear phagocytes, when they are primed and activated, can produce IL-12, IL-10, IL-6, IL-1, GM-CSF, IL-8 and TNF-α depending on the inciting stimulus and site of infection and inflammation (Fig. 1). If control of cytokine production is left unchecked, excessive amounts of TNF-α, IL-1 and IFN-γ can result in serious medical problems including shock and respiratory distress [34]. Both IL-12 and IFN-γ are necessary cytokines for an appropriate Th1 response to intracellular pathogens; IFN-γ is a very important cytokine in stimulating macrophage responses. IFN-γ itself is important in regulating the synthesis of IL-12, which in turn strongly induces differentiation of naive CD4+ cells toward Th1 cell type and enhances CTL and NK cell activity. Th1 cells scan in turn produce IFN-γ to further promote macrophage activity. Although it appears as though IFN-γ is required for IL-12 production, evidence for IL-12 production independent of IFN-γ stimulation has been reported in IFN-γ receptor-deficient murine cells challenged with *L. monocytogenes* and *T. gondii in vitro* [35, 36]. Others have shown that IL-12 is composed of a p35 chain constitutively produced by many cell types and a macrophage regulated p40 chain that requires both IFN-γ and a second stimulus from microbial products for optimal IL-12 synthesis [37, 38].

Mononuclear phagocytes as well as dendritic cells are important MHC class II expressing APC that efficiently present antigens to CD4+ T cells (Fig. 2) [39, 40]. Mononuclear phagocytes, like neutrophils, also ingest and kill bacteria and generate reactive oxygen metabolites but less efficiently than the neutrophils.

Dendritic cells are particularly potent APCs that, in humans, initiate T helper proliferation and cytokine release as well as induce cytolytic T cell responses [41, 42]. Dendritic cells present certain antigens more efficiently than B cells or macrophages, and they produce more IL 12 than macrophages [43, 44].

Development of antigen presenting cells in the fetus and neonate

As early as the 4th week of gestation, macrophages are found in the yolk sac followed by the liver and bone marrow (Table 1) [45]. Cytokine production by neonatal monocytes appears to be moderately impaired with respect to IL-6, TNF-α and GM-CSF, and relatively intact for IL-1 [46]. In addition, there is some evidence that IL-12 production is diminished in monocytes from umbilical cord blood which in turn results in a decrease of IFN-γ and Th1 response [47]. Since the mononuclear phagocyte system is perhaps the most primitive, it is the earliest to develop and plays an important part in antigen presentation. With the exception of diminished cutaneous delayed hypersensitivity reactions due to impaired chemotaxis, monocyte activity in the neonate has been reported to be qualitatively equal to and quantitatively equal to or greater than that of the adult [48]. When monocytes migrate from the circulation into tissues, they differentiate into macrophages and lose their myeloperoxidase activity. After migration into the tissues, macrophages do not recirculate and have an approximate life span of 4-12 weeks. Production of reactive oxygen metabolites, phagocytosis of particles and inhibition of viral replication by the neonatal monocyte are similar to that of monocytes of adults [49, 50]. Unfortunately, less is known about these functions of neonatal tissue macrophages because of difficulty isolating them. Few studies, however, suggest that phagocytosis and generation of oxygen metabolites are modestly impaired in the neonate [51].

Dendritic cells are present in the fetus. The fetus makes TGF-1 but this differs in its function in the fetus and adults [52].

Dendritic cells, mononuclear phagocytes, and Toxoplasma gondii infection

In vitro studies of human dendritic cells demonstrated a potent IL-12 response to either live *T. gondii* or parasite antigens but only in the presence of previously *T. gondii*-exposed T cells [53]. Contact between the T cell and dendritic cells was important for optimal IL-12 production and suggested the need for a receptor-ligand interaction in regulating the dendritic cells response. In murine models, this receptor is CD40 on dendritic cells, which is stimulated by the T cell ligand CD40L [54-56]. *In vivo* stimulation with *T. gondii* antigens induces rapid CD40L-independent production of IL12 by dendritic cells and their redistribution to T cell areas of the thymus [57]. Dendritic cells in human umbilical cord blood are functionally competent and resemble in their immature/resting state CD11c⁻ DC in peripheral blood [58].

During the earliest stages of *T. gondii* infection, parasite components stimulate macrophage release of IL-12, TNF-α and IL-1B [59]. Production of these cytokines appears to be the same in newborns with congenital toxoplasmosis and their mothers when stimulated with *T. gondii* antigens or other non-specific stimuli. (Mack et al., in preparation). These pro-inflammatory cytokines form the milieu in which parasite antigens interact with MHC molecules in the context of co-stimulatory molecules and T cell receptors (TCR) leading to a strong Th1 response. The details of this response and signaling pathways involved in the initial production of IFN-γ and IL-12 in response to microbial stimuli have been reviewed recently [59]. Data derived from experiments that utilized knockout mice, antibody blocking experiments and SCID mouse models have shown that this is a T cell independent process resulting in early IFN-γ production and stimulation of monocyte microbicidal function. In SCID mouse models, IFN-γ can be produced in the absence of B and T lymphocytes and is regulated by IL-12, IL-10 and TNF-α [28, 60]. Antibodies to IFN-γ, IL-12 TNF-α and NK cells result in increased susceptibility to parasite infection [37, 61, 6 2]. Protection against parasite invasion can be restored by replacing the deficient cytokine [37, 62-64]. Interestingly, the protective effects of treatment with recombinant IL-12 is blocked by antibodies to IFN-γ or NK cells and in IFN-γ knockout models suggesting that this cytokine acts via IFN-γ produced by NK cells [35]. *T. gondii* lysates alone reportedly also can stimulate IL-12 production from mouse dendritic cells in the absence of IFN-γ and independent of CD40/CD40L interaction with T cells [57]. In addition, production of the p40 chain of IL-12 appears to be regulated in part by an IFN-γ consensus sequence binding protein (ICSBP) such that ICSBP knockout mice are unable to produce sufficient

IL-12 and show impaired resistance to infection with this parasite [65]. These studies combined indicate that IFN-γ is essential for an optimal cell-mediated immune response to *T. gondii*.

As previously mentioned, the activation of monocytes and NK cells are important in the early stages of *T. gondii* infection by limiting the early extent of parasite replication and directing the Th1 cell response. Human mononuclear phagocytes are able to eliminate the majority of *T. gondii* that infect or invade them but not all and IFN-γ (plus TNF-α) leads to enhanced mononuclear phagocyte microbicidal capacity [66, 67]. In addition, parasite-human monocyte interactions can influence the subsequent T-cell response via altering the expression of co-stimulatory molecules, CD80 (B7.1) and CD86 (B7.2) [68].

IL-10 produced by Th2 cells, B cell and macrophages inhibits IFN-γ production from NK and T-cells via its effect on macrophages [69]. IL-10 blocks the activation of macrophages resulting in decreased IL-12, inhibition of microbicidal NO metabolite production and down-regulation of the Th1 response [70]. It has also been proposed that IL-10 production can avert an overwhelming Th1 response and that *T. gondii* may effectively induce immunosuppression by increasing IL-10 and thereby evade the murine host immune response [71, 72]. IL-4 similarly inhibits macrophage activity by potentiating IL-10 activity and directing CD4$^+$ Th differentiation toward the Th2 response [73]. Data derived from experiments using IL-4 knockout mice has shown that IL-4 too may be important in preventing an overwhelming Th1 response and thus, a mechanism for downmodulating an overabundant host immune response [74]. Similar evasion of the host immune response may be seen with TGF-β through influence on NO production, IL-10 potentiation and IL-12 inhibition as well as MHC molecule down-regulation in *T. gondii* infection [61, 73, 75, 76]. The *Nramp* gene in mice also appears to play a role in protection against toxoplasmosis perhaps through macrophage killing of *T. gondii* [67, 77, 78].

PMN

Neutrophilic granulocytes are a subset of phagocytic cells that ingest and kill bacteria. Once neutrophils [79] are released from the bone marrow, they circulate in peripheral blood until they are attracted to a site of infection or injury. Chemotactic factors and adhesion molecules help coordinate the recruitment of neutrophils to these sites. Phagocytosis often requires the help of opsonins (antibody or complement) and is followed by ingestion and exposure to oxygen-dependent killing of organisms. Neutrophils produce leukotrienes (LTB4) in addition to the inflammatory mediators, IL-1, TNF-α and IL-8 [80, 81].

PMN development in the fetus/neonate

The fetus and newborn have an impaired ability to mount a sustained neutrophil response to infection primarily due to limited bone marrow reserve and near maximal rate of production. In the fetus, precursors are initially detected in the yolk sac, liver, spleen and bone marrow after macrophages are seen at approximately 4 weeks gestation. By 14-16 weeks gestation, mature neutrophils are present. Neutrophils constitute fewer than 10% of circulating leukocytes up to 22-24 weeks gestation and 50-60% at term [48]. Studies with neonatal rats have shown that the neutrophil bone marrow reserves are only 20-30% of adult levels and that these stores are easily depleted in response to inflammatory stimuli [82]. In addition, human neutrophil adhesion ability is estimated to be only 40-45% of that seen in adults and results in diminished binding and migration into tissues [83, 84]. Diminished chemotaxis is also noted in the newborn and in children up to 1-2 years of age [85, 86]. Oxygen-dependent microbicidal mechanisms for the most part, however, appear relatively intact [87, 88]. Mature neutrophils circulate for approximately 8-10 hours and then migrate into the tissues where they die after 24 hours.

PMN and T. gondii infection

In the earliest stages of *T. gondii* infection, neutrophils (as well as macrophages, NK cells and dendritic cells) release cytokines such as IL-12, TNF-α, and IFN-γ [89].

Eosinophils

Eosinophils are granulocytes involved in immune responses to allergic states, some parasite infections, and some autoimmune and malignant diseases. Proliferation of eosinophils involves IL-3, GM-CSF and IL-5 [90].

Development of eosinophils in the fetus and neonate

IgE binds eosinophil cell surface markers resulting in the release of peroxidase [91]. In human cord blood studies, the FcεRI surface marker is expressed relatively early in differentiation whereas the CD23/FcεRII surface marker expression suggests eosinophil activation [79, 92]. In the fetus, eosinophils comprise 10-20% of the total granulocytes at 18-30 weeks gestation, and in the neonate peak numbers occur 3-4 weeks after birth [92].

Eosinophils and T. gondii infection

Eosinophilia (i.e. sometimes quite marked with as many as 50% peripheral blood eosinophils and substantial numbers of CSF eosinophils) can be marked in human congenital *T. gondii* infection (unpublished), but the reasons for this are not known. Murine (i.e. rat) eosinophils have been reported to have microbicidal capacity against antibody coated *T. gondii* [93].

Specific immunity/ Cell-mediated and humoral

T-cells and cell-mediated immunity [6]

T lymphocytes are thymus-derived cells that recognize protein antigens and regulate the immune response by acting as effector cells against intracellular pathogens. These cells depend on non-lymphoid accessory cells to initiate the recognition phase of the T cell response and to provide a co-stimulatory signal for full T cell activation. Initiation of this response occurs when antigen presenting cells (APC), such as mononuclear phagocytes or dendritic cells, display foreign peptides on their surface. These specialized APCs provide T cells with peptide bound to self-molecules derived from genes of the major histocompatibility complex (MHC). Class I MHC molecules associate with beta-2 microglobulin and present peptides cleaved from proteins processed within the cytoplasm of APC (Fig. 2). In contrast, class II MHC molecules associate with peptides originally derived from extracellular proteins internalized via endocytosis prior to transport to the cell surface (Fig. 2). The internalized proteins are then broken down, producing peptide products for display on the APC surface membrane. The genetic region encoding the human leukocyte antigens (HLA) is known as the human MHC and corresponds to the murine H-2 gene locus (Fig. 3) [40, 94].

T cell signalling is mediated by a number of membrane proteins and accessory molecules, including the T cell antigen receptor (TCR). The TCR is structurally related to immunoglobulin, containing a variable region that binds antigen and a conserved region anchored to the membrane. Gene rearrangement of the variable region forms a unique antigen recognition site that provides incredible diversity of the TCR. In lymphoid organs, the TCR exists as a heterodimer predominately of the alpha-beta form while the gamma-delta TCR form is more abundant in mucosal tissues. In addition, the TCR associates with a T cell membrane protein complex, CD3, which is thought to be intimately involved in signal transduction within the cell.

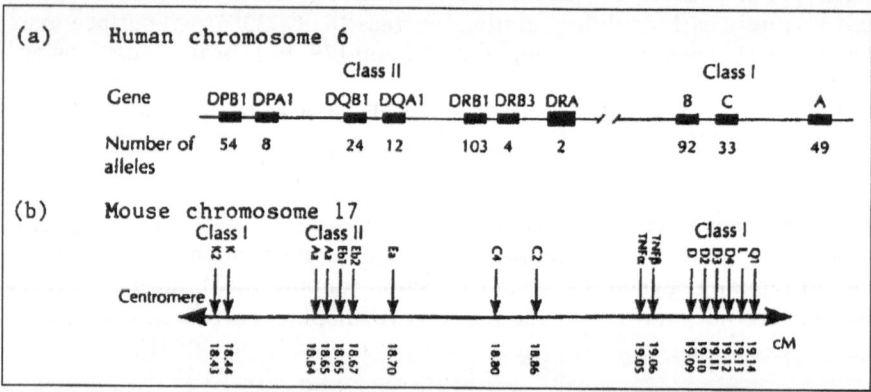

Fig. 3. (a) Map of location of polymorphic HLA Class I and Class II genes in the human MHC on chromosome 6. The number of known alleles of each gene, whether identified serologically or by sequence analysis, is indicated. From [179] and [180], with modifications based on data from [181]. (b) Schematic diagram indicating the location of these MHC loci on mouse chromosome 17. Control of resistance to cyst burden following peroral infection with *T. gondii* had been mapped previously to a region of mouse chromosome 17 of approximately 140 kb. From McLeod et al. [40], and Brown et al. [94] with permission

T cells may be separated into subsets based on their functionally distinct cell membrane proteins. For instance, CD4+ cells are usually T helper cells, recognize class II MHC molecules bearing peptide and produce IL-2. CD4+ T cells also produce IFN-γ and thus stimulate macrophage activity and enhance the production of antibody by B cells. Alternatively, CD8+ cells are usually cytolytic T lymphocytes (CTL), recognize class IMHC molecules (Fig. 2) and also can produce IFN-γ. These cells lyse other cells expressing foreign antigen in the context of peptide associated with MHC class I and eliminate pathogens that infect and live intracellularly. In addition to identification of specific cell subtypes, these cell surface proteins play an important role in the activation and function of T cells. Upon encountering an APC with antigen bound to the proper MHC class, the TCR in association with CD3 forms a receptor complex that signals T cell activation. T cell activation involves the stimulation of a naïve T cell to proliferate in response to its own growth-promoting cytokines, principally IL-2, and the up-regulation of the IL-2 receptor (IL-2R). This proliferation results in clonal expansion and the production of enough antigen-specific T cells to mount an appropriate immune response. In the case of the CTL, encountering an antigen bound to class I MHC activates the cell via the TCR/CD3 complex. This response is enhanced by CD2 (LFA-2), LFA-1 and CD28 on the T cell and in association with their respective counter receptors LFA-3, CD54 and B7 on the APC. Once activated, the cytolytic T cell produces perforins and serine esterases that mediate cytolysis [95, 96]. Antibody blocking experiments have shown that the CD4 and CD8 molecules are not absolutely essential for a T cell response. Instead, they are thought to facilitate the T cell response by increasing the avidity of the TCR that has a low affinity for the APC peptide-MHC complex. Upon activation, T cells differentiate into helper T cells or cytolytic T cells, which activate a cascade of immune response through the production of interleukins and interferon gamma (IFN-γ) (Table 3) [97].

The CD4+ T helper (Th) immune response illustrates the important modulatory effects of T cell cytokines. CD4+ Th cells mobilize different effect or functions, Th1 or Th2, based on the cytokines produced [98]. Th1 cells respond to IL-12 and IFN-γ by producing cytokines that activate macrophages and provide optimal protection against intracellular pathogens (phagocyte-dependent host response). In murine models, Th1 cells produce IL-2, IFN-γ and control IgG2a production. Th2 cells , on the other hand, respond to IL-4 to enhance B cell maturation and antibody production (phagocyte-independent host response). Th2 responses are toxic to complex pathogens and simultaneously inhibit macrophages. Th2 cells have been shown in mice to produce IL-4, IL-5, and IL-10 as well as to control IgG1 and IgE production.

In addition to cytokines produced by T cells, there is a co-stimulatory signal produced by APCs that is required for T cell clonal expansion and optimal cytokine production [68, 99]. The most important co-stimulatory signal identified to date is the interaction between CD28 (homologous to CTLA-4) found on T cells and its counter receptor, CD80 (B7.1) and CD86 (B7.2) found on the APC [68, 100, 101]. In human T cell studies, IL-12 synergizes with the B7/CD28 complex resulting in cell proliferation and cytokine production [102].

Table 3. The source and actions of cytokines important for *T. gondii* infection

Cytokines	Major sources	Actions in *T. gondii* infection	Effect ont murine Acute	Toxoplasmosis Chronic
IFN-γ	CD4· T cells CD8· T cells NK cells	Inhibits parasite growth by: (i) Induction of ROI and RNI by macrophages (ii) Eicosinoid production via 5-lipoxygenase pathway in macrophages (iii) Induction of IDO and tryptophan starvation by various cell types	Protective Exogenous IFN-γ prolongs survival in infected mice	Protective Neutralisation of IFN-γ increases cyst rupture and severity of encephalitis in infected mice
TNF-α	Macrophages	Acts in synergy with IL-12 to induce NK cell production of IFN-γ	Protective Neutralisation of TNF-α increases mortality in infected mice	Protective Neutralisation of TNF-α increases cyst rupture and severity of encephalitis in infected mice
IL-12	Macrophages	Acts in synergy with TNF-α to induce IFN-γ production by NK cells and CD4· and CD8· T cells	Protective Exogenous IL-12 prolongs survival in infected mice	Not required Neutralisation of IL-12 has no effect on survival or cyst numbers
IL-2	CD4· T cells	Increased production of IFN-γ by NK cells Enhanced cytotoxicity of CD8· T cells	Protective Exogenous IL-2 prolongs survival in infected mice	Protective Exogenous IL-1 decreases cyst numbers in brain
IL-4	CD4· T cells	Down regulation of Th1 associated, pro-inflammatory cytokines	Protective Increased mortality in infected IL-4 gene knockout mice compared with wild type mice	Detrimental Increased cyst numbers and severity of encephalitis in infected IL-4 gene knockout mice compared with wild type mice
IL-10	CD4· T cells	Inhibits IL-12 synthesis by acrophages. Down regulation of TH1 associated, pro-inflammatory cytokines	Protective Increased mortality infected IL-10 gene knockout mice compared with wild type mice	Not known
TGF-β	Macrophages	Antagonises the actions of IFN-γ	Unclear Neutralisation of TGF-β delayed time to death. Exogenous TGF-β led to earlier death in SCID mice	Not known

From Roberts F., MD Thesis, Glasgow University (with permission)

The relevance of this co-stimulation is emphasized by the finding that occupancy of the TCR in the absence of a co-stimulatory signal results in a state of T cell unresponsiveness [103, 104]. The cell is unable to produce IL-2 even when subsequently exposed to the appropriate antigen and the required co-stimulatory signal. This state of unresponsiveness is similar to *in vivo* T cell clonal anergy. It is suggested that the manipulation of co-stimulatory molecules by intracellular pathogens may represent a strategy to avoid detection thereby inducing anergy or immunosuppression [68].

While some of the progeny of antigen-stimulated lymphocytes develop into effector cells, others are destined to become memory cells. These cells remain quiescent until stimulated by specific antigen. The factors responsible for inducing and maintaining the responsiveness of memory cells are not known; however, they do not appear to require all of the co-stimulatory signals needed by the naïve T cell to respond. Distinct cell surface proteins distinguish naïve and memory T cells and it is estimated that approximately 40% of human CD4$^+$ T cells have memory function and express CD45RO protein. The remaining 60% of CD4$^+$ T cells are considered naïve and express CD45RA on their cell surface. It is unclear if similar surface proteins appear on the CD8$^+$ memory or naïve T cells. Memory cells are more readily activated to proliferate than naive T cells and are able to produce IL-4 and IFN-γ, but have reduced capacity to produce IL-2 [105].

In addition, there is yet another avenue down which antigen stimulated lymphocytes may travel. This is known as apoptosis and is a form of regulated, physiologic cell death. Apoptosis is considered to be an important homeostatic mechanism of the immune system and is thought to contribute to maintenance of a fairly constant lymphoid pool [106]. Another form of apoptosis is known as activation-induced cell death and is thought to play an important role in recognition of self-antigens and induction of tolerance to some foreign antigens.

T cell development/function in the neonate and fetus

Before the thymus is colonized with precursor T cells, lymphoid cells are found in the yolk sac and liver of the human fetus at 7 weeks gestation [107]. These cells express the CD7 surface marker characteristic of prothymocytes found in the bone marrow; however, no other surface markers indicating further maturation of the T cell lineage is found. Thymocyte differentiation is marked by the migration of prothymocytes from the bone marrow and liver to the subcapsular region of the thymus at about 8.5 weeks gestation. These cells have neither undergone TCR rearrangement nor expression and are referred to as type I thymocytes (CD7$^+$ CD3$^-$ CD4$^-$ CD8$^-$). Once in this environment, they begin to express CD3 and undergo TCR gene rearrangement with subsequent expression of intact protein [108]. This process is analogous to B cell clonal development and immunoglobulin gene rearrangement. The $\gamma\delta$ receptor is the first TCR to be expressed during fetal life followed by the $\alpha\beta$ receptor. Epitope mapping studies describe the $\gamma\delta$-TCR as interacting with MHC at a distinctly different site than the $\alpha\beta$-TCR. This observation suggests

that the molecular nature of the αβ-TCR is fundamentally different from the
γδ-TCR [109]. At this stage they become type II thymocytes. If gene rearrangement fails to yield an intact protein, alternate rearrangement may occur at
the other allele. A functional TCR product, however, blocks additional rearrangement at the other allele demonstrating the process of allelic exclusion.
The mechanisms for generating diversity of the TCR include gene rearrangement as well as imprecise recombinase enzymes and the activity of terminal
deoxytranferase (TdT). The recombinase allows for various numbers of
nucleotides to be lost during segment rearrangement whereas TdT is able to
add nucleotides at random to the adjoining segments. These mechanisms in
combination with the occasional duplication of nucleotides (P-nucleosides)
at segment junctions result in the tremendous diversity of TCR specificity.
The 8 weeks old fetus, however, demonstrates limited diversity in the V, D and
J region of the TCRβ chain reportedly due to decreased activity of the TdT
enzyme. By 16 weeks gestation, the TdT enzyme activity has increased to near
adult levels, allowing for minimal restriction of TCR diversity [110]. Pairing
the two heterodimers (γδ, αβ) of the TCR together further increases diversity.
From these observations, limitation of the TCR repertoire is not a major difference from adults in the neonate but may be so in the fetus prior to mid-
gestation.

By 12-14 weeks gestation, the thymus supports type II and III thymocytes
making up the cortex and medulla, respectively. Type II thymocytes not only
express CD3 and a functional TCR, they also exhibit high levels of CD4 and
CD8 cell surface markers (CD7+ CD3+ CD4+ CD8+). Around this time they
undergo a positive selection process that allows only self-MHC restricted cells
to survive [111, 112]. In addition, some cells also undergo negative selection
via apoptosis when the TCR in conjunction with CD4 or CD8 reacts too strongly to self-peptide bound by MHC. This clonal deletion process or tolerance
is important to the developing immune system as it involves the deletion of
self-reactive T cells during their maturation in the thymus thereby circum-
venting the problem of potential self-reactivity [113]. The process of negative
selection is demonstrated in mice using experimentally introduced self-antigens and proteins of tumor viruses that result in the elimination of that particular reactive T cell during thymic development [114-116]. Positive and
negative selection interact in combination with unproductive gene rearrangement to result in the majority of thymic precursors dying rather than becoming mature thymocytes [111, 117]. This preserves the developing T cells that
express self-MHC restriction and foreign antigen-specific TCRs.

Type III thymocytes are those cells located in the medulla and express CD7,
CD3 and either CD4 or CD8. These CD4+ or CD8+ T cells emigrate from the
thymus and are found in the fetal liver and spleen around 14 weeks gestation
[118]. Like peripheral CD4+ T cells, CD4+CD8- thymocytes can produce IL-2
and enhance B cell production of antibody. Similarly, CD4-CD8+ thymocytes
mimic their peripheral CD8+ T cell counterparts in their ability to mediate
cytolytic activity after antigen priming.

The last trimester demonstrates the most rapid increase in thymic cellularity and this increased cellularity continues until 10 years of age when the

thymus begins to involute sparing the medulla relative to the cortex (type III > type II thymocytes). The number of circulating fetal T cells gradually increases from the second trimester until about 6 months of age when a decline to adult levels is observed. The CD4:CD8 ratio during fetal life is high and this persists until 4 years of age when the ratio approaches adult levels [119]. Most circulating neonatal CD4⁺ T cells express the CD45RA⁺ surface marker similar to that of naïve adult T cells with a limited exposure to antigen. This number appears to decline with conversion to CD45RO⁺ phenotype with age and exposure to antigenic stimuli [120]. There is also some evidence that neonatal CD8⁺ T cells also lack cell surface markers associated with CTL memory cell activation [121]. Anywhere from 0 to 100% of adult CTL activity is reported at 15-22 weeks gestation and 50-100% activity is reported in presensitized neonatal CTL *in vitro*, which may reflect the absence of memory T cells [122].

The presentation of antigens is critically important to activation and generation of an appropriate T cell response. By 12 weeks gestation, the major APCs present are mononuclear phagocytes B cells, dendritic cells), as are the class I and II MHC molecules [123, 124]. There are reports of effective and defective fetal monocyte/macrophage antigen presentation [123-125]. CD8⁺ CTL are also reported to produce a vigorous response to non-matched transplanted tissue. These data together suggest that fetal and neonatal APC function and expression of surface MHC is grossly intact.

Cytokines are the key immune-modulators of the T cell immune response. Neonatal T cells have intact IL-2 mediated response indicated by their expression of IL-2 and IL-2R as effectively as adult T cells [126, 127]. Their ability to proliferate and respond to *in vitro* stimuli, however, is more similar to the adult naïve T cell [128]. This is thought to be more a function of the intrinsically naïve and immature nature of the cell rather than dysfunction since the response improves with an increase in proportion of memory T cells. The production of other cytokines (i.e. IFN-γ, IL-4) by the neonatal immune system is slightly or markedly reduced [129]. Cell culture studies suggest that in humans, IL-10 inhibits T cell IFN-γ production by suppression of NK and accessory cell stimulation [130]. Overall, fetal and neonatal T cell function is impaired compared to the adult. Reduced cytokine production and the relative deficiency of memory T cells may contribute in part to this impairment. T cell responses in neonates are biased toward a Th2 profile [131]. Mechanisms for this polarization are not yet defined. Neonatal T cells have altered thresholds of responsiveness to signaling and more rapid degradation and thus biological effects of cytokines [131].

T cells and T. gondii infection

Resistance to *T. gondii* in the immunocompetent host is mediated primarily by CD4+ and CD8+ T lymphocytes [132]. Although CD8+ cells are the major effector cells in mice, their induction and optimal function is dependent on CD4+ cells, most likely Th1 cells, through the effects of IL-12 and IL-2 [9, 133, 134]. In humans, CD4+ and CD8+ T cells have been reported to be cytotoxic for *T. gondii* infected cells [135]. Cytolytic T cells of mice do not appear to cause apoptosis of the parasite when they cause apoptosis of the infected cell [136, 137].

Interestingly, *T. gondii* infection causes marked involution of the thymus in the human fetus and this was also shown to be the case in animal models in adult animals [138, 139], (Fig. 4). The responsible mechanisms and implications of this finding for outcome of congenital infection when this happens to the developing fetal thymus have not been determined.

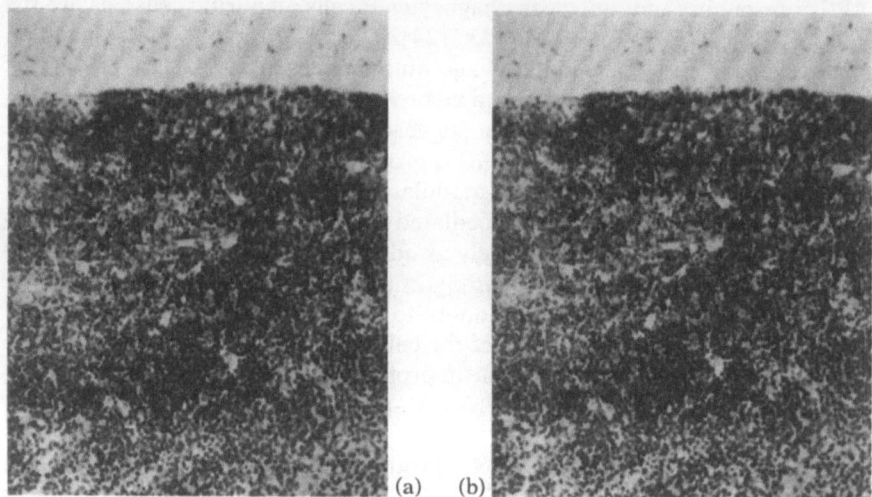

(a)   (b)

Fig. 4. Thymus tissue from an SWR/J mouse infected with the Me49 strain of *T. gondii* (a) 13 days earlier, and (b) from an uninfected control mouse. In the normal thymus, the richly cellular cortex is demarcated from the less cellular medulla (original magnification x128). In the atrophic thymus from the *Toxoplasma* infected mouse, a depletion of cells is evident in the cortex without a demarcation between the cortex and the medulla (original magnification x128). Similar changes have been described in the fetal human thymus of congenitally infected individuals. From McLeod et al. [139] (with permission)

Hohfeld et al. [140] reported that peripheral blood from the congenitally infectected fetus has a smaller % CD3 and CD4 T cells, an absolute decrease in the number of CD4 cells and a lower CD4:CD8 ratio. LeColier [141] described an increase in fetal CD8+T cells (3-6 weeks after acquisition of maternal infection) and a decrease in CD4+ T cells (7-13 weeks after acquisition of maternal infection), findings similar to those of acutely infected adults, but Foulon [142] did not confirm these results.

In humans, control of *T. gondii* infection is associated in part with an early response of T cells with αβ-TCR [143]. NK cells as well as αβ T cells respond to the early invasion of the parasite and are an important source of IFN-γ. Unprimed newborn αβ T cells proliferate when incubated with *T. gondii* infected macrophages suggesting that they recognize traditionally processed parasite antigen. In addition, other studies have reported T cell unresponsiveness to *T. gondii* in congenital infection [144, 145]. McLeod et al. [144] reported normal blastogenesis and production of IL-2 and IFN-γ of newborn mononuclear leukocytes to the mitogens conanavalinA and phytohemagglutinin and in mixed leukocyte culture but not to *Toxoplasma*-lysate antigens (TLA). The unresponsiveness to TLA was no longer present for most children when medications were discontinued at 1 year of age (Fig. 5), [144, 146], but for some children the magnitude of response remained less than that of adults [3]. Children infected earlier in gestation and with more severe disease had the most impaired immune responses. Inability to produce IL-2 and IFN-γ correlated with lymphocyte unresponsiveness, although another study [147] identified elevated levels of IFN-γ in peripheral blood as a nonspecific marker of the congenital infection. There was no clonal deletion, suppression or uniformly predominant Th2 cytokine response (although this was present for some infants) to explain the immunologic unresponsiveness to *Toxoplasma gondii* antigens in our study.

In contrast to McLeod et al.'s finding of normal blastogenic response to ConA and in MLR, Hara et al. [145] reported both αB and γδ T cells from infants with severe congenital infection were unresponsive to CD3 as a mitogen, TLA, and live *Toxoplasma* infected cells when they were one month of age. At 5 months old, they exhibited selective anergy to TLA and *Toxoplasma* infected cells. Interestingly, by 1 year of age γδ T cells were shown to proliferate and secrete interferon when exposed to parasite infected cells where as the αβ T cells remained unresponsive to *Toxoplasma* antigens, perhaps contributing to their increased susceptibility to ocular reactivation. This suggests that the γδ T cell unresponsiveness appeared to be lost earlier than the αβ T cell unresponsiveness in infected infants [145].

Studies using murine models have shown that host protection is mediated largely by IFN-γ produced by CD8+ cells, CD4+ Th1 cells and NK cells, through activation of macrophages, and inhibitory-down modulating Th2 cytokine production [26]. Although the CD4+ T cell response to *T. gondii* infection is preferentially of the Th1 type, in the immunocompetent host, pregnancy is thought to be associated with a hormonally-influenced increase in Th2 cytokines [148, 149]. The Th2 response is associated with the down-regulation of the Th1 response, NK cells and CD8+ cells. The down-regulation of the Th1 response is thought to be a protective measure in pregnancy as it reduces the exposure of the fetus to potentially harmful pro-inflammatory cytokines (i.e. IL-2, IFN-γ).

Interestingly, the predominance of the Th2 immunologic response increases the susceptibility to *T. gondii* infection in pregnant mice. This is likely due to decreases in the production of IFN-γ, IL-2 and TNF-α, all of which contribute to protection against *T. gondii* infection [150]. Pregnant mice deficient in IL-4, a Th2 product, showed an improved survival following *T. gondii* infection compared to non-pregnant mice [148]. IL-10 deficient mice show similar decreased mortality [71]. In addition, the high levels of progesterone during pregnancy can increase IL-4 production and also may be a contributing factor in susceptibility to *T. gondii* [151]. Some reports even suggest that since *T. gondii* is such a potent inducer of a Th1 mediated response, it could promote abortion by altering the preferred Th2 cytokine pattern during pregnancy [152]. Interestingly, it is postulated that pregnant immuno-competent mice have an increased mortality post-partum due to a rebound response as they shift from a predominantly hormonally induced Th2 to a vigorous and possibly lethal Th1 response [148].

There are two mechanisms by which CD8+ lymphocytes act to limit *T. gondii* infection. The first is through production of IFN-γ and the second is through the direct cytolytic effect on the parasite by the T cells. The role of IFN-γ is demonstrated by the ablation of CD8+ cell mediated resistance by anti-IFN-γ in mice [153]. Although CD4+ cells secrete a higher level of IFN-γ than NK cells do, it is thought that *T. gondii* infected cells express parasite peptides presented in an MHC class I restricted manner that preferentially stimulate CD8+ T cells and IFN-γ activity *in vivo* [152]. The production of IFN–γ by the NK cells is necessary but not sufficient for protection against *T. gondii* [37, 63]. IFN-γ is not only important for the promotion of the Th1 response and inhibition of the Th2 response; it also effects tachyzoite growth in somatic cells and macrophages. The second mechanism for CD8+ T cells activity is through direct cytolytic effect on *T. gondii*-infected host cells but not on the parasite itself [135, 154-156]. These effector cells are class I MHC restricted and require interaction with target cells as well as expansion due to IL-2 [157].

The observation that the most severely affected neonates have acquired their *T. gondii* infection in the first trimester is consistent with reports of T cells having a limited ability for antigen recognition during this time [110]. Severe cases are often acquired in early gestation when host defenses are relatively primitive and tolerance more pronounced. Tolerance is a significant problem in congenital toxoplasmosis and results in T cells that are incapable of distinguishing *T. gondii* from self. These newborns have little to no lymphocyte blastogenic response to *Toxoplasma* lysate antigen (TLA) and poor production of IL-2 and IFN-γ [137]. The severity of clinical manifestations also appeared to correlate with lower lymphocyte proliferation although this is likely the result of multiple types of immune dysfunction. Similar effects are seen in congenital HSV [158] and CMV [159] supporting the assumption that early exposure in gestation and ontogeny of T cells results in the recognition of foreign antigen as self and tolerance to that antigen.

Co-stimulatory molecules play a crucial role in the T cell response to *T. gondii* infection. T cell proliferation in response to *T. gondii* is dependent on the initiation of CD80 and the up-regulation of CD86 expression on APC and subsequent IFN-γ and IL-2 production [68]. These co-stimulatory signals act to enhance the antigen-specific T cell response. CD40 and CD40 ligand also appear to be essential for protection against toxoplasmosis. Interestingly,

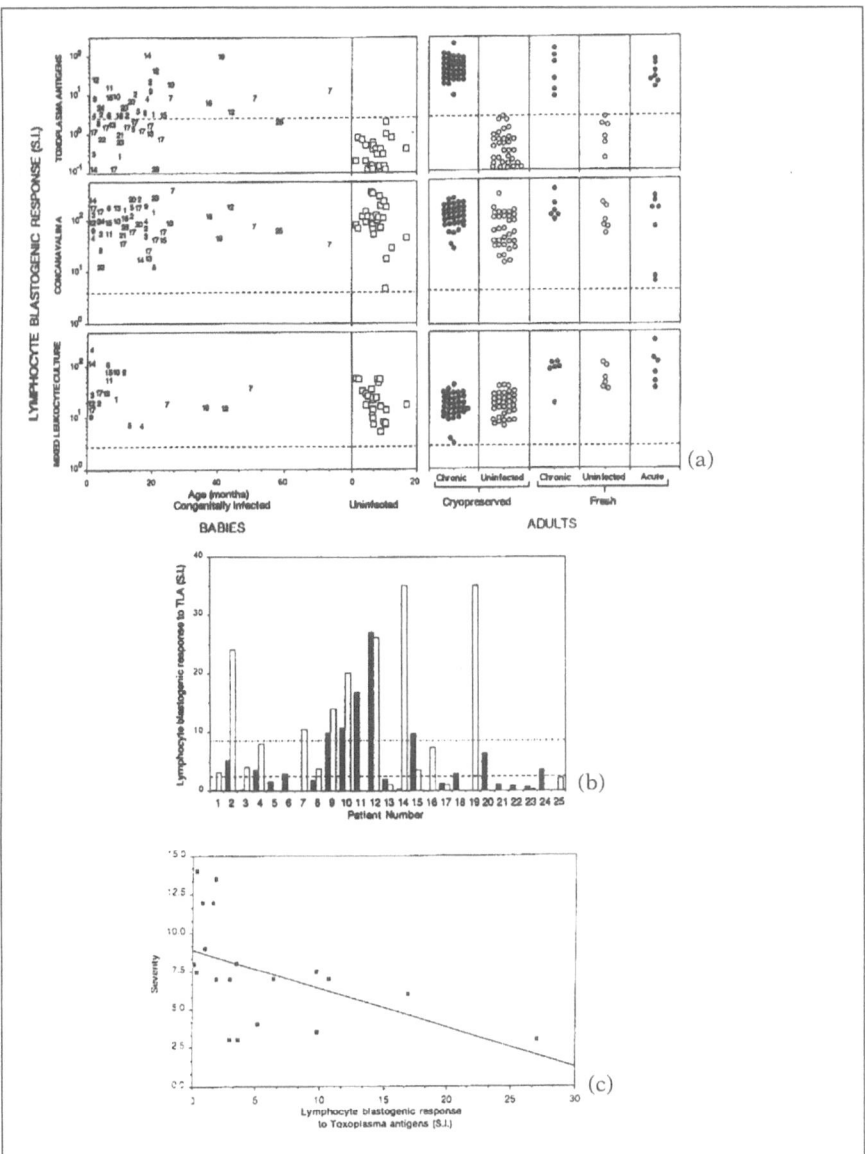

Fig. 5. Lymphocyte blastogenic responses in infants with congenital toxoplasmosis. (a) *Toxoplasma* lysate antigens (*top*), Concanavalin A (*center*) and mixed leukocyte culture (*bottom*). The dashed lines demarcate positive and negative responses; (b) Lymphocyte response of all study children to *Toxoplasma* lysate antigens. Infants older than 13.5 months are represented by solid bars and those children older than 15.6 months by open bars. The horizontal dashed line at S.I. = 2.5 demarcates positive and negative responses. The horizontal dashed and dotted line at S.I. = 8 indicate the lowest responses of lymphocytes from infected adults; (c) Correlation of lymphocyte blastogenic response to *Toxoplasma* lysate antigen and severity score. Correlation between diminished transformation and severity was significant (P = 0.002). Patient numbers are those used in publications from the US National Collaborative Study Group. (a-c) From McLeod et al. [144] (with permission)

other intracellular organisms (*Leishmania* and *Mycobacterium* species) fail to increase and can decrease the expression of certain of these co-stimulatory molecules [160, 161]. This demonstrates the ability of intracellular organisms to have a significant effect on immunity by avoiding recognition and inducing anergy through the regulation of co-stimulation.

IFN-γ is a major cytokine involved in the host protective response to *T. gondii*; however, in the neonate its production, as with IL-4, is markedly reduced [162, 163]. Interestingly, the diagnosis of *T. gondii* infection is suspected in the fetus with elevated levels of IFN-γ [164]. If blocked by anti-IFN-γ antibody, the protective effects of IFN-γ are disrupted in mice [165]. Administration of recombinant IFN-γ decreases mortality and prolongs survival in *T. gondii* infected mice [166]. The production of IL-6 in term newborns is only slightly diminished whereas in preterm newborns it is 25% of adult levels [167]. The role of TNF-α may depend on amount of a TNF-α produced relative to other cytokines and perhaps other aspects of host genetics of TNF, or other factors, as it has been shown to be both protective and associated with increased mortality in murine models [64, 168].

Recent data suggest another subversion of the host cell immune system that involves the resistance of *T. gondii* infected cells to multiple stimulators of apoptosis [169]. *T. gondii* is thought to likely block either the activation or function of three proteases that cleave repair enzymes. Heat shock protein 65 expression has also been shown to protect *T. gondii* infected macrophages from apoptosis [170]. Similarly, the self-produced TNF-α protects *Leishmania* infected macrophages from apoptosis [171].

Humoral Immunity [15]

Humoral immunity is mediated by blood borne immunoglobulins, expressed on or secreted by B lymphocytes. Like the TCR, immunoglobulins associate with antigens and transmit signals to the interior of cells. Once stimulated, B cells differentiate and proliferate into specific antibody secreting plasma cells. B cells may also participate in antigen presentation to CD4+ T cells via MHC Class II recognition. In studies using murine models, there are three types of responses (T1-type 1, T1-type 2 and T-dependent) to antigen stimulation. T1-type 1 antigen binds to B cells and is independent of the thymus and T cells. T1-type 2 antigens are primarily polysaccharides and require a few T cells for optimal antibody production. The T-dependent antigen responses, however, are the majority and require B cell and T cell interactions. With the exception of IgM, T-dependent antibody production depends on the CD40 B cell molecule binding to the CD40-ligand on T cells [172]. Similar interactions with B7/CD28 and LFA-1/CD54 ligand pairs are also seen [173].

B cell development in the fetus and neonate

Pre-B cells are in the fetal liver by 8 weeks gestation and in the fetal bone marrow by 13 weeks ADDIN ENRfu [174]. By 10 weeks gestation, IgM but not IgG is expressed and antigen exposure at this stage delivers a tolerogenic signal [168]. Between 10-12 weeks, IgA, IgG and IgD appear and by 22 weeks, the number of B cells in lymphoid organs is similar to the adult [169]. Maternal IgG transport across the placenta is seen at 8 weeks of gestation and by term, the neonatal contribution of IgG exceeds the maternal level by 5-10% [170]. By 10-12 months of age, the IgG is completely derived from the infant. The concentration of IgM reaches 60% of adults at 12 months of age. IgA concentrations are approximately 20% of adult levels by 12 months of age and continue to rise through adolescence. Secretory IgA, however, is undetectable at birth, first seen at 2 months of age and reaches adult values by 6-8 years of age [171]. T cell help for B cells in the neonate is not grossly deficient since B cell production of antibody is similar or only slightly reduced [172, 173]. In addition, there appears to be no difference in antibody synthesis from pre-term B cells and those from term neonates.

Humoral immunity and T. gondii infection

Protective immune responses to *T. gondii* infection are primarily via cell-mediated immune mechanisms; however, there is evidence in mice that antibodies produced after exposure to *Toxoplasma* antigens may enhance survival and reduce the number of *Toxoplasma* brain cysts. Antibody and complement lyse extracellular parasites and opsinization of parasites leads to their intracellular destruction within nonactivated macrophages where the parasite cannot inhibit fusion of phagosomes and lysosomes. Humoral immunity does not completely prevent initial invasion or establishment of latent [174]. It is interesting, nonetheless, that immunocompetent pregnant women transmit *T. gondii* transplacentally if it is their initial infection, but do not usually do so if they were infected prior to pregnancy. Human IgG crosses the placenta, but transplacental humoral immunity in mice is not relevant to human infection, as mice do not transfer IgG across the placenta.

Immunogenetics

Possible racial differences, concordance of monozygotic and discordance of infection and disease manifestations in dizygotic twins, varying maternal transmission, and murine models all indicate that immunogenetics influence acquisition and outcome of toxoplasmosis. These studies and evidence were reviewed recently [40]. Blackwell [175] (Fig. 6) recently summarized methods for identification of candidate gene regions for human susceptibility to parasitic infections: (i) by analysis of regions showing synteny (e.g., conservation with regions of the murine genome known to be involved in disease susceptibility; (ii) through knowledge of types of immune responses important in development of innate and acquired protective immune responses (e.g. Fig 6 is a representative example for tuberculosis, leprosy, and Leishmaniasis), and (iii) through total genome scans using multicase families to test for genetic linkage between disease susceptibility and microsatellite markers. Recently, we have found an association between HLA DQ3 and the development of hydrocephalus in human infants with congenital toxoplasmosis and used human HLA transgenic mice to confirm the role of these HLA Class II molecules in protection against toxoplasmosis [3], which should prove to be a powerful tool for studying immunogenetics of susceptibility to congenital toxoplasmosis.

Susceptibility genes : Mouse - Human Homology

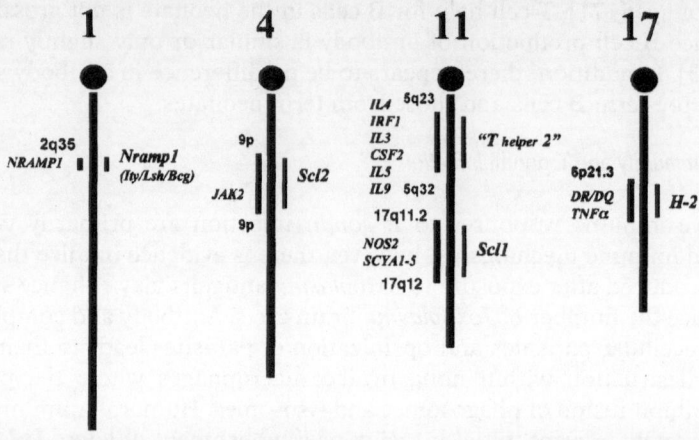

Fig. 6. Genes that have influenced susceptibility to a variety of infections. Locations on mouse chromosomes and homologous human genes are indicated. To date, although only human MHC genes have been proven to be important in outcome of human congenital toxoplasmosis [3], it is likely that at least certain of these other genes also will be found to be important. From Blackwell [175] (with permission)

Immune system and the brain and eye

We have recently reviewed the natural history and experimental approaches to acute acquired and congenital ocular toxoplasmosis [176], and we and others have began to examine influence of various murine and human genes on this congenital infection. *T. gondii* infection of the central nervous system and immune responses that protect or are pathogenic in the central nervous system also were recently reviewed [177, 178]. There is little information about the pathogenic mechanisms involved in the unique central nervous system and the eye lesions of congenital toxoplasmosis.

Summary

Incomplete development of the fetal and newborn immune system is described (Table 2). This immaturity of the immune system contributes to manifestations of congenital toxoplasmosis. Our understanding of the mechanisms whereby this occurs is just beginning.

Acknowledgements

This work was supported by NIH R01 TMP AI 23748. Rima McLeod is the Jules and Doris Stein RPB Professor at the University of Chicago. We thank V. Aitchison and E. Holnfels for their help in preparation of this manuscript, the patients in our study of congenital toxoplasmosis and all the members of the Toxoplasmosis Study Group for providing the stimulus to our consideration of what it is about fetal infection that renders individuals with congenital toxoplasmosis susceptible to more prominent and prolonged manifestations of infections. We also gratefully acknowledge many helpful and interesting discussions with colleagues and Dan McGehee for his encouragement.

References

1. Boyer K.a.M R (1998) Toxoplasmosis: Principles and Practice of Pediatric Infectious Disease. In : Long P (ed) *Principles and Practice of Pediatric Infectious Disease.*Prober, Churchill Livingstone New York, pp. 1421-1448
2. Deckert-Schluter M et al (1994) Activation of the innate immune system in murine congenital Toxoplasma encephalitis. J Neuroimmunol 53(1):47-51
3. Mack D JJ, Roberts F, Roberts C, Estes R, David C, Grumet FC, McLeod R (1999) HLA-Class II Genes Modify Outcome of Infection. (in preparation)
4. Versteeg R (1992) NK cells and T cells: mirror images? Immunol Today 13(7):244-247
5. Schlossman S, BL, Gilks W, Harlan J, Kishimoto T, Morimoto C, Ritz J, Shaw S, Silverstein R, Springer T, Tedder T, Todd R (1994) Leukocyte Typing. 5ᵗʰ ed. S S Oxford University Press
6. Abbas AK, Lichtman AH, Pober JS (1997) Cellular and molecular immunology. 3rd ed. Saunders text and review series. Saunders, Philadlephia: xii, 494 , 8 of plates
7. Raulet DH (1992) Immunology. A sense of something missing [news; comment]. Nature 358(6381):21-22
8. Moretta L et al (1992) Allorecognition by NK cells: nonself or no self? Immunol Today 13(8):300-306
9. Seder RA et al (1993) Interleukin 12 acts directly on CD4⁻ T cells to enhance priming for interferon gamma production and diminishes interleukin 4 inhibition of such priming. Proc Natl Acad Sci USA, 90(21):10188-10192
10. Bancroft GJ (1993) The role of natural killer cells in innate resistance to infection. Curr Opin Immunol, 5(4):503-510
11. Lanier LL (1997) Natural killer cells: from no receptors to too many. Immunity, 6(4):371-378
12. Moretta A et al (1997) Major histocompatibility complex class I-specific receptors on human natural killer and T lymphocytes. Immunol Rev 155:105-117
13. Agrawal S et al (1999) Cutting Edge: MHC Class I Triggering by a Novel Cell Surface Ligand Costimulates Proliferation of Activated Human T Cells. J Immunol 162(3): 1223-1226
14. Phillips JH et al (1992) Ontogeny of human natural killer (NK) cells: fetal NK cells mediate cytolytic function and express cytoplasmic CD3 epsilon delta proteins. J Exp Med 175(4):1055-1056
15. Lewis DB, Wilson CB (1995) Developmental Immunology and Role of Host Defenses in Neonatal Susceptibility. In : Remington JS, Klein RB (eds) Infections of the Fetus and Newborn Infant. WB Saunders Company: Philadelphia. pp. 20-98
16. Boehmer (1997) Aspects of lymphocyte developmental biology. Immunology Today,18(6): 260-262
17. Lanier LL, Phillips JL (1992) Natural killer cells. Curr Opin Immunol 4(1):38-42

18. Yabuhara A, Kawai H, Komiyama A (1990) Development of natural killer cytotoxicity during childhood: marked increases in number of natural killer cells with adequate cytotoxic abilities during infancy to early childhood. Pediatr Res 28(4):316-322

19. Qian JX et al (1997) Decreased interleukin-15 from activated cord versus adult peripheral blood mononuclear cells and the effect of interleukin-15 in upregulating antitumor immune activity and cytokine production in cord blood. Blood 90(8): 3106-3117

20. Shore SL et al (1977) Antibody-dependent cellular cytotoxicity to target cells infected with herpes simplex viruses: functional adequacy in the neonate. Pediatrics 59(1):22-28

21. Pabst HF, Kreth HW (1980) Ontogeny of the immune response as a basis of childhood disease. J Pediatr 97(4):519-534

22. Sancho L et al (1991) Two different maturational stages of natural killer lymphocytes in human newborn infants. J Pediatr 119(3): 446-454

23. Baley JE, Schacter BZ (1985) Mechanisms of diminished natural killer cell activity in pregnant women and neonates. J Immunol 134(5):3042-3048

24. Subauste CS, Dawson L, Remington JS (1992) Human lymphokine-activated killer cells are cytotoxic against cells infected with *Toxoplasma gondii*. J Exp Med 176(6):1511-1519

25. Dannemann BR et al (1989) Assessment of human natural killer and lymphokine-activated killer cell cytotoxicity against *Toxoplasma gondii* trophozoites and brain cysts. J Immunol 143(8):2684-2691

26. Suzuki Y et al (1988) Interferon-gamma: the major mediator of resistance against *Toxoplasma gondii*. Science 240(4851):516-518

27. Denkers EY et al (1993) Emergence of NK1.1+ cells as effectors of IFN-gamma dependent immunity to Toxoplasma gondii in MHC class I-deficient mice. J Exp Med 178(5): 1465-1472

28. Hunter CA et al (1994) Production of gamma interferon by natural killer cells from *Toxoplasma gondii*-infected SCID mice: regulation by interleukin-10, interleukin- 12, and tumor necrosis factor alpha. Infect Immun 62(7):2818-2824

29. Hunter CA et al (1997) The role of the CD28/B7 interaction in the regulation of NK cell responses during infection with *Toxoplasma gondii*. J Immunol 158(5):2285-2293

30. Beaman MH, Araujo FG, Remington JS (1994) Protective reconstitution of the SCID mouse against reactivation of toxoplasmic encephalitis. J Infect Dis 169(2):375-383

31. Lindberg RE, Frenkel JK (1977) Toxoplasmosis in nude mice. J Parasitol 63(2):219-221

32. Hughes HP et al (1988) Absence of a role for natural killer cells in the control of acute infection by *Toxoplasma gondii* oocysts. Clin Exp Immunol, 72(3):394-399

33. van Furth R, Raeburn JA, van Zwet TL (1979) Characteristics of human mononuclear phagocytes. Blood 54(2):485-500

34. Glauser MP et al (1991) Septic shock: pathogenesis [see comments]. Lancet 338(8769): 732-736

35. Scharton-Kersten TM et al (1996) In the absence of endogenous IFN-gamma, mice develop unimpaired IL-12 responses to *Toxoplasma gondii* while failing to control acute infection. J Immunol, 157(9):4045-4054

36. McDyer JF, Wu CY, Seder RA (1998) The regulation of IL-12: its role in infectious, autoimmune, and allergic diseases. J Allergy Clin Immunol 102(1):11-15

37. Gazzinelli RT et al (1994) Parasite-induced IL-12 stimulates early IFN-gamma synthesis and resistance during acute infection with *Toxoplasma gondii*. J Immunol 153(6): 2533-2543

38. Ma X et al (1996) The interleukin 12 p40 gene promoter is primed by interferon gamma in monocytic cells. J Exp Med 183(1):147-157

39. Abbas AK, Lichtman AH, Pober JS (1991) Cellular and Molecular Immunology. Saunders, Philadelphia.

40. McLeod RJJ, Estes R, Mack D (1996). *Toxoplasma gondii*. In : Gross U (ed) in Current Topics in Microbiology and Immunology. Springer-Verlag, Berlin Heidelberg, pp. 95-112

41. Roth R, Spiegelberg HL (1996) Activation of cloned human CD4+ Th1 and Th2 cells by blood dendritic cells. Scand J Immunol 43(6):646-651

42. Bhardwaj N et al (1996) IL-12 in conjunction with dendritic cells enhances antiviral CD8+ CTL responses in vitro. J Clin Invest 98(3):715-722

43. Bhardwaj N et al (1992) Dendritic cells are potent antigen-presenting cells for microbial superantigens. J Exp Med 175(1):267-273

44. Cella M et al (1996) Ligation of CD40 on dendritic cells triggers production of high levels of interleukin-12 and enhances T cell stimulatory capacity: T-T help via APC activation. J Exp Med 184(2):747-752

45. Kelemen E, Janossa M (1980) Macrophages are the first differentiated blood cells formed in human embryonic liver. Exp Hematol 8(8):996-1000

46. English BK et al (1992) Decreased granulocyte-macrophage colony-stimulating factor production by human neonatal blood mononuclear cells and T cells. Pediatr Res 31(3): 211-216

47. Lee SM et al (1996) Decreased interleukin-12 (IL-12) from activated cord versus adult peripheral blood mononuclear cells and upregulation of interferon-gamma, natural killer, and lymphokine-activated killer activity by IL-12 in cord blood mononuclear cells. Blood 88(3):945-954

48. Christensen RD (1989) Hematopoiesis in the fetus and neonate. Pediatr Res 26(6):531-535

49. Speer CP et al (1985) Oxidative metabolism in cord blood monocytes and monocyte-derived macrophages. Infect Immun 50(3):919-921

50. Conly ME, Speert DP (1991) Human neonatal monocyte-derived macrophages and neutrophils exhibit normal nonopsonic and opsonic receptor-mediated phagocytosis and superoxide anion production. Biol Neonate 60(6):361-366

51. Wilson CB, Haas JE (1984) Cellular defenses against *Toxoplasma gondii* in newborns. J Clin Invest 73(6):1606-1616

52. Lin RY (1996) The role of the fetal fibroblast and transforming growth factor-beta in a model of human fetal wound repair. Semin Pediatr Surg 3:165-174

53. Seguin R, Kasper LH (1999) Sensitized lymphocytes and CD40 ligation augment interleukin-12 production by human dendritic cells in response to *Toxoplasma gondii* [In Process Citation]. J Infect Dis 179(2):467-474

54. Ridge JP, Di Rosa F, Matzinger P (1998) A conditioned dendritic cell can be a temporal bridge between a CD4+ T-helper and a T-killer cell [see comments]. Nature 393(6684): 474-478

55. Schoenberger SP et al (1998) T-cell help for cytotoxic T lymphocytes is mediated by CD40-CD40L interactions [see comments]. Nature 393(6684):480-483

56. DeKruyff RH, Gieni RS, Umetsu DT (1997) Antigen-driven but not lipopolysaccharide-driven IL-12 production in macrophages requires triggering of CD40. J Immunol 158(1):359-366

57. Sousa CR et al (1997) In vivo microbial stimulation induces rapid CD40 ligand-independent production of interleukin 12 by dendritic cells and their redistribution to T cell areas [see comments]. J Exp Med 186(11):1819-1829

58. Sorg RV, K.G.a.P.W. (1998) Functional competence of Dendritic Cells in human umbilical cord blood. Bone Marrow Transplantation 22(Suppl 1.):552-554

59. Denkers EY, Gazzinelli RT (1998) Regulation and function of T-cell-mediated immunity during *Toxoplasma gondii* infection. Clin Microbiol Rev 11(4):569-588

60. Johnson LL (1992) SCID mouse models of acute and relapsing chronic *Toxoplasma gondii* infections. Infect Immun 60(9):3719-3724

61. Hunter CA et al (1995) Studies on the role of interleukin-12 in acute murine toxoplasmosis. Immunology 84(1):16-20

62. Johnson LL (1992) A protective role for endogenous tumor necrosis factor in *Toxoplasma gondii* infection. Infect Immun 60(5):1979-1983

63. Gazzinelli RT et al (1993) Interleukin 12 is required for the T-lymphocyte-independent induction of interferon gamma by an intracellular parasite and induces resistance in T-cell-deficient hosts [see comments]. Proc Natl Acad Sci USA, 90(13):6115-6119

64. Chang HR, Grau GE, Pechere JC (1990), Role of TNF and IL-1 in infections with *Toxoplasma gondii*. Immunology 69(1):33-37

65. Scharton-Kersten T et al (1997) Interferon consensus sequence binding protein-deficient mice display impaired resistance to intracellular infection due to a primary defect in interleukin 12 p40 induction. J Exp Med 186(9):1523-1534

66. Channon JY, Kasper LH (1996) *Toxoplasma gondii*-induced immune suppression by human peripheral blood monocytes: role of gamma interferon. Infect Immun 64(4):1181-1189

67. McLeod R et al (1980) Effects of human peripheral blood monocytes, monocyte-derived macrophages, and spleen mononuclear phagocytes on *Toxoplasma gondii*. Cell Immunol 54(2):330-350
68. Subauste CS, de Waal Malefyt R, Fuh F (1998) Role of CD80 (B7.1) and CD86 (B7.2) in the immune response to an intracellular pathogen. J Immunol 160(4):1831-1840
69. Moore KW et al (1993) Interleukin-10. Annu Rev Immunol 11:165-190
70. Gazzinelli RT et al (1992) IL-10 inhibits parasite killing and nitrogen oxide production by IFN- gamma-activated macrophages. J Immunol 148(6):1792-1796
71. Gazzinelli RT et al (1996) In the absence of endogenous IL-10, mice acutely infected with *Toxoplasma gondii* succumb to a lethal immune response dependent on CD4⁺ T cells and accompanied by overproduction of IL-12, IFN-gamma and TNF-alpha. J Immunol 157(2):798-805
72. Neyer LE et al (1997) Role of interleukin-10 in regulation of T-cell-dependent and T-cell- independent mechanisms of resistance to *Toxoplasma gondii*. Infect Immun 65(5): 1675-1682
73. Oswald IP et al (1992) IL-10 synergizes with IL-4 and transforming growth factor-beta to inhibit macrophage cytotoxic activity. J Immunol 148(11):3578-3582
74. Roberts CW et al (1996) Different roles for interleukin-4 during the course of *Toxoplasma gondii* infection. Infect Immun 64(3):897-904
75. Bermudez LE, Covaro G, Remington J (1993) Infection of murine macrophages with *Toxoplasma gondii* is associated with release of transforming growth factor beta and downregulation of expression of tumor necrosis factor receptors. Infect Immun 61(10): 4126-4130
76. Luder CG et al (1998) Down-regulation of MHC class II molecules and inability to up-regulate class I molecules in murine macrophages after infection with *Toxoplasma gondii*. Clin Exp Immunol 112(2):308-316
77. McLeod R et al (1989) Genetic regulation of early survival and cyst number after per-oral *Toxoplasma gondii* infection of A x B/B x A recombinant inbred and B10 congenic mice. J Immunol 143(9):3031-3034
78. Blackwell JM, Roberts CS, Roach TI, Alexander J (1994) Influence of macrophage resis-tance gene Lsh/S/Ity/Bcg (candidate NRamp on Toxoplasma gondii infection in mice). Clin Exp Immunol 97:107-112
79. Capron M et al (1997) Differentiation of eosinophils from cord blood cell precursors: kinetics of Fc epsilon RI and Fc epsilon RII expression. Int Arch Allergy Immunol 113(1-3):48-50
80. Lewis RA, Austen KF, Soberman RJ (1990) Leukotrienes and other products of the 5-lipoxygenase pathway. Biochemistry and relation to pathobiology in human diseases. N Engl J Med 323(10):645-655
81. Huber AR et al (1991) Regulation of transendothelial neutrophil migration by endoge-nous interleukin-8 [published errata appear in Science 1991 Nov 1:254(5032):631 and 1991 Dec 6:254(5037):1435]. Science 254(5028):99-102
82. Erdman SH et al (1982) Supply and release of storage neutrophils. A developmental study. Biol Neonate, 41(3-4):132-137
83. Anderson DC et al.(1991) Diminished lectin-, epidermal growth factor-, complement binding domain-cell adhesion molecule-1 on neonatal neutrophils underlies their impaired CD18-independent adhesion to endothelial cells in vitro. J Immunol 146(10): 3372-3379
84. Anderson DC et al (1984) Impaired motility of neonatal PMN leukocytes: relationship to abnormalities of cell orientation and assembly of microtubules in chemotactic gra-dients. J Leukoc Biol 36(1):1-15
85. Hill HR (1987) Biochemical, structural, and functional abnormalities of polymorpho-nuclear leukocytes in the neonate. Pediatr Res 22(4):375-382
86. Klein RB et al (1977) Decreased mononuclear and polymorphonuclear chemotaxis in human newborns, infants, and young children. Pediatrics, 60(4):467-472
87. Newburger PE (1982) Superoxide generation by human fetal granulocytes. Pediatr Res, 16(5):373-376.
88. Ambruso DR et al (1984) Oxidative metabolism of cord blood neutrophils: relationship to content and degranulation of cytoplasmic granules. Pediatr Res 18(11):1148-1153

89. Marshall AJ, Denkers EY (1998) *Toxoplasma gondii* triggers granulocyte-dependent cytokine-mediated lethal shock in D-galactosamine-sensitized mice. Infect Immun, 66(4):1325-1333
90. Saito H et al (1988) Selective differentiation and proliferation of hematopoietic cells induced by recombinant human interleukins. Proc Natl Acad Sci USA, 85(7):2288-2292
91. Khalife J et al (1986) Role of specific IgE antibodies in peroxidase (EPO) release from human eosinophils. J Immunol 137(5):1659-1664
92. Forestier F et al (1986) Hematological values of 163 normal fetuses between 18 and 30 weeks of gestation. Pediatr Res, 20(4):342-346
93. Ridel PR et al (1988) Protective role of IgE in immunocompromised rat toxoplasmosis. J Immunol 141(3):978-983
94. Brown CR et al (1995) Definitive identification of a gene that confers resistance against *Toxoplasma* cyst burden and encephalitis. Immunology 85(3):419-428
95. Stanley K, Luzio P (1988) Perforin. A family of killer proteins [news]. Nature 334(6182): 475-476
96. Masson D, Tschopp J (1987) A family of serine esterases in lytic granules of cytolytic T lymphocytes. Cell 49(5):679-685
97. Roberts MD (1999) Thesis Department of Pathology, Glasgow
98. Romagnani S (1996) Th1 and Th2 in human diseases. Clin Immunol 80(3 Pt 1):225-235
99. Gimmi CD et al (1991) B-cell surface antigen B7 provides a costimulatory signal that induces T cells to proliferate and secrete interleukin 2. Proc Natl Acad Sci USA, 88(15): 6575-6579.
100. Freeman GJ et al (1993) Murine B7-2, an alternative CTLA4 counter-receptor that costimulates T cell proliferation and interleukin 2 production. J Exp Med 178(6):2185-2192
101. Linsley PS, Ledbetter JA (1993) The role of the CD28 receptor during T cell responses to antigen. Annu Rev Immunol 11:191-212
102. Kubin M, Kamoun M, Trinchieri G (1994) Interleukin 12 synergizes with B7/CD28 interaction in inducing efficient proliferation and cytokine production of human T cells. J Exp Med 180(1):211-222
103. Schwartz RH (1990) A cell culture model for T lymphocyte clonal anergy. Science, 248(4961):1349-1356
104. Schwartz RH (1992) Costimulation of T lymphocytes: the role of CD28, CTLA-4, and B7/BB1 in interleukin-2 production and immunotherapy. Cell 71(7):1065-1068
105. Mackay CR (1993) Immunological memory. Adv Immunol 53:217-265
106. Vaux DL, Strasser A (1996) The molecular biology of apoptosis. Proc Natl Acad Sci USA, 93(6):2239-2244
107. Haynes BF et al (1988) Analysis of expression of CD2, CD3, and T cell antigen receptor molecules during early human fetal thymic development [published erratum appears in J Immunol 1989 Feb 15:142(4):1410]. J Immunol 141(11):3776-3784
108. Davis MM (1988) Molecular genetics of T-cell antigen receptors. Hosp Pract (Off Ed) 23(5):157-164, 169-170
109. Schild H et al (1994) The nature of major histocompatibility complex recognition by gamma delta T cells. Cell 76(1):29-37
110. George JF Jr, Schroeder HW Jr (1992) Developmental regulation of D beta reading frame and junctional diversity in T cell receptor-beta transcripts from human thymus. J Immunol 148(4):1230-1239
111. Blackman M, Kappler J, Marrack P (1990) The role of the T cell receptor in positive and negative selection of developing T cells. Science 248(4961):1335-1341
112. Alam SM et al (1996) T-cell-receptor affinity and thymocyte positive selection [see comments]. Nature 381(6583):616-620
113. Robey EA et al (1992) The level of CD8 expression can determine the outcome of thymic selection. Cell 69(7):1089-1096
114. Nossal GJ (1994) Negative selection of lymphocytes. Cell 76(2):229-239
115. Kisielow P et al (1988) Tolerance in T-cell-receptor transgenic mice involves deletion of nonmature CD4+8+ thymocytes. Nature 333(6175):742-746
116. Kappler JW et al (1988) Self-tolerance eliminates T cells specific for Mls-modified products of the major histocompatibility complex. Nature 332(6159):35-40
117. von Boehmer H, Teh HS, Kisielow P (1989) The thymus selects the useful, neglects the useless and destroys the harmful. Immunol Today 10(2):57-61

118. Asma GE, Van den Bergh RL, Vossen JM (1983) Use of monoclonal antibodies in a study of the development of T lymphocytes in the human fetus. Clin Exp Immunol, 53(2):429-436

119. Erkeller-Yuksel FM et al (1992) Age-related changes in human blood lymphocyte subpopulations. J Pediatr 120(2 Pt 1):216-222

120. De Paoli P, Battistin S, Santini GF (1988) Age-related changes in human lymphocyte subsets: progressive reduction of the CD4 CD45R (suppressor inducer) population. Clin Immunol Immunopathol 48(3):290-296

121. Azuma M et al (1993) Requirements for CD28-dependent T cell-mediated cytotoxicity. J Immunol 150(6):2091-2101

122. Rayfield LS, Brent L, Rodeck CH (1980) Development of cell-mediated lympholysis in human foetal blood lymphocytes. Clin Exp Immunol 42(3):561-570

123. Oliver AM et al (1989) The distribution and differential expression of MHC class II antigens (HLA-DR, DP, and DQ) in human fetal adrenal, pancreas, thyroid, and gut. Transplant Proc, 21(1 Pt 1):651-652

124. Harvey JE, Jones DB (1990) Distribution of LCA protein subspecies and the cellular adhesion molecules LFA-1, ICAM-1 and p150,95 within human foetal thymus. Immunology 70(2):203-209

125. Khalili H, DR, Chang MY (1997) The defective antigen-presenting activity of murine fetal macrophage cell lines. Immunology 4:487-493

126. Hayward AR, Kurnick J (1981) Newborn T cell suppression: early appearance, maintenance in culture, and lack of growth factor suppression. J Immunol 126(1):50-53

127. Wilson CB et al (1986) Decreased production of interferon-gamma by human neonatal cells. Intrinsic and regulatory deficiencies. J Clin Invest 77(3):860-867

128. Pirenne H et al (1992) Comparison of T cell functional changes during childhood with the ontogeny of CDw29 and CD45RA expression on CD4+ T cells. Pediatr Res 32(1): 81-86

129. Lewis DB et al (1991) Cellular and molecular mechanisms for reduced interleukin 4 and interferon-gamma production by neonatal T cells. J Clin Invest 87(1):194-202

130. D'Andrea A et al (1993) Interleukin 10 (IL-10) inhibits human lymphocyte interferon-gamma production by suppressing natural killer cell stimulatory factor/IL-12 synthesis in accessory cells. J Exp Med 178(3):1041-1048

131. Kos FJ, Engleman EG (1996) Immune regulation: a critical link between NK cells and CTLs. Immunol Today 17(4):174-176

132. Gazzinelli R et al (1992) Simultaneous depletion of CD4+ and CD8+ T lymphocytes is required to reactivate chronic infection with *Toxoplasma gondii*. J Immunol 149(1): 175-180

133. Gazzinelli RT et al (1991) Synergistic role of CD4+ and CD8+ T lymphocytes in IFN-gamma production and protective immunity induced by an attenuated *Toxoplasma gondii* vaccine. J Immunol 146(1):286-292

134. Trinchieri G (1993) Interleukin-12 and its role in the generation of TH1 cells. Immunol Today 14(7):335-338

135. Montoya JG et al (1996) Human CD4+ and CD8+ T lymphocytes are both cytotoxic to *Toxoplasma gondii*-infected cells. Infect Immun 64(1):176-181

136. Brown C, ER, McLeod R (1995) Fate of an intracellular parasite during lysis of its host cell by CD8+ lymphocytes. Keystone meeting, Keystone, CO

137. Nash PB et al (1998) *Toxoplasma gondii*-infected cells are resistant to multiple inducers of apoptosis. J Immunol 160(4):1824-1830

138. Huldt (1973) Effect of *Toxoplasma gondii* on the thymus. Nature 244(5413): 301-303

139. McLeod R et al (1984) Immune response of mice to ingested *Toxoplasma gondii*: a model of toxoplasma infection acquired by ingestion. J Infect Dis 149(2):234-244

140. Hohfeld PF, Marion S, Thulliez P, Marcon P, Daffos F (1990) *Toxoplasma gondii* infection during pregnancy: T lymphocyte subpopulations in mothers and fetuses. Pedatr Infect Dis J 9:878-881

141. Lecolier B et al (1989) T-cell subpopulations of fetuses infected by *Toxoplasma gondii* [letter]. Eur J Clin Microbiol Infect Dis 8(6):572-573

142. Foulon W et al (1990) Detection of congenital toxoplasmosis by chorionic villus sampling and early amniocentesis. Am J Obstet Gynecol 163(5 Pt 1):1511-1513

143. Subauste CS et al (1998) Alpha beta T cell response to *Toxoplasma gondii* in previously unexposed individuals. J Immunol 160(7):3403-3411
144. McLeod R et al (1990) Phenotypes and functions of lymphocytes in congenital toxoplasmosis. J Lab Clin Med 116(5):623-635
145. Hara T et al (1996) Human V delta 2+ gamma delta T-cell tolerance to foreign antigens of *Toxoplasma gondii*. Proc Natl Acad Sci USA, 93(10):5136-5140
146. Mack DM, Holfels E, McLeod R (1999) Immune Responses in human congenital toxoplasmosis. (in preparation).
147. Raymond J et al (1990) Presence of gamma interferon in human acute and congenital toxoplasmosis [published erratum appears in J Clin Microbiol 1990 28(12):2853]. J Clin Microbiol 28(6):1434-1437
148. Alexander J et al (1998) The role of IL-4 in adult acquired and congenital toxoplasmosis. Int J Parasitol 28(1):113-120
149. Wegmann TG et al (1993) Bidirectional cytokine interactions in the maternal-fetal relationship: is successful pregnancy a TH2 phenomenon? [see comments]. Immunol Today 14(7):353-356
150. Alexander J et al (1997) Mechanisms of innate resistance to *Toxoplasma gondii* infection. Philos Trans R Soc Lond B Biol Sci 352(1359):1355-1359
151. Piccinni MP et al (1995) Progesterone favors the development of human T helper cells producing Th2-type cytokines and promotes both IL-4 production and membrane CD30 expression in established Th1 cell clones. J Immunol 155(1):128-133
152. Gazzinelli RT, Denkers EY, Sher A (1993) Host resistance to *Toxoplasma gondii*: model for studying the selective induction of cell-mediated immunity by intracellular parasites. Infect Agents Dis 2(3):139-149
153. Suzuki Y, Remington JS (1990) The effect of anti-IFN-gamma antibody on the protective effect of Lyt- 2+ immune T cells against toxoplasmosis in mice. J Immunol 144(5):1954-1956
154. Yano A et al (1989) Antigen presentation by *Toxoplasma gondii*-infected cells to CD4+ proliferative T cells and CD8+ cytotoxic cells. J Parasitol 75(3):411-416
155. Parker SJ, Roberts CW, Alexander J (1991) CD8⁺ T cells are the major lymphocyte subpopulation involved in the protective immune response to *Toxoplasma gondii* in mice. Clin Exp Immunol 84(2):207-212
156. Purner MB et al (1996) CD4-mediated and CD8-mediated cytotoxic and proliferative immune responses to *Toxoplasma gondii* in seropositive humans. Infect Immun 64(10):4330-4338
157. Black CM et al (1989) Effect of recombinant tumour necrosis factor on acute infection in mice with *Toxoplasma gondii* or *Trypanosoma cruzi*. Immunology 68(4):570-574
158. Sullender WM et al (1987) Humoral and cell-mediated immunity in neonates with herpes simplex virus infection [published erratum appears in J Infect Dis 155(4):838]. J Infect Dis 155(1):28-37
159. Gehrz RC et al (1987) HLA class II restriction of T helper cell response to cytomegalovirus (CMV). I. Immunogenetic control of restriction. J Immunol 138(10):3145-3151
160. Lang T et al (1994) Leishmania donovani-infected macrophages: characterization of the parasitophorous vacuole and potential role of this organelle in antigen presentation. J Cell Sci 107(Pt 8):2137-2150
161. Saha B et al (1994) Macrophage-T cell interaction in experimental mycobacterial infection. Selective regulation of co-stimulatory molecules on *Mycobacterium*-infected macrophages and its implication in the suppression of cell- mediated immune response. Eur J Immunol 24(11):2618-2624
162. Himeno K, Hisaeda H (1996) Contribution of 65-kDa heat shock protein induced by gamma and delta T cells to protection against *Toxoplasma gondii* infection. Immunol Res 15(3):258-264
163. Moore KJ, Matlashewski G (1994) Intracellular infection by *Leishmania donovani* inhibits macrophage apoptosis. J Immunol 152(6):2930-2937
164. Huskinson J et al (1989) *Toxoplasma* antigens recognized by immunoglobulin G subclasses during acute and chronic infection. J Clin Microbiol 27(9):2031-2038
165. Noelle RJ, Ledbetter JA, Aruffo A (1992) CD40 and its ligand, an essential ligand-receptor pair for thymus- dependent B-cell activation. Immunol Today 13(11):431-433
166. Clark EA, Lane PJ (1991) Regulation of human B-cell activation and adhesion. Annu Rev Immunol 9:97-127

167. Gathings WE, Lawton AR, Cooper MD (1977) Immunofluorescent studies of the development of pre-B cells, B lymphocytes and immunoglobulin isotype diversity in humans. Eur J Immunol 7(11):804-810
168. Yellen AJ et al (1991) Signaling through surface IgM in tolerance-susceptible immature murine B lymphocytes. Developmentally regulated differences in transmembrane signaling in splenic B cells from adult and neonatal mice. J Immunol 146(5):1446-1454
169. DeBiagi M, Andreani M, Centis F (1985) Immune characterization of human fetal tissues with monoclonal antibodies. Prog Clin Biol Res 193:89-94
170. Kohler PF, Farr RS (1966) Elevation of cord over maternal IgG immunoglobulin: evidence for an active placental IgG transport. Nature 210(40):1070-1071
171. Burgio GR et al (1980) Ontogeny of secretory immunity: levels of secretory IgA and natural antibodies in saliva. Pediatr Res 14(10):1111-1114
172. Andersson U et al (1981) Humoral and cellular immunity in humans studied at the cell level from birth to two years of age. Immunol Rev 57:1-38
173. Splawski JB, Lipsky PE (1991) Cytokine regulation of immunoglobulin secretion by neonatal lymphocytes. J Clin Invest 88(3):967-977
174. McLeod R et al (1988) Subcutaneous and intestinal vaccination with tachyzoites of *Toxoplasma gondii* and acquisition of immunity to peroral and congenital toxoplasma challenge. J Immunol 140(5):1632-1637
175. Blackwell JM (1998) Genetics of host resistance and susceptibility to intramacrophage pathogens: a study of multicase families of tuberculosis, leprosy and leishmaniasis in north-eastern Brazil. Int J Parasitol 28(1):21-28
176. Roberts F.a.R.M. (1999) Pathogenesis of Toxoplasmic Retinochoroiditis. Parasitology Today 15(2):51-57
177. Suzuki Y (1997) Cells and cytokines in host defense of the central nervous system. In: Peterson R (ed) In Defense of the Brain, Blackwell Science, Malden, 56-73
178. Montoya G, Remington JS (1997) Toxoplasmosis of the Central Nervous System. In: Peterson R (ed). In Defense of the Brain. Blackwell Science, Malden, pp. 163-188
179. Hill AVS, Willis AC, Aidoo M, Allsopp CE, Gotch FM, Gai XM, Takiguchi M, Greenwood BM, Townsend AR (1992) Molecular analysis of the association of HLA-B53 and resistance to severe malaria. Nature 360:434-439
180. McLeod R, Arbuckle D, Skamene E (1995) Immunogenetics in the analysis of resistance to intracellular pathogens. Curr Opin Immunol 7:539-552
181. Bodner JG, Albert ED, Bodmer WF, Dupont B, Erlich HD, Mach B, Mayr WR, Patnam P, Sasazuld T (1994) Nomenclature report: nomenclature for factors of the HLA system. Tissue Antigens 44:1-18

1.5. The immunology of *Toxoplasma gondii* infection in the immune-competent host

J. ALEXANDER, C.W. ROBERTS, W. WALKER, G. REICHMANN, C.A. HUNTER

Introduction

The protozoan parasite *Toxoplasma gondii* (*T. gondii*) is one of the most common parasites of humans, with clinical toxoplasmosis constituting a major risk to immuno-compromised individuals, pregnant women and unborn children [1]. *T. gondii* infection is common in most warm blooded vertebrates and infects approximately 15-80% of the world's human population depending on ethnicity or geographical location [2]. The sexual stage of the life cycle takes place in the intestine of the definitive host, the cat. Transmission to the intermediate host can occur in several ways – ingestion of infective sporulated oocysts released in cat faeces, or by the ingestion of meat containing the long-lived tissue cyst stage which allows direct transmission from one intermediate host to another. Vertical transmission results in congenital infection or more unusually, infection can be acquired as a result of receiving transplants from infected individuals or occasionally as a result of a laboratory accident.

In immuno-competent individuals, infection with *T. gondii* normally results in an early mild to subclinical phase of infection, associated with the rapidly dividing tachyzoite stage of the life cycle which has the ability to invade and multiply in virtually any nucleated cell of the host. The rapid onset of immunity limits parasite growth and induces conversion to the dormant cyst stage which contains slow growing bradyzoites. Infected individuals are thought to harbour tissue cysts for life, particularly within skeletal and heart muscle and the central nervous system. This persistence of the parasite results in continual stimulation of the immune response and results in a state of immunity to reinfection which is presumed to be life-long. However, in patients who develop defects in T cell function, *T. gondii* can cause significant disease. This group of susceptible individuals includes organ transplant recipients, patients with certain cancers and patients with AIDS in whom *T. gondii* is the single largest cause of cerebral mass lesions [3, 4]. In these patients, it appears that reactivation of latent tissue cysts, rather than recently acquired infection, is the cause of disease [3, 4]. Clinical toxoplasmosis is a consequence of tachyzoite replication and this stage of the parasite can be effectively treated with pyrimethamine and sulphadiazine. However, the bradyzoite stage found within the tissue cysts and associated with the chronic stage of infection, is generally refractory to treatment. Thus, even after treatment the cyst stage persists and is responsible for the high incidence of relapse observed in AIDS patients with toxoplasmic encephalitis and in congenitally infected individuals with retinochoroiditis.

While the inability of patients with defects in T cell function to maintain *T. gondii* as a latent infection provides clear insights as to the immunological mechanisms which constitute protective immunity, it is not the main focus of the present article and is covered elsewhere in this volume. Herein, we review the innate and adaptive mechanisms of immunity against this organism operating in normal individuals. While appropriate studies in humans are for the most part comparatively limited, a wealth of information on the immune response against *T. gondii* has recently been published using murine models of infection. This information has proved very useful in determining the immunoregulatory controls operating against *T. gondii* infection [5, 6]. However, toxoplasmosis can manifest differently in mice making it difficult on occasions to extrapolate directly from this experimental model to humans. We shall, therefore, compare and contrast, where appropriate, the immunological responses in experimental models and humans following infection with *T. gondii*.

Host and parasite factors affecting susceptibility to *T. gondii*

As *T. gondii* persists in numerous cell types and tissues, and as different stages of the parasite life cycle are involved at different phases of disease the immune response against *T. gondii* is inevitably complex. It is therefore not surprising that studies in experimental models as well as in humans have demonstrated a disease spectrum. The severity of disease resulting from infection with *T. gondii* is under the influence of various parasite and host related factors. Despite a sexual life cycle stage only 3 major clonal lineages of *T. gondii* have been identified with little recombination between these lineages [7, 8]. These findings indicate that the protective immune response generated following infection with *T. gondii* is very effective, rapid and long lasting and prevents infection of animals with multiple strains of *T. gondii*. The recognition that the three major clonal lineages of *T. gondii* correlated with virulence of the parasite in mice was an important step in our understanding of the role of parasite derived factors in the pathogenesis of infection. The type 1 lineage is associated with acute virulence in mice [9], whereas the type 2 lineage induces chronic pathology in susceptible strains of mice and the type 3 lineage is the least virulent [4, 10]. In addition, acute virulence in mice is associated in part with polymorphisms in the major tachyzoite surface antigen SAG1 [10, 11]. In humans, the type 1 lineage is most frequently associated with congenital infection whereas the type 2 lineage is more common in patients in whom the disease has reactivated [4]. Additional parasite factors involved in the outcome of infection include the fact that oocysts are more virulent than tissue cysts [2], while the frequency of tissue cyst passage and the inoculum size of the initial infection can also affect disease severity [12]. Although only an experimental phenomenon, the route of infection can also greatly alter disease severity [13, 14]. Of particular interest are the recent reports that *T. gondii* has superantigen activity in the mouse inducing preferential expansion of Vβ5+ CD8+ T cells, the first parasite for which this phenomenon has been demonstrated [15-17]. There is the intriguing possibility that different clonal lineages of *T. gondii* may differ in their ability to act as superantigens and so provide a basis for the differences in virulence. However, the significance of this activity is uncertain and recent studies have demonstrated that *T. gondii* does not possess superantigen activity with regard to human lymphocytes though it does have mitogenic activity [18, 19].

Numerous host factors have been described which influence the severity of infection. The influence of human genes in controlling *T. gondii* infection is demonstrated by the variation in disease susceptibility in different ethnic groups as well as in HLA typing studies. Furthermore, the concordance of disease manifestations in monozygotic, but not dyzygotic twins, following congenital infection also supports a role for host genetic factors (reviewed by McLeod et al [20]). Studies in mice, using inbred congenic and recombinant mouse strains, have characterized the contribution of host genetics to different facets of infection. In humans, the development of Toxoplasmic Encephalitis (TE) is associated most commonly with a loss of T cell function due to AIDS, malignancy or immunosuppressive therapy. A similar phenotype can be identified in the mouse by depletion of CD4+ and CD8+ T cells [21, 121]. Thus, it is not surprising that genetic susceptibility to TE in both humans and mice is associated with differences in their class I genes. Analysis of the genetic basis of resistance to development of TE has revealed that differences in the genes within the H-2D region correlate with resistance or susceptibility to development of TE and that resistance to TE, in mice infected with the Me49 strain, is correlated absolutely with the L^d gene [22]. That resistance maps to this MHC class I gene suggests that it is a defect in the CD8+ T cell response that results in susceptibility to TE. Interestingly, Remington and colleagues have correlated the HLA phenotype of patients with AIDS with susceptibility to TE [23]. Other host factors which influence severity of infection, undoubtedly through their effect on immunological status, include age, sex and pregnancy [24]). Thus, for example, the incidence of toxoplasmic lymphadenopathy has been shown to be greater in males than females under the age of 15, but greater in females than males over the age of 25 [25].

Early response to *T. gondii*

In recent years experiments using severe combined immune deficient (SCID) mice which lack T and B lymphocytes have demonstrated an extremely important role for the innate immune response in the control of early *T. gondii* infection (reviewed by Alexander and Hunter [5]; Alexander et al [26]; Denkers and Gazzinelli [6]). Upon infection with live or sensitisation with dead *T. gondii*, inflammatory macrophages produce IL-12 which in turn stimulates NK cell production of IFN-γ [27, 28]. However, recent studies have implicated dendritic cells as an earlier source of IL-12 *in vivo* [29]. Neutrophils have also been proposed to be an alternative early source of IL-12 [30], and the ability of CD4+ T cells to produce IFN-γ may also contribute to the innate response [31]. While IL-12 is the critical initiator of NK cell IFN-γ production this activity is greatly augmented by cytokines including IL-1, TNF-α, IL-15 and particularly IL-18 [27, 32-34]. Similarly, costimulation of NK cells via CD28 enhances IL-12 mediated production of IFN-γ [34, 35] and resistance to *T. gondii* in SCID mice [33]. Thus, treatment of *T. gondii*–infected SCID mice with neutralising antibodies against IFN-γ, TNF-α or IL-12 [36-39] results in earlier mortality. Similarly exogenous IL-12 [28, 40] or rIFN-γ [39, 41] though not rTNF-α [39], prolongs the life of infected SCID mice. Conversely, administration of neutralising antibodies against TGF-β or IL-10 [40, 42] results in prolonged time to death in SCID mice. Whereas TGF-β has an inhibitory effect on NK cell production of IFN-γ [42, 43], IL-10 probably directly antagonises macrophage functions particularly TNF-α, IL-1, IL-12 and nitric oxide production [44-46]. Consequently, as would be predicted, SCID IL-10-/- mice infected with *T. gondii* survive for longer than infected IL-10+/+ controls [47].

In murine models, activation of NK cells (as measured by NK cell cytolysis of tumor target cells), is one of the first events to occur following infection with *T. gondii* [48, 49]. Similarly, enhancement of human NK cell activity by *T. gondii* lysates has been demonstrated *in vitro* as measured by proliferation, increased lytic activity for target cells and IFN-γ production [50]. Although IL-2 activated human NK cells have been reported to lyse targets infected with *T. gondii* [51], this does not appear to be the case with murine NK cells [36] and it is the ability of NK cells to produce IFN-γ early in the course of infection that results in resistance to *T. gondii*. Live parasites are not required to induce the accessory cell dependent activation of NK cells: antigen preparations of *T. gondii* can activate murine NK cells *in vivo* [52] and stimulate human and mouse NK cells to produce IFN-γ *in vitro* [27, 50].

In addition to NK cells [50], stimulation of peripheral blood mononuclear cells (PBMC's) from seronegative individuals with parasite or antigen pulsed antigen presenting cells results in the expansion of γδ and αβ T cells [18, 19, 53]. Human γδ T cells were found to be cytotoxic for *T. gondii* in a MHC unrestricted manner and produced IFN-γ, IL-2 and TNF-α but not IL-4 [53]. The involvement of γδ T cells early in infection is particularly appropriate given the association of these cells with the intestinal mucosa, the normal portal of entry of *T. gondii* into the host and significantly this cell population has also been identified as playing a protective role against *T. gondii* in the mouse gut epithelia [41]. αβ CD4+, but not CD8+ T cells also produce significant amounts of IFN-γ following *in vitro* stimulation with parasites [18]. Increased IFN-γ production by human αβ and γδ T cells was associated with upregulation of CD80 and CD86 expression by *T. gondii* infected lymphocytes [54]. This upregulation of the co-stimulatory molecules could only be induced by viable parasites. Earlier studies in SCID mice also demonstrated that *T. gondii* infection increased CD28, the receptor for CD80 and CD86 on NK cells. Significantly, blocking of CD28/CD80 and CD86 interactions with monoclonal antibodies inhibited both murine NK cell [33] and human T cell IFN-γ production [54]. It would seem likely, though it has yet to be demonstrated, that upregulation of CD80 and CD86 would also enhance human NK cell production to further promote the generation of an early protective response.

The adaptive T cell response

The pro-inflammatory cytokines associated with the early response, IL-12 and IFN-γ, have also been clearly demonstrated as playing influential roles in the development of the adaptive immune response during toxoplasmosis (reviewed by Alexander and Hunter [5]; Denkers and Gazzinelli [6]). IL-12 and IFN-γ trigger the expansion of the Th1 subset of CD4+ lymphocytes which in turn produces IL-2 which drives the expansion of CD8 lymphocytes [55-57], perhaps in conjunction with macrophage derived IL-15 [58]. IL-12 has also been shown to promote type 1 (IFN-γ producing) cytolytic CD8+ T cell development [59], again emphasising the important role of the innate immune system in directing the evolution of the adaptive immune response. Adoptive transfer and *in vivo* depletion studies in various mouse strains confirm the paramount importance of CD8+ T cells in mediating immunity in this species, not only during acute infection but also in preventing high cyst burdens and toxoplasmic encephalitis [56, 60-63]. It has been suggested that CD8+ T cells may mediate their effect through IFN-γ production [64]. However, CD8+ T cells have been shown to lyse infected cells in a class I restricted manner in humans [65] as well as mice [55]. Despite an early study which demonstrated that depletion of CD4+ T cells during chronic infection in the mouse reactivates infection in the central nervous system [121] the role of the CD4+ T cell populations during murine *T. gondii* infection remains controversial (reviewed Alexander and Hunter [5]) with both protective and pathological effects being described.

In humans a more precise role for CD4+ T cells in protective responses has been identified in studies using both CD4+ and CD8+ T cell lines which have been generated using cells derived from individuals with chronic *T. gondii* infections [65-72]. An early study found that a CD8+ T cell clone could kill *T. gondii* infected cells in a class I dependent manner while a CD4+ clone proliferated in response to homologous infected cells [65]. Other studies have demonstrated the ability of CD4+ T cell lines to produce IFN-γ and IL-2 in response to stimulation with soluble tachyzoite antigen and *Toxoplasma* infected APC's [19, 66]. CD4+ T cell clones are also capable of killing autologous cells either pulsed with tachyzoite antigen or infected with tachyzoites [68, 69]. One study found that individual CD4+ and CD8+ T cell lines were effective against cells infected with strains representative of any of the 3 major *T. gondii* sub-types (C56, Me49 and RH) [70]. The production of IFN-γ by *T. gondii*-specific CD4+ T cells has been shown to up-regulate class II expression on target cells and thus promote their killing [69]. CD4+ T cells lines generated from chronically infected healthy individuals have been shown not only to produce cytokines normally associated with TH1 cells (IL-2 and IFN-γ), but also simultaneously to produce the TH2 associated cytokines IL-4 , IL-5 and IL-10 [71]. However, a futher study found that stimulation of freshly isolated peripheral blood mononuclear cells (PBMC's) from chronically infected individuals produced IL-2 and IFN-γ but not IL-4 or IL-5 [73]. It is likely that the apparent discrepancy between these two studies may reflect differences between freshly isolated lymphocytes and T cell clones propagated *in vitro* for relatively long periods of time. Collectively the weight of evidence would suggest at least as important a protective role for CD4+ as CD8+ T cells in humans. In fact while both CD4 and CD8-mediated specific cytotoxic and proliferative responses as well as IFN-γ production can be elicited from the peri-pheral blood leucocytes of seropositive individuals a recent study would suggest these are primarily CD4 dominated responses [72].

T cells from chronically infected humans recognise a number of *T. gondii* antigens [67] including synthetic peptides derived from the ROP2 protein of *T. gondii* [74] and toxoplasma-specific CD4+ lines were found to be cytotoxic for target cells expressing not only ROP1, SAG1, SAG3 and GRA6 but antigens (presumably common) derived from the related non-pathogenic coccidian *Besnoita jellesoni* [75]. These observations suggest possible targets for future vaccine development.

The humoral response

While much recent research on *T. gondii* infection has focused on cell mediated immunity, acquired infection is also associated with strong antibody responses. Indeed, previous studies of human subjects have found that uninfected individuals possess low titre natural antibodies of the IgM and IgG isotypes that are reactive with *T. gondii* [76], indicating some form of innate humoral immunity to this parasite. These antibodies are multireactive, have opsonizing activity *in vitro* and are thought to be the result of polyclonal stimulation of CD5+ B cells, possibly by gastrointestinal bacteria. Early after infection there are high levels of low affinity circulating IgM which can be used diagnostically to distinguish acute infection [77]. As the infection enters the chronic phase isotype switching occurs and high levels of complement fixing parasite-specific IgG can be detected in the serum. Detection of these antibodies form the basis of the diagnostic Sabin-Feldman dye test which is still used to confirm infection of individuals exposed to the parasite [78]. This response in humans is almost entirely against tachyzoite specific antigens with little recognition of cyst stage antigens [79]. *T. gondii*-specific IgG antibodies in infected individuals are predominantly of the IgG1 isotype (associated with Th1 responses in humans) and studies with SCID-human mice have shown that both the human recall response and initial vaccination-induced response to *T. gondii* antigen consists of IgG1 antibodies [80]. These findings are consistent with mouse studies where infection induces large serum titres of Th1-associated IgG2a antibodies [81-83]. While these findings illustrate that the humoral immune response reflects the strong Th1 response associated with infection the role of antibody in protection remains unclear. Obviously within the host cell the parasite is safe from the effects of antibodies. However, secretory IgA may protect mucosal surfaces from parasite invasion [84] and it has been suggested that candidate vaccines against *T. gondii* should ideally induce protection at this site [85]. In addition, it has been shown that antibodies can opsonize extracellular tachyzoites for phagocytosis by macrophages. Under such conditions lysosome fusion with the parasitophorous vacuole takes place and death of the parasite ensues (Jones *et al.* 1975). Consequently several, but by no means all [87], studies have demonstrated that mortality following *T. gondii* infection in laboratory models can be reduced by the passive transfer of antibodies [88, 89]. Nevertheless, studies in antibody deficient mice [90, 91] have demonstrated that T cell mediated immunity is of paramount importance in controlling infection. However, it may be significant that one study has demonstrated that the presentation of antigen by B cells can differentially regulate CD4+ T cells [92].

Although levels of antibody fall after the immune response controls the parasite, they remain elevated for the life of the host. Continued presence of cysts and occasional release of tachyzoites may lead to chronic stimulation of the immune response and maintain the high antibody levels that are characteristic of the chronic stage of infection. The stimulation of a strong antibody response allows the identification of individuals who have been exposed to *T. gondii* and can be used to distinguish whether an individual has a recently acquired infection or is chronically infected. This is an important tool which allows physicians to assess the likelihood of transmission of congenital disease and whether immune-compromised individuals are at risk of disease or if an individual suspected of toxoplasmosis has active disease [77].

Anti-*Toxoplasma* effector mechanisms

Numerous studies have identified IFN-γ as the primary mediator of anti-parasite effector mechanisms against *T. gondii* although other cytokines including TNF-α, IL-1β, IL-12, IFNα, IFNβ [28, 42, 64, 93-96] have been shown either to induce anti-toxoplasma activity themselves or augment the activity of IFN-γ. However, it is clear that several anti-microbial mechanisms may be involved in limiting parasite growth depending on the cell type examined and the species from which they are derived. Early studies identified the ability of human monocytes and granulocytes to generate toxic oxygen metabolites as playing a role in controlling *T. gondii* growth [97-100]. Support for these observations was provided by studies with monocytes from patients with chronic granulamatous disease (CGD), which fail to undergo a respiratory burst and have limited microbial activity against *T. gondii*. Nevertheless, IFN-γ does enhance the ability of CGD monocytes to control *T. gondii* growth indicating that alternate microbial mechanisms must also operate. Similarly, P47-phox mice, which lack an inducible oxidative burst [101], can control acute and chronic *T. gondii* infection and their macrophages can limit parasite growth *in vitro*. Indeed, superoxide dismutase activity has been detected in *T. gondii* extracts

[102] and a gene coding for this enzyme sequenced from the RH strain of *T. gondii*. The presence of this enzyme activity could serve to protect the parasite from superoxide molecules. Thus, while the production of toxic oxygen radicals is undoubtedly one of the anti-parasitic mechanisms operating during *T. gondii* infection, current evidence would suggest it is not the major effector mechanism.

IFN-γ, with TNF-α and IL-1 as co-factors, is thought to mediate its anti-parasitic effects in the murine model primarily by upregulating the expression of macrophage and microglial inducible nitric oxide synthase (iNOS) [64, 103] and the production of NO [104]. NO is believed not only to be directly toxoplasmacidal [104] but also to promote tachyzoite to bradyzoite transformation by inhibition of mitochondrial respiration [105]. Nevertheless, control of early parasite growth in mice seems to be independent of nitric oxide production as mice deficient in inducible nitric oxide synthase (iNOS) and tumour necrosis factor receptor were able to control early growth of *T. gondii*, although they later succumbed to infection [106]. Nitric oxide does, however, seem to be important in controlling persistent infection as treating mice 22-25 days post infection with iNOS metabolic inhibitors resulted in disease reactivation [26]. However, recent studies with iNOS deficient mice have shown that vaccine based immunity does not require NO, suggesting that long-term immunity after acute infection does not rely on NO-based killing mechanisms [107]. Obviously the precise role of NO in controlling *T. gondii* infection in the mouse awaits to be resolved but several lines of evidence would indicate that it does play a crucial role in the maintenance of the chronic phase of infection [26, 106, 108]. While human astrocytes activated by IFN-γ and IL-1β also produce NO and inhibit *T. gondii* multiplication [109], a role for RNI has not been demonstrated in human macrophages. Alternatively, IFN-γ has been shown to limit *T. gondii* replication in human fibroblasts [110], macrophages [111], glioblastoma cells [112] and retinal pigment epithelial cells [94] by inducing the enzyme indolamine oxygenase, thus starving the parasite of tryptophan. Nevertheless, this effector mechanism has not been shown to be active in mice [113].

Several other studies have indicated that tachyzoite multiplication can be inhibited by a variety of alternative mechanisms. For example, IFN-γ activated murine astrocytes inhibit *T. gondii* replication independent of RNI or tryptophan starvation [114]. In addition, human endothelial cells can be activated by IFN-γ to inhibit *T. gondii* growth in a reactive oxygen intermediate, IDO and RNI independent manner [115]. Also in IRF-/- mice (Interferon Regulatory Factor), the control of parasite growth is mediated by IL-12, apparently acting through CD4+ T cells, independent of IFN-γ and NO production [116]. Further studies have also shown a role for 5-lipoxygenase arachadonic acid metabolites in human macrophage, IFN-γ induced, anti-toxoplasma activity [117]. Collectively, these observations suggest that multiple, as well as some as yet uncharacterised, anti-microbial mechanisms are controlling the growth of *T. gondii*.

Concluding remarks

Immunological control of *T. gondii* infection is complex and dependent on many host and parasite factors. This review has highlighted important similarities as well as differences in the immune responses of mice and humans to this parasite. The suitability of using the mouse as an experimental model of *T. gondii* has often been questioned and an argument for using other species such as rats and sheep supported [118]. This is due to the often quoted extreme vulnerability of mice to infection compared with humans. We would argue that this viewpoint is somewhat disingenuous. Certainly many inbred laboratory mouse strains are exquisitely susceptible to *T. gondii* infection as measured by mortality, cyst burden and encephalitis. Nevertheless, many mouse strains are highly resistant using the same criteria. Selecting the appropriate mouse strain(s) can often circumvent perceived problems. Thus while *T. gondii* can often be transmitted from a chronic infection to the foetus during pregnancy in mice, a rare event during human pregnancy, this does not occur using the BALB/c mouse strain [119]. Also, as discussed above there are obvious correlations between the virulence of *T. gondii* clonal lineages in mice and the severity of disease they produce in humans. Nevertheless species differences do exist and these not only emphasise the versatility of *T. gondii*, but may provide valuable insights into fundamental differences in the immunological mechanisms operating in humans and mice. The potential of transgenic mice which express immunologically functional human molecules and SCID-human mice which may allow experimental manipulation of a "human" immune system is now being explored [80, 120].

References

1. Cook GC (1990) *Toxoplasma gondii* infection: a potential danger to the unborn fetus and AIDS sufferer. Q J Med 74:3
2. Jackson MH, Hutchison WM (1989) The prevalence and source of *Toxoplasma infection* in the
3. Luft BJ, Remington JS (1992) Toxoplasmic encephalitis in AIDS. Clin Infect Dis 15:211-222
4. Ambroise-Thomas P, Pelloux H (1993) Toxoplasmosis-congenital and in immuno-compromised patients: a parallel. Parasitol Today 9:61-62
5. Alexander J, Hunter CH (1998) Immunoregulation during Toxoplasmosis. Mol Immunol 70:81-102
6. Denkers EY, Gazzanelli R (1998) Regulation and function of T-cell-mediated immunity during *Toxoplasma gondii* infection. Clin Microbiol Rev 11:569-588
7. Sibley LD, Howe DK (1996) Genetic Basis of Pathogenicity in Toxoplasmosis. Curr Top Microbiol Immunol 219:3-16
8. Darde ML (1996) Biodiversity in *Toxoplasma gondii*. Curr Top Microbiol Immunol 219:27-41
9. Sibley LD, Boothroyd JC (1992) Virulent strains of *Toxoplasma gondii* comprise a single clonal lineage. Nature 350:82-85
10. Howe DK, Sibley LD (1995) *Toxoplasma gondii* is comprised of 3 clonal lineages: correlation of parasite genotype with human disease. J Inf Dis 13:322-356
11. Rinder H, Thomschkle A, Darde ML, Loscher T (1995) Specific DNA polymorphisms discriminate between virulence and non-virulence to mice in nine *Toxoplasma gondii* isolates. Mol Biochem Parasitol 69:123-126
12. Araujo FG, Williams DM, Grumet FC, Remington JS (1976) Strain dependent differences in murine susceptibility to *Toxoplasma gondii*. Infect Immun 13:1528-1530
13. Blackwell JM, Roberts CW, Alexander J (1993) Influence of genes within the MHC on mortality and brain cyst development in mice infected with *Toxoplasma gondii*: kinetics of immune regulation in BALB H-2 congenic mice. Parasit Immunol 15:317-324

14. Brown CR, McLeod R (1994) Mechanisms of survival of mice during acute and chronic *Toxoplasma gondii* infection. Parasitol Today 10:290-292
15. Denkers EY, Caspar P, Sher A (1994) *Toxoplasma gondii* possesses a super antigen that selectively expands murine T cell receptor Vβ5-bearing CD8+ lymphocytes. J Exp Med 180:985-994
16. Denkers EY, Caspar P, Hieny S, Sher A (1996) *Toxoplasma gondii* infection induces specific nonresponsiveness in lymphocytes bearing the Vbeta5 chain of the mouse T cell receptor. J Immunol 156:1089-1094
17. Denkers EY (1996) A *Toxoplasma gondii* superantigen. Biological effects and implications for the Host-Parasite Interaction. Parasitol Today 12:362-366
18. Subauste, CS, de Waal Malefyt R, Fuh F (1998) Role of CD80 (B7.1) and CD86 (B7.2) in the immune response to an intracellular pathogen. J Immunol 160:1831-1840
19. Purner MB, Berens RL, Tomavo S, Lecordier L, Cesbron-Delauw MJ, Kotzin BL, Curiel TJ (1998) Stimulation of human lymphocytes obtained from *Toxoplasma gondii*-seronegative persons by proteins derived from *T. gondii*. J Infect Dis 177:746-753
20. McLeod R, Johnson J, Estes R, Mack D (1996) Immunogenetics in Pathogenesis and protection against Toxoplasmosis. Curr Top Microbiol Immunol 219:95-112
21. Gazzinelli RT, Xu Y, Hieny S, Cheever A, Sher A (1992) Simultaneous depletion of CD4+ and CD8+ T lymphocytes is required to reactivate chronic infection with *Toxoplasma gondii*. J Immunol 149:175-180
22. Brown CR, Hunter CA, Estes RG, Beckmann J, Forman J, David C, Remington JS, McLeod R (1995) Definitive identification of a gene that confers resistance against *Toxoplasma* cyst burden and encephalitis. Immunol 85:419-428
23. Suzuki Y, Wong SY, Grumet FC, Fessel J, Montoya JG, Zolopa AR, Patmore A, Schumacher-Perdreau F, Schrappe M, Koppen S, Ruf B, Brown BW, Remington JS (1996) Evidence for genetic regulation of susceptibility to toxoplasmic encephalitis in AIDS patients. J Infect Dis 173:265-268
24. Roberts CW, Satoskar A, Alexander J (1996) The influence of sex steroids and pregnancy associated hormones on the development and maintenance of immunity to parasite infection. Parasitol Today 12:382-388
25. Beverley JKA, Fleck DG, Kwantes W, Ludlam G (1976) Age-sex distribution of various diseases with particular reference to toxoplasmic lymphadenopathy. J Hyg 76:215-228
26. Alexander J, Scharton-Kersten TM, Yap G, Roberts CW, Liew FY, Sher A (1997) Mechanisms of innate resistance to *Toxoplasma gondii* infection. Phil Trans R Soc Lond B. 352:1355-1359
27. Sher A, Oswald IP, Hieny S, Gazzinelli R (1993) *Toxoplasma gondii* induces a T-independent IFN-γ response in natural killer cells that requires both adherent accessory cells and tumor necrosis factor-α. J Immunol 150:3982-3989
28. Gazzinelli RT, Denkers EY, Sher A (1993). Host resistance to *Toxoplasma gondii*: model for studying the selective induction of cell-mediated immunity by intracellular parasites. Infect Agents Dis 2:139-149
29. Reis e Sousa BC, Hieny S, Scharton-Kersten T, Jankovic D, Charset H, Germain RN, Sher A (1997) *In vivo* microbial stimulation induces rapid CD40 ligand-independent production of interleukin 12 by dendritic cells and their redistribution to T cell areas. J Exp Med 186:1819-1829
30. Denkers EY, Marshall AJ (1998) Neutrophils as a source of immunoregulatory cytokines during microbial infection. The Immunologist 6:116-20
31. Scharton-Kersten T, Nakajima H, Yap G, Sher A, Leonard, WJ (1998) Infection of mice lacking the common cytokine receptor γ-chain (γc) reveals an unexpected role for CD4+ T lymphocytes in early IFN-γ-dependent resistance to *Toxoplasma gondii*. J Immunol 160:2565-2569
32. Hunter CA, Chizzonite R, Remington JS (1995) Interleukin 1β is required for the ability of IL-12 to induce production of IFN-γ by NK cells: A role for IL-1β in the T cell independent mechanism of resistance against intracellular pathogens. J Immunol 155:4347-4354
33. Hunter CA, Ellis-Neyer L, Gabriel K, Kennedy M, Linsley P, Remington JS (1997) The role of the CD28/B7 interaction in the regulation of NK cell responses during infection with *Toxoplasma gondii*. J Immunol 158, 2285-2293
34. Walker W, Aste-Amezaga M, Kastelein RA, Trinchieri G, Hunter CA (1999) Interleukin-18 and CD28 use distinct molecular mechanisms to enhance natural killer cell production of IL-12-induced interferon-gamma. J Immunol (in press)
35. Nandi D, Gross, JA, Allison JP (1994) CD28-mediated costimulation is necessary for optimal proliferation of murine NK cells. J Immunol 152:3361
36. Hunter CA, Subauste CS, Van Cleave VH, Remington JS (1994) Production of gamma interferon by natural killer cells from *Toxoplasma gondii*-infected SCID mice: regulation by interleukin-10, interleukin-12, and tumor necrosis factor alpha. Infect Immun 62:2818-2824
37. Johnson LL (1992) SCID mouse models of acute and relapsing chronic *Toxoplasma gondii* infections. Infect Immun 60:3719-3724
38. Gazzinelli RT, Wysocka M, Hayashi S, Denkers EY, Hieny S, Caspar P, Trinchieri G, Sher A (1994) Parasite-induced IL-12 stimulates early IFN-γ synthesis and resistance during acute infection with *Toxoplasma gondii*. J Immunol 153:2533-2543

39. Hunter CA, Suzuki Y, Subauste CS, Remington JS (1996). Cells and cytokines in resistance to *Toxoplasma gondii*. Curr Top Microbiol Immunol 219:113-125
40. Hunter CA, Abrams JS, Beaman MH, Remington JS (1993) Cytokine mRNA in the central nervous system of SCID mice infected with *Toxoplasma gondii*: importance of T-cell-independent regulation of resistance to *T. gondii*. Infect Immun 61:4038-4044
41. McCabe RE, Luft BJ, Remington JS (1984) Effect of murine interferon gamma on murine toxoplasmosis. J Infect Dis 150:961-962
42. Hunter CA, Bermudez L, Beernink H, Waegell W, Remington JS (1995) Transforming growth factor-β inhibits interleukin-12-induced production of interferon-γ by natural killer cells: A role for transforming growth factor-β in the regulation of T-cell independent resistance to *Toxoplasma gondii*. Eur J Immunol 25:994-1000
43. Bellone G, Aste-Amezaga M, Trinchieri G, Rodeck U (1995) Regulation of NK cell functions by TGF-β1. J Immunol 155:1066-1073
44. D'Andrea A, Aste-Amezaga M, Valiante NM, Ma X, Kubin M, Trinchieri G (1993) Interleukin 10 inhibits human lymphocyte interferon-γ production by suppressing natural killer cell stimulatory factor/IL-12 synthesis in accessory cells. J Exp Med 178:1041-1048
45. Rennick D, Berg D, Holland G (1992) Interleukin 10: an overview. Prog Growth Factor Res 4:207-227
46. Fiorentino DF, Zlotnik A, Mosmann TR, Howard M, O'Garra A (1991) IL-10 inhibits cytokine production by activated macrophages. J Immunol 146:3815-3822
47. Neyer LE, Grunig G, Fort M, Remington JS, Rennick D, Hunter CA (1997) Role of interleukin-10 in regulation of T cell dependent and T cell independent mechanisms of resistance to *Toxoplasma gondii*. Infect Immun 65:1675-1682
48. Goyal M, Ganguly NK, Mahajan RC (1988) Natural killer cell cytotoxicity against *Toxoplasma gondii* in acute and chronic toxoplasmosis. Med Sci Res 16:375-377
49. Hauser WE, Sharma SD, Remington JS (1982). Natural killer cells induced by acute and chronic *Toxoplasma* infection. Cell Immunol 69:330-346
50. Sharma SD, Verhoef J, Remington JS (1984) Enhancement of human natural killer cell activity by subcellular components of *Toxoplasma gondii*. Cell Immunol 86:317-326
51. Subauste CS, Dawson L, Remington JS (1992) Human lymphokine-activated killer cells are cytotoxic against cells infected with *Toxoplasma gondii*. J Exp Med 176:1511-1519
52. Hauser WE, Sharma SD, Remington JS (1983) Augmentation of NK cell activity by soluble and particulate fractions of *Toxoplasma gondii*. J Immunol 131:458-463
53. Subauste CS, Chung JY, Do D, Koniaris AH, Hunter CA, Montoya JG, Porcelli S, Remington JS (1995) Preferential activation and expansion of human peripheral blood gamma delta T cells in response to *Toxoplasma gondii* in vitro and their cytokine production and cytotoxic activity against *T. gondii*-infected cells. J Clin Invest 96:610-619
54. Subauste CS, Fuh F, de Waal Malefyt R, Remington JS (1998) αβ T cell response to *Toxoplasma gondii* in previously unexposed individuals. J Immunol 160:3403-3411
55. Denkers EY, Sher A, Gazzinelli RT (1993) T cell interactions with *Toxoplasma gondii*: implications for processing of antigen for class I-restricted recognition. Res Immunol 14:51-57
56. Gazzinelli RT, Hakim FT, Hieny S, Shearer GM, Sher A (1991) Synergistic role of CD4+ and CD8+ lymphocytes in IFN-γ production and protective immunity induced by an attenuated *Toxoplasma gondii* vaccine. J Immunol 146:286-292
57. Gazzinelli RT, Amichay D, Scharton-Kersten T, Grunvald E, Farber JM, Sher A (1996) Role of macrophage-derived cytokines in the induction and regulation of cell mediated immunity to *Toxoplasma gondii* Curr Top Microbiol Immunol 219:127-140
58. Khan IA, Kasper LH (1996) IL-15 augments CD8+ T cell-mediated immunity against *Toxoplasma gondii* infection in mice. J Immunol 157:2103-2108
59. Croft M, Carter L, Swain SL, Dutton RW (1994) Generation of polarised antigen-specific CD8 effector populations: reciprocal action of interleukin IL-4 and IL-12 in promoting type 2 versus type 1 cytokine profiles. J Exp Med 180:1715-1728
60. Brown CR, David CS, Khare SJ, McLeod R (1994) Effects of human class I transgenes on *Toxoplasma gondii* cyst formation. J Immunol 152:4537-41
61. Khan IA, Ely KH, Kasper LH (1991) A purified parasite antigen (P30) mediates CD8+ T cell immunity against fatal *Toxoplasma gondii* infection in mice. J Immunol 47:3501-3506
62. Subuaste CS, Koniaris AH, Remington JS (1991) Murine CD8+ cytotoxic T lymphocytes lyse *Toxoplasma gondii*-infected cells. J Immunol 147:3955-3959
63. Parker SJ, Roberts CW, Alexander J (1991) CD8+ T cells are the major lymphocyte subpopulation involved in the protective immune response to *Toxoplasma gondii* in mice. Clin Exp Immunol 84:207-212
64. Gazzinelli RT, Hieny S,Wynn TA, Wolf S, Sher A (1993) Interleukin 12 is required for the T-lymphocyte-independent induction of interferon-γ by an intracellular parasite and induces resistance in T-cell deficient hosts. Proc Nat Acad Sci USA 90:6115-6119
65. Yano A, Aosai F, Ohta M, Hasekura H, Sugane K, Hayashi S (1989) Antigen presentation by *Toxoplasma gondii*-infected cells to CD4+ proliferative T cells and CD8+ cytotoxic cells. J Parasitol 75:411-416

66. Saavedra R, Herion P (1991) Human T-cell clones against *Toxoplasma gondii*: production of interferon-gamma, interleukin-2, and strain cross-reactivity. Parasitol Res 77:379-385
67. Khan IA, Smith KA, Kasper LH (1990) Induction of antigen-specific human cytotoxic T cells by *Toxoplasma gondii*. J Clin Invest 85:1879-1886
68. Curiel TJ, Krug EC, Purner MB, Poignard P, Berens RL (1993) Cloned human CD4+ cytotoxic T lymphocytes specific for *Toxoplasma gondii* lyse tachyzoite-infected target cells. J Immunol 151:2024-2031
69. Yang TH, Aosai F, Norose K, Ueda M, Yano A (1995) Enhanced cytotoxicity of IFN-gamma-producing CD4+ cytotoxic T lymphocytes specific for *T. gondii*-infected human melanoma cells. J Immunol 154:290-298
70. Montoya JG, Lowe KE, Clayberger C, Moody D, Do D, Remington JS, Talib S, Subauste CS (1996) Human CD4+ and CD8+ T lymphocytes are both cytotoxic to *Toxoplasma gondii*-infected cells. Infect Immun 64:176-181
71. Prigione I, Facchetti P, Ghiotto F, Tasso P, Pistoia V (1995) *Toxoplasma gondii*-specific CD4+ T cell clones from healthy, latently infected humans display a Th0 profile of cytokine secretion. Eur J Immunol 25:1298-1305
72. Purner MB, Berens RL, Nash PB, van Linden A, Ross E, Kruse C, Krug EC, Curiel TJ (1996) CD4-mediated and CD8-mediated cytotoxic and proliferative immune responses to *Toxoplasma gondii* in seropositive humans. Infect Immun 64:4330-4338
73. Gazzinelli R, Bala S, Stevens R, Baseler M, Wahl L, Kovacs J, Sher A (1995) HIV infection suppresses type 1 lymphokine and IL-12 responses to *Toxoplasma gondii* but fails to inhibit the synthesis of other parasite-induced monokines. J Immunol 155:1565-1567
74. Saavedra R, Becerril MA, Dubeaux C, Lippens R, De Vos MJ, Herion P, Bollen A (1996) Epitopes recognized by human T lymphocytes in the ROP2 protein antigen of *Toxoplasma gondii*. Infect Immun 64:3858-3862
75. Purner MB, Krug EC, Nash P, Cook DR, Berens RL, Curiel TJ (1995) Cross-reactivity of human *Toxoplasma*-specific T cells; implications for development of a potential immunotherapeutic or vaccine. J Infect Dis 171:984-991
76. Konishi E (1993) Naturally occurring antibodies that react with protozoan parasites. Immunol Today 9:361
77. Remington JS, McLeod R, Desmonts G (1994) Toxoplasmosis. In: Infectious Diseases of the Fetus and Newborn Infant. Remington JS, Klein JO (eds)
78. Sabin A, Feldman HA (1948) Dyes as microchemical indicators of new immunity phenomenon affecting a protozoan parasite (*Toxoplasma*). Science 108:660
79. Smith JE, McNeil G, Zhang YW, Dutton S, Biswas-Hughes G, Appleford P (1996) Serological recognition of *Toxoplasma gondii* cyst antigens. Curr Top Microbiol Immunol 67-72
80. Walker W, Roberts CW, Brewer JM, Alexander J (1995) Antibody responses to *Toxoplasma gondii* antigen in human peripheral blood lymphocyte-reconstituted severe-combined immunodeficient mice reproduce the immunological status of the lymphocyte donor. Eur J Immunol 25:1426-1430
81. Burke JM, Roberts CW, Hunter CA, Murray M, Alexander J (1994) Temporal differences in the expression of mRNA for IL-10 and IFN-γ in the brains and spleens of C57BL/10 mice infected with *Toxoplasma gondii*. Parasite Immunology 16:305-314
82. Roberts CW, Ferguson DJP, Jebbari H, Satoskar A, Bluethmann H, Alexander J (1996) Different roles for interleukin-4 during the course of *Toxoplasma gondii* infection. Infect Immun 64:897-904
83. Nguyen TDBG, Van Broeck J, Vercammen M, Nguyen TN, Delmee M, Turneer, M, Wolf SF, Coutelier JP (1998) Acute and chronic phases of *Toxoplasma gondii* infection in mice modulate the host immune responses. Infect Immun 66:2991-2995
84. Mineo JR, McLeod R, Mack D, Smith J, Khan IA, Ely KH, Kasper LH (1993) Antibodies to *Toxoplasma gondii* major surface protein (SAG1 P30) inhibit infection of host cells are produced in murine intestine after peroral infection. J Immunol 150:3951
85. Araujo FG (1994) Immunization against *Toxoplasma gondii*. Parasitol Today 10:358-360
86. Jones TC, Len L, Hirsch JG (1975) Assessment *in vitro* of immunity against *Toxoplasma gondii*. J Exp Med 141:466-482
87. Gill HS, Prokesh O (1970) Chemotherapy of experimental *Toxoplasma gondii* (RH strain) infection. Indian J Med Res 58:1197-1200
88. Krakenbuhl JL, Ruskin J, Remington JS (1972) The use of killed vaccines in immunization against an intracellular parasite *Toxoplasma gondii*. J Immunol 108:425-431
89. Johnson AM, McDonald PJ, Neoh SH (1983) Monoclonal antibodies to *Toxoplasma gondii* cell membrane surface antigens protect mice from toxoplasmosis. J Protozool 30:351-356
90. Brinkmann V, Remington JS, Sharma SD (1987) Protective immunity in toxoplasmosis: correlation between antibody response, brain cyst formation, T-cell activation, and survival in normal and B-cell-deficient mice bearing the H-2^k haplotype. Infect Imm 55:990-994
91. Frenkel JK, Taylor DW (1982) Toxoplasmosis in immunoglobulin M-suppressed mice. Infect Immun 38:360-367

92. Brinkmann V, Sharma SD, Remington JS (1986) Different regulation of the L3T4-T cell subset by B cells in different mouse strains bearing the H-2ᴷ haplotype. J Immunol 9:2991-2997
93. Sibley LD, Adams LB, Y Fukutomi Y, Krahenbuhl JL (1991) Tumor necrosis factor-α triggers antitoxoplasmal activity of IFN-γ primed macrophages. J Immunol 147:2340-2345
94. Chandrasekharam NN, Pardhasaradhi K, Martins MC, Detrick B, Hooks JJ (1996) Mechanisms of interferon-induced inhibition of *Toxoplasma gondii* replication in human retinal pigment epithelial cells. Infect Imm 64:4188-4196
95. Schmitz JL, Carlin JM, Borden EC, Byrne GI (1989) Beta interferon inhibits *Toxoplasma gondii* growth in human monocyte-derived macrophages. Infect Immun 57:3254-3256
96. Wilson CB, Westall J (1985) Activation of neonatal and adult human macrophages by alpha, beta and gamma interferons. Infect Immun 49:351-356
97. Murray HW, Cohn ZA (1979) Macrophage oxygen-dependent anti-microbicidal activity. I. Susceptibility of *Toxoplasma gondii* to oxygen intermediates. J Exp Med 150:938-949
98. Murray HW, Juangbhanich CW, Nathan CF, Cohn ZA (1979) Macrophage oxygen-dependent anti-microbicidal activity. II. The role of oxygen intermediates. J Exp Med 150:950-964
99. Murray HW, Rubin BY, Carriero SM, Harris AM, Jaffee EA (1985) Human mononuclear phagocyte antiprotozoal mechanisms: oxygen dependent vs. oxygen-independent activity against intracellular *Toxoplasma gondii*. J Immunol 134:1982-1988
100. Wilson CB, Remington JS (1979) Activity of human blood leukocytes against *Toxoplasms gondii*. J Infect Dis 140:890-895
101. Jackson SH, Gallin JI, Holland SM (1995) The p47 phox mouse knock-out model of chronic granulomatous disease. J Exp Med 182:751-758
102. Sibley LD, Lawson R, Weidner E (1986) Superoxid dismutase and catalase in *Toxoplasma gondii*. Mol Biochem Parasitol 19:83-87
103. Jun CD, Kim SH, Soh CT, Kang SS, Chung HT (1993) Nitric oxide mediates the toxoplasmastatic activity of murine microglial cells in vitro. Immunol Invest 22:487-501
104. Langermans JAM, Van der Hulst MEB, Nibbering PH, Hiemstra PS, Fransen L, Van Furth R (1992) IFN-γ induced L-arginine-dependent toxoplasmastatic activity in murine peritoneal macrophages is mediated by endogenous tumor necrosis factor-α. J Immunol 148:568-574
105. Bohne W, Heesemann J, Gross U (1994) Reduced replication of *Toxoplasma gondii* is necessary for induction of bradyzoite specific antigens: a possible role for nitric oxide in triggering stage conversion. Infect Immun 62:1761-1767
106. Scharton-Kersten TM, Yap G, Magram J, Sher A (1997) Inducible nitric oxide is essential for host control of persistent but not acute infection with the intracellular pathogen, *Toxoplasma*
107. Khan IA, Matsuura T, Kasper LH (1998) Inducible nitric oxide synthase is not required for long-term vaccine-based immunity against *Toxoplasma gondii*. J Immunol 161:2994-3000
108. Hayashi S, Chan CC, Gazzinelli R, Roberge FG (1996) Contribution of nitric oxide to the host parasite equilibrium in toxoplasmosis. J Immunol 15:1476-1481
109. Peterson PK, Gekker G, Hu S, Chao CC (1995) Human astrocytes inhibit intracellular multiplication of *Toxoplasma gondii* by a nitric oxide-mediated mechanism. J Infect Dis 171:516-518
110. Pfefferkorn ER, Eckel M, Rebhun S (1986) Interferon-γ suppresses the growth of *Toxoplasma gondii* in human fibroblasts through starvation for tryptophan. Mol Biochem Parasitol 20:215-224
111. Murray HW, Szurol-Sudol A, Wellner D, Oca MJ, Granger AM, Libby DM, Rothermel CD, Rubin BY (1989) Role of tryptophan degradation in respiratory burst independent antimicrobial activity of gamma interferon-stimulated human macrophages. Infect Immun 57:845-849
112. Daubener W, Remscheid C, Nockemann S, Pilz K, Seghrouchini S, Mackenzie C, Hadding U (1996) Anti-parasite effector mechanism in human brain tumor cells: role of interferon-γ and tumor necrosis factor-α. Eur J Immunol 26:487-492
113. Schwartzman JD, Gonias SL, Pfefferkorn ER (1990) Murine gamma interferon fails to inhibit *Toxoplasma gondii* growth in murine fibroblasts. Infect Immun 58:833-834
114. Halonen SK, Chiu FC, Weiss LM (1998) Effect of cytokines on growth of *Toxoplasma gondii* in murine astrocytes. Infect Immun 66:4989-4993
115. Woodmann JP, Dimier IH, Bout DT (1991) Human endothelial cells are activated by IFN-γ to inhibit *Toxoplasma gondii* replication. J Immunol 147:2019-2023
116. Khan IA, Matsuura T, Fonseka S, Kasper LH (1996) Production of nitric oxide (NO) is not essential for protection against acute *Toxoplasma gondii* infection in IRF-1-/- mice. J Immunol 156:636-646
117. Yong EC, Chi EY, Henderson WR (1994) *Toxoplasma gondii* alters eicosanoid release by human mononuclear phagocytes: role of leukotrienes in interferon-γ-induced antitoxoplasma activity. J Exp Med 180:1637-1648
118. Innes EA (1997) Toxoplasmosis: comparative species susceptibility and host immune response. Comp Immunol Microbiol Infect Dis 20:131-138

119. Roberts CW, Alexander J (1992) Studies on a murine model of congenital toxoplasmosis: vertical disease transmission only occurs in BALB/c mice infected for the first time during pregnancy. Parasitology 104:19-23
120. Brown CR, David CS, Khare SJ, McLeod R (1994) Effects of human class I transgenes on *Toxoplasma gondii* cyst formation. J Immunol 152:4537-4541
121. Vollmer TL, Waldor MK, Steinman L, Conley FK (1987) Depletion of T-4· lymphocytes with monoclonal antibody reactivates toxoplasmosis in the central nervous system: a model of superinfection in AIDS. J Immunol 138:3737-41

1.6. Biological diagnosis of congenital toxoplasmosis: methods

H. Pelloux, P. Ambroise-Thomas

Introduction

The biological techniques used, for diagnosis, in the field of congenital toxo-plasmosis are numerous and very different from each other. This is due to the fact that each step of the diagnosis (acquired immunity or not, determination of seroconversion, ante-natal diagnosis, diagnosis at birth and follow-up of the child) has its own particularities and needs one type of methods. For instance, the determination of a toxoplasmic seroconversion is based on the results of serological methods, while the ante-natal diagnosis performed in amniotic fluid relies on the detection of the parasite (entire parasite or DNA) [1]. Furthermore, in each category of methods (serological methods, detection of the parasite, etc...), many different kits or different techniques are available [2]. This has induced the publication of a huge number of articles devoted to the biological diagnosis of congenital toxoplasmosis. Our goal, in this chapter, is not to give a complete list of the kits and techniques available and employed, what would be quite impossible (a complete book would not be enough to cite all the references related to this topic), but to make an over-view of these methods, focusing on their advantages, drawbacks, and on the kind of biological samples they can be applied on. The interpretation of the results will be developed in other chapters of this book. Serological methods, and parasite detection techniques will be successively presented and discus-sed.

Serological methods

Toxoplasma antigens

The *Toxoplasma* antigens used in serological methods are of paramount importance for the definition of the parameters useful for the interpretation of results, such as earliness of antibodies appearance, antibodies kinetics or cut-off value [3]. Two groups of toxoplasmic antigens can be identified and used in serological methods. Membrane antigens are recognised by antibo-dies which are produced early after infection. These antibodies directed against peripheral antigens are those detected when using techniques in which complete *Toxoplasma* tachyzoites are used as target antigen, such as Immunofluorescence or Agglutination tests [4]. Cytoplasmic antigens (and possibly, to some extent, exoantigens), often mixed with membrane (such as P30 protein) antigens, are used in Enzyme-Linked Immuno Assay, the most widely used method for *Toxoplasma* serology to date. In such technique, the antigen mix is not standardised from one kit to another and, consequently, the results obtained can hardly be compared. The cut-off value, the kinetics, the sensitivity and specificity are different for each kit, thus medical biologists should be aware of the characteristics of the kit they use [5].

Antibodies isotypes: G, M, A, E

Among the different isotypes of anti-*T. gondii* antibodies that can be detected, some are more widely (and for a long time) used (IgG, IgM) than others (IgA, IgE). Furthermore, the kinetics of appearence of these isotypes are very different, and individual variations may occur, what led some authors to develop a computerized help to interpret serological data [6]. However, some basic guidelines can be given.

IgG

The search for anti-*T. gondii* IgG is the most widely used approach to determine the presence or not of a specific immunity. This is due to the fact that specific IgG are always present in case of toxoplasmic infection (expect in the first days of it), even if they are not the main effectors of anti-toxoplasmic immunity, and that IgG detection remains positive all life long in immunocompetent patients. Thus, presence of IgG before pregnancy ensures that there is no risk of congenital toxoplasmosis for the fetus [7].

IgM

IgM is the second, after IgG, most widely detected isotype of *T. gondii* antibodies. If IgM appear earlier than IgG, they also disappear earlier. This makes IgM an early and sensitive marker of acute infection in the mother, and congenital infection in the child [8-10]. However, depending on the technique used, IgM may persist for a long time after infection, what makes the interpretation of serological results somewhat difficult, even when using the most recent tests, such as immunocapture ones [3, 11-14].

IgA

The detection of anti-toxoplasmic IgA is less widely used than these of IgG or IgM. The reported advantage of IgA detection was the described disappearence of IgA a few months after infection, what would lead to an easier datation of seroconversion and its use as a marker of congenital infection [15, 16]. However, these advantages or drawbacks are highly dependent on the kit used

[17], and several studies showed that specific IgA could persist a long time after infection [18, 19].

IgE

IgE detection is quite rarely used. It has been used mainly for the study of toxoplasmic reactivations in immunocompromised patients, but could be a marker of acute infection [20-22].

"Classical techniques"

Dye test

The Dye test is the oldest (and for some authors the "gold standard") technique described for the serological diagnosis of toxoplasmosis. Briefly, the serum to test is challenge with living tachyzoites of *T. gondii* and, after incubation, the percentage of died parasites is measured. Its high sensitivity allows the detection of very low levels of antibodies, but it is not automatized and needs to obtain living tachyzoites from mouse ascitis [23]. Thus, to date, only very few laboratories still perform the Dye test.

IFAT

As the dye test, the ImmunoFluorescent Antibodies Technique detects antibodies against the entire tachyzoite of *T. gondii*. Briefly, the parasites are fixed on a slide, and the serum to test is incubated with it. If antibodies are present, they are revealed by an antidody conjugated with fluorescein [24-26]. This technique allows the expression of the results in international units for IgG, since a calibrated gold standard can be included in the reaction (WHO reference serum). IgM can also be detected using IFAT, with a lower sensitivity than more recent techniques, but it can be useful for datation of toxoplasmic seroconversions since IFAT IgM become negative approximately 3 months after infection. False positive results may occur due to the presence of rheumatoid factors [25].

ELISA

The Enzyme-Linked Immunosorbent Assay is the technique that made the toxoplasmic serology easier to perform. It is the most widely used to date. This technique (which has different forms: sandwich, double sandwich, immunocapture, etc.) detects antibodies directed against antigens obtained after lysis of the parasite. The results of each kit are highly dependent on the antigens used, and on the revelation system. The ELISA kits are automatized and can now allow to express, to some extent, the results using international units. However, the commercial kits available are different from each other, and thus the cut-offs and antibodies kinetics are sometimes difficult to compare since the *Toxoplasma* antigens and the detection techniques are not standardised [5, 27, 28].

Agglutination

Numerous agglutination methods are used in the field of toxoplasmic serology. Entire tachyzoites, red cells or latex particles coated with *T. gondii* antigens can be agglutinated in presence of specific antitoxoplasmic antibodies. Some of these techniques are performed in highly specialized laboratories and allow a precise datation of the seroconversion [4], while others are very easy to perform and can be used as screening (non quantitative tests) [29-31]. One of these techniques, (ImmunoSorbent Agglutination Assay) allows a very sensitive and early detection of IgM [8].

Others

Other techniques, although used in some laboratories or countries, are less widely used and published. For instance, flow cytometry has been described as useful to detect anti-*T. gondii* antibodies in patients' sera [32]. Complement fixation test is used in some studies [19]. The use of skin-test to determine the presence or not of an anti-*Toxoplasma* immunity has been studied and published [33].

Improvement of these methods: IgG avidity

Recently, an important improvement of IgG detection has been described in the field of toxoplasmic serology: the determination of IgG avidity. Briefly, the principle of the method is that IgG against an recently acquired infection have a lower avidity than those directed against an older infection. This technique allows a better determination of the date of the toxoplasmic infection in the pregnant woman, when this is difficult using only the "classical" detection of IgG, IgM or IgA [34-36].

Detection of antibodies directed against characterized antigens, or neosynthetized (newborn) antibodies

The techniques described in the previous section can be quantitative or not, but none of them allows the determination of the antigen the antibodies are directed against. For instance, if a mother and her newborn have the same titers of anti-*T. gondii* antibodies, it is impossible to know if mother's or newborn's antibodies are directed against the same toxoplasmic antigens. That means that it is impossible to know if the newborn's antibodies are transmitted from the mother (no congenital infection) or synthetised by the baby (congenitally infected). That is why techniques such as Enzyme-Linked Immuno Filtration Assay and Western blot, which allow the comparison of the serological profiles, are useful in the field of congenital toxoplasmosis.

ELIFA

The application of Enzyme-Linked Immunofiltration Assay to the diagnosis of congenital toxoplasmosis was described by Pinon et al [37]. It allows a higher sensitivity than "classical" serological methods to affirm the absence or presence of congenital toxoplasmosis in newborns and infants, by comparing their immunological profile (which toxoplasmic antigen their antibodies are directed against) with those of their mother [38, 39]. The method is, briefly, a counter immuno-electrophoresis (migration of the antigens in front of the serum) revealed by an enzyme-linked assay. Its use is limited to a vey small number of laboratories since the system is not commercially available.

Western blot

The goal of western blot use is the same, in the field of congenital toxoplasmosis, as that of ELIFA. However, western blot is more widely used than ELIFA because the material is easier to get. After birth, the profiles of the child and the mother can be compared. Here again, the sensitivity and the specificity of the technique are higher than those of the "classical" techniques [38]. Briefly, the technique consists first in an electrophoresis of toxoplasmic antigens, followed by a transfer on a membrane and then an incubation with the sera, the antibodies being revealed by an enzymatic system.

Parasite detection

The methods which are related to the parasite detection are numerous and very different, considering the biological targets and indications. Some are old (staining), others are more recent, such as Polymerase Chain Reaction (PCR), and represent a great improvement in the diagnosis of toxoplasmosis, even if technical drawbacks must not be forgotten.

Staining

Staining is the oldest and the simplest method to detect *T. gondii*. However, it cannot be used in all the samples available in which *T. gondii* detection is interesting, since its sensitivity is lower than that of techniques such as culture or PCR.

Giemsa staining

This technique allows to identify *T. gondii*, as well as other protozoan parasites. It is mainly used on tissue biopsies or fluids [39].

ImmunoFluorescence microscopy

Indirect IF can also be used to detect *T. gondii* directly in samples such as bronchoalveolar lavage, or biopsies. The primary (anti-*T. gondii*) antibodies and the fluorescein marked one can be the same as used in the revelation of cell cultures [40].

Histopathology and immunohistochemistry

Detection using immunoperoxidase or alkaline-phosphatase are mainly used in anatomo pathology studies, such as autopsies or studies on biopsies from immunocompromised patients or fetus after abortion. The quality of the results obviously depends on the characteristics of the anti-*T. gondii* antibody used [41, 42]. Some staining methods are important in this field, even if they do not directly detect *T. gondii*, because they allow to describe the tissue lesions (necrosis, inflammation, etc.) related to the presence of *Toxoplasma* cysts and/or tachyzoites, and/or the presence of other pathogens. These are, for instance, hematoxylin-eosin-saffron, peridic acid-schiff [41]. The determination of the presence of cysts is important in case of reactivation of latent infection, in immunocompromised patients. Histopathology is, in such case, the only way to affirm the reactivation, by showing the rupture of dormant cysts.

Mouse inoculation

Mouse inoculation is the oldest technique to allow culture of *T. gondii* from medical samples. It is still the "reference method" for culture in many laboratories. It is still performed, even in association with PCR, because it is sensitive and allows to easily isolate the strain of *T. gondii* present in the patient's sample. Briefly, the technique consists in an intra-peritoneal inoculation of the samples in Swiss female white mice. A toxoplasmic serology is performed in the mice 3 and 6 weeks after inoculation. The eventual presence of *Toxoplasma* cysts (if the sample contained parasites) is checked by microscopic examination of mice brains. Although the sensitivity of mouse inoculation is quite satisfying, and its specificity obviously perfect, the major drawback of the technique is the delay (3 to 6 weeks after inoculation) of the results. This is an important problem, particularly when the medical management of the toxoplasmosis requires a quick therapeutic decision, such as in case of prenatal diagnosis of congenital toxoplasmosis using amniotic fluid sampling. However, in such cases, mouse inoculation can be performed associated with more recent and quick methods [1, 43].

In vitro cultures

Considering the major drawback of mouse inoculation, the delay for results, techniques of *in vitro* cultures were developed. These methods use human cell lines which can be grown easily *in vitro*. Different cell types can be used, but all of them allow to obtain results faster than when using mouse inoculation. As for mouse inoculation, the biological specificity of the method can not be discussed, since the growth of *Toxoplasma* in these cultures is the consequence of the presence of living parasites in the sample which was sealed [7]. The only cause of "false positive" is not biological, but technical: this could be the result of poor manipulation in the laboratory, leading to contamination of cells or media with parasites. False positive or false negative results can also be due to difficulties in the detection of parasites in cell cultures, when a microscopic detection (using immuno fluorescent assay, for example) is performed. The intrepretation is not always easy, and the identification of parasites sometimes subjective. However, the results are obtained in a few days, in comparison with few weeks for mouse inoculation, even if the sensitivity of *in vitro* culture, in comparison to these of murine culture, can be discussed [43, 44].

MRC5 cells

This type of cell cultures is the most widely used [45]. MRC5 cells are human embryonic lung fibroblasts wich are easy to obtain, since they are commercialised and used for other applications, such as diagnostic in virology. MRC5 are adherent cells, easy to handle, which form a monolayer in culture wells of flasks.

THP1

The cell lines different from MRC5 cells are less used. THP1 cells are monocytic non adherent cells, which have been used by several teams for *in vitro* culture of *Toxoplasma*. However, when using non-adherent cells, the detection of *T. gondii* growth must be performed with methods such as cytofluorometry [46].

Antigen detection

Some research protocols for the detection of *T. gondii* antigens have been described. However, these works have remained in the field of research. They have no wide routine use practically, because of the complexity of *Toxoplasma* antigens, and because the protocols are not yet standardized [47, 48].

PCR and molecular biology techniques

As described previously in this chapter, none of the techniques used for the direct detection of *T. gondii* is at the same time sensitive, specific, quick, reproducible, automatized and easy to use. That is why, when molecular biology techniques, and more precisely Polymerase Chain Reaction, were developed in the field of microbiology, specific sequences and primer sets were defined for *T. gondii*. PCR represents a real improvement for the biological diagnosis of toxoplasmosis, even if all the defined goals are not achieved. One of the main difficulties of PCR for toxoplasmosis is the lack of standardisa-

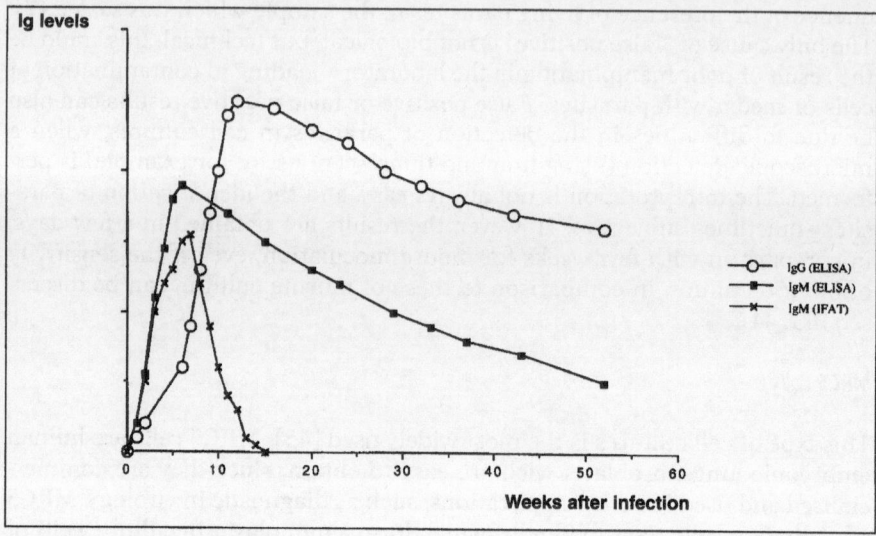

Fig. 1. Examples of IgG or IgM kinetics

tion (no commercial kits are available), and consequently the fact that these techniques are not available for non-specialized laboratories. However, the strong advantage for PCR is its high sensitivity and specificity [49].

Target sequences

Several target sequences (primers pairs and probes) were described (P30, TGR1E, ARNr, B1 gene) and used for diagnosis but also for strain characterisation [50]. Among them, the B1 gene sequence is now the most widely used, even if, inside this gene, different targets have been described, what is the reflect of the lack of a "gold standard" sequence accepted by all authors [49, 51-54].

Methodological problems (extraction, revelation, etc.)

The goal of this chapter is not to describe all the parameters of the technique, but we will focus on some of the most important points. Like for all diagnostic PCRs, the fact that the technique is performed in *ad hoc* room, to avoid carry-over contaminations, is of main importance. The inclusion in the protocol of a decontamination kit (UNG), also to avoid contaminations, and an internal control sequence, to detect polymerase inhibitors, are key steps of the technique. Furthermore, the DNA extraction method and the technique of detection of amplified products (gels, or enzymatic systems in microwell plates) are also of importance. Together, all this different parameters induce great discrepancies in the PCR protocols used by the different teams. When comparison on the same samples are performed, differences concerning the results appear clearly. This demonstrates the fact that, to date, PCR for toxoplasmosis should not be performed by non specialised labs [55, 56].

Samples: which technique to use?

For the biological diagnosis of toxoplasmosis (in the congenital, but also in immunocompromised patients), one of the main issues is to determine which biological method to apply on the different samples. This question is of paramount importance, and needs a close collaboration between physicians and biologists, to avoid wrong sampling that can be the cause of anxiety and lesions for the patient.

Sera

Obviously, serological methods have to be performed on sera. However, one can wonder if antigen detection will be, in the future, a routine technique applied to sera. When PCR for toxoplasmosis was first described, some studies focused on the value of this technique for detection of toxoplasmic DNA in sera. But the results were not satisfying. The use of fetal blood for antenatal diagnosis of fetal infection (serology and detection of parasite) has been proposed for several years. However, fetal blood sampling has now been abandoned by most of the teams because of the use of very sensitive techniques, such as PCR, on amniotic fluid, the sampling of which is easier and safer [1].

Fluids: amniotic fluid, cerebrospinal fluid, aqueous humor and others

Serological methods have been used on these different fluids, but to date they are no more used, since the techniques of detection of *T. gondii*, such as PCR, have become more useful, particularly in amniotic fluid. However, the evaluation of intraocular secretion of anti-*T. gondii* antibodies remains useful for the diagnosis of retinochoroiditis, even if PCR can be associated [57, 58].

Placenta, tissues, biopsies

In tissue samples, serological techniques have obviously no usefulness. The most important techniques are those of detection of *T. gondii*, such as staining, mouse inoculation, *in vitro* culture and PCR. However, one must be aware of the potential difficulties for DNA extraction in such bloody samples [59].

Conclusion

This overview clearly emphazises that numerous biological techniques are available in the field of congenital toxoplasmosis. For the medical biologist, (and to some extent for physicians who have to discuss the results with the patients), the problem is to choose the best methods depending on the step of the diagnosis and the sample used, and to be able to know perfectly well its advantages and drawbacks. This choice is of paramount importance for a good management of the toxoplasmic infection, and thus for the health of the pregnant woman and her child.

References

1. Hohlfeld P, Daffos F, Costa JM, Thulliez P, Forestier F, Vidaud M (1994) Prenatal diagnosis of congenital toxoplasmosis with a polymerase-chain-reaction test on amniotic fluid. N Engl J Med 331:695-699
2. Petithory JC, Ambroise-Thomas P, De Loye J, Pelloux H, Goullier-Fleuret A, Milgram M, Buffard C, Garin JP (1996) Serodiagnosis of toxoplasmosis: a comparative study of a series of control sera using various currently available tests and expression of the results in international units. WHO Bull 74:291-298
3. Candolfi E, Kien T (1990) Les nouvelles données de l'interprétation de la sérologie de la toxoplasmose par l'évaluation comparée d'anciennes et de nouvelles techniques sérologiques. Spectra Biol 90:55-62
4. Dannemann BR, Vaughan WC, Thulliez P, Remington JS (1990) Differential agglutination test for diagnosis of recently acquired infection with Toxoplasma gondii. J Clin Microbiol 28:1928-1933
5. Derouin F, Garin YJF, Buffard C, Berthelot F, Petithory JC (1994) Multicentre study on serological testing for toxoplasmosis using various commercial ELISA reagents. WHO Bull 72:249-256
6. Nagy S, Hayde M, Panzenböck B, Adlassnig KP, Pollack A (1997) Toxopert-1: knowledge-based automatic interpretation of serological tets for toxoplasmosis. Comp Meth Prog Biomed 53:119-133
7. Wong SY, Remington JS (1994) Toxoplasmosis in pregnancy. Clin Infect Dis 18:853-862
8. Desmonts G, Naot Y, Remington JS (1981) Immunoglobulin M-immunosorbent agglutination assay for diagnosis of infectious diseases: diagnosis of acute congenital and acquired Toxoplasma infection. J Clin Microbiol 14:486-491
9. Eaton RB, Petersen E, Seppänen H, Tuuminen T (1996) Multicenter evaluation of fluorometric enzyme immunocapture assay to detect Toxoplasma-specific immunoglobulin M in dried blood filter paper specimens from newborns. J Clin Microbiol 34:3147-3150
10. Jenum P, Stray-Pedersen B (1998) Development of specific immunoglobulins G, M and A following primary Toxoplasma gondii infection in pregnant women. J Clin Microbiol 36:2907-2913
11. De Champs C, Pelloux H, Cambon M, Fricker-Hidalgo H, Goullier-Fleuret A, Ambroise-Thomas P (1997) Evaluation of the second generation IMx Toxo IgG antibody assay for detection of antibodies to Toxoplasma gondii in human sera. J Clin Lab Anal 11:214-219
12. Jenum P, Stray-Pedersen B, Melby KK, Kapperud G, Whitelaw A, Eskild A, Eng J (1998) Incidence of Toxoplasma gondii infection in 35,940 pregnant women in Norway and pregnancy outcome for infected women. J Clin Microbiol 36:2900-2906
13. Liesenfield O, Press C, Montoya JG, Gill R, Isaac-Renton JL, Hedman K, Remington JS (1997) False-positive results in immunoglobulin M (IgM) Toxoplasma antibody tests and importance of confirmatory testing : the Platelia Toxo IgM test. J Clin Microbiol 35:174-178
14. Pelloux H, Fricker-Hidalgo H, Goullier-Fleuret A, Ambroise-Thomas P (1997) Detection of anti-Toxoplasma Immunoglobulin M in pregnant women. J Clin Microbiol 35:2187
15. Decoster A, Darcy F, Caron A, Vinatier D, Houze de l'Aulnoit D, Vittu G, Niel G, Heyer F, Lecolier B, Delcroix M, Monnier JC, Duhamel M (1992) Anti-P30 IgA antibodies as prenatal markers of congenital toxoplasma infection. Clin Exp Immunol 87:310-315
16. Stepick-Biek P, Thulliez P, Araujo FG, Remington JS (1990) IgA antibodies for diagnosis of acute congenital and acquired toxoplasmosis. J Inf Dis 162:270-273
17. Decoster A, Gontier P, Dehecq E, Demory JL, Duhamel M (1995) Detection of anti-Toxoplasma immunoglobulin A antibodies by Platelia-toxo IgA directed against P30 and by IMX Toxo IgA for diagnosis of acquired and congenital toxoplasmosis. J Clin Microbiol 33:2206-2208
18. Gorgievski-Hrisoho M, Germann D, Matter L (1996) Diagnostic implications of kinetics of immunoglobulin M and A antibody responses to Toxoplasma gondii. J Clin Microbiol 34:1506-1511
19. Gross U, Bohne W, Schröder J, Roos T, Heesemann J (1993) Comparison of a commercial enzyme immunoassay and an immunoblot technique for detection of immunoglobulin A antibodies to Toxoplasma gondii. Eur J Clin Microbiol Infect Dis 12:636-639

20. Montoya JG, Remington JS (1995) Studies on the serodiagnosis of toxoplasmic lymphadenitis. Clin Inf Dis 20:781-789
21. Pinon JM, Foudrinier F, Mougeot G, Marx C, Aubert D, Toupance O, Niel G, Danis M, Camerlynck P, Remy G, Frottier J, Jolly D, Bessieres MH, Richard-Lenoble D, Bonhomme A (1995) Evaluation of risk and diagnostic value of quantitative assays for anti-*Toxoplasma gondii* immunoglobulin A (IgA), IgE, and IgM and analytical study of specific IgG in immunodeficient patients. J Clin Microbiol 33:878-884
22. Wong SY, Hadju MP, Ramirez R, Thulliez P, McLeod R, Remington JS (1993) Role of specific immunoglobulin E in diagnosis of acute *Toxoplasma* infection and toxoplasmosis. J Clin Microbiol 31:2952-2959
23. Sabin AB, Feldman HA (1948) Dyes as microchemical indicators of a new immunity phenomenon affecting a protozoan parasite (toxoplasma). Science 108:660-663
24. Ambroise-Thomas P (1963) L'immunofluorescence dans le diagnostic direct et indirect des parasitoses : application à la toxoplasmose. Thèse médecine, Lyon, 160 p, 115 réf.
25. Ambroise-Thomas P, Francesio J, Simon J, Micouin C, Pierson Y (1980) Les facteurs rhumatoïdes cause de non-spécificité de l'immuno-fluorescence anti-IgM dans la toxoplasmose. Ann Biol Clin (Paris) 38:315-319
26. Ambroise-Thomas P, Garin JP, Rigaud A (1966) Amélioration de la technique d'immuno-fluorescence par l'emploi de contre colorants. Application à la toxoplasmose. Presse Méd 74:2215-2216
27. Petithory JC, Reiter-Owona I, Berthelot F, Milgram M, De Loye J, Petersen E (1996) Performance of European laboratories testing serum samples for *Toxoplasma gondii*. Eur J Clin Microbiol Infect Dis 15:45-49
28. Petithory JC, Milgram M, Janot C, Maisonneuve P, Miguérès ML, Charlier N, Fromage M, Berthelot F, Leblanc A (1998) Réévaluation de 40 trousses de reactifs pour la détection des anticorps anti-toxoplasme de type IgG. Rev Fr Lab 301:59-64
29. Dunford P, Johnson J (1991) Detection of toxoplasma-specific immunoglobulin-G: assessment of a slide agglutination test. Med Lab Sci 48:137-141
30. Galanti LM, Dell'Omo J, Wanet B, Guarin JL, Jamart J, Garrino MG, Masson PL, Cambiaso CL (1997) Particle counting assay for anti-toxoplasma IgG antibodies. Comparison with four automated commercial enzyme-linked immunoassays. J Immunol Meth 207:195-201
31. Yamamoto YI, Hoshino-Shimizu S, Camarguo ME (1991) A novel IgM-indirect hemagglutination test for the serodiagnosis of acute toxoplasmosis. J Clin Lab Anal 5:127-132
32. Cozon G, Roure C, Lizard G, Greenland T, Larget-Piet D, Gandilhon F, Peyron F (1993) An improved assay for the detection of *Toxoplasma gondii* antibodies in human serum by flow cytometry. Cytometry 14:569-575
33. Rougier D, Ambroise-Thomas P (1985) Detection of toxoplasmic immunity by multipuncture skin test with excretory-secretory antigens. Lancet I:121-123
34. Hedmann K, Lappalainen M, Seppâla I, Mäkelä O (1989) Recent primary toxoplasma infection indicated by a low avidity of specific IgG. J Inf Dis 159:736-740
35. Jenum P, Stray-Pedersen B, Gundersen AG (1997) Improved diagnosis of primary *Toxoplasma gondii* infection in early pregnancy by determination of antitoxoplasma immunoglobulin G avidity. J Clin Microbiol 35:1972-1977
36. Pelloux H, Guy E, Angelici MC, Aspock H, Bessières MH, Blatz R, Del Pezzo M, Girault V, Gratzl R, Holberg-Petersen M, Johnson J, Krüger D, Lappalainen M, Naessens A, Olsson M (1998) A second European collaborative study on polymerase chain reaction for *Toxoplasma gondii* involving 15 teams. FEMS Microbiol Lett 165:231-237
37. Pinon JM, Thoannes H, Gruson N (1985) An enzyme-linked immunofiltration assay used to compare infant and maternal antibody profiles in toxoplasmosis. J Immunol Meth 77:15-23
38. Chumpitazi BFF, Boussaid A, Pelloux H, Racinet C, Bost M, Goullier-Fleuret A (1995) Diagnosis of congenital toxoplasmosis by immunoblotting and relationship with other methods. J Clin Microbiol 33:1479-1485
39. Pinon JM, Chemla C, Villena I, Foudrinier F, Aubert D, Puygauthier-Toubas D, Leroux B, Dupouy D, Quereux C, Talmud M, Trenque T, Potron G, Pluot M, Remy G, Bonhomme A (1996) Early neonatal diagnosis of congenital toxoplasmosis: value of comparative enzyme-linked immunofiltration assay immunological profiles and anti-*Toxoplasma gondii* immunoglobulin M (IgM) or IgA immunocapture and implications for postnatal therapeutic strategies. J Clin Microbiol 34:579-583
39.bis Bottone EJ (1991) Diagnosis of acute pulmonary toxoplasmosis by visualization of invasive and intracellular tachyzoites in giemsa-stained smears of bronchoalveolar lavage fluid. J Clin Microbiol 29:2626-2627
40. Sundermann CA, Estridge BH, Branton MS, Brigman CR, Lindsay DS (1997) Immunohistochemical diagnosis of *Toxoplasma gondii*: potential for cross-reactivity with *Neospora caninum*. J Parasitol 83:440-443

41. Brouland JP, Audouin J, Hofman P, Le Tourneau A, Basset D, Rio B, Zittoun R, Diebold J (1996) Bone marrow involvement by disseminated toxoplasmosis in acquired immunodeficiency syndrome: the value of bone marrow trephine biopsy and immunohistochemistry for the diagnosis. Hum Pathol 27:302-306
42. Jautzke G, Sell M, Thalmann U, Janitschke K, Gottsckalk J, Schürmann D, Ruff B (1993) Extracerebral toxoplasmosis in AIDS. Histological and immunohistological findings based on 80 autopsy cases. Path Res Pract 189:428-436
43. Fricker-Hidalgo H, Pelloux H, Muet F, Racinet C, Bost M, Goullier-Fleuret A, Ambroise-Thomas P (1997) Prenatal diagnosis of congenital toxoplasmosis: comparative value of fetal blood and amniotic fluid using serological techniques and cultures. Prenat Diag 17:831-835
44. Derouin F, Mazeron MC, Garin YJ (1987) Comparative study of tissue culture and mouse inoculation methods for demonstration of *Toxoplasma gondii*. J Clin Microbiol 25:1597-1600
45. Derouin F, Garin YJF (1992) Isolement de *Toxoplasma gondii* par culture cellulaire chez les sujets infectés par le VIH. Presse Méd 21:1853-1856
46. Tirard V, Niel G, Rosenheim M, Katlama C, Ciceron L, Ogunkolade W, Danis M, Gentilini M (1991) Diagnosis of toxoplasmosis in patients with AIDS by isolation of the parasite from the blood. N Engl J Med 324:634
47. Derouin F, Thulliez P, Candolfi E, Daffos F, Forestier F (1988) Early prenatal diagnosis of congenital toxoplasmosis using amniotic fluid samples and tissue culture. Eur J Clin Microbiol Infect Dis 7:423-425
48. Hafid J, Tran Man Sung R, Raberin H, Akono ZY, Pozzetto B, Jana M (1995) Detection of circulating antigens of *Toxoplasma gondii* in human infection. Am J Trop Med Hyg 52:336-339
49. Weiss JB (1995) DNA probes and PCR for diagnosis of parasitic infections. Clin Microbiol Rev 8:113-130
50. Cristina N, Liaud MF, Santoro F, Oury B, Ambroise-Thomas P (1991) A family of repeated DNA sequences in *Toxoplasma gondii*: cloning, sequence analysis, and use in strain characterization. Exp Parasitol 73:73-81
51. Dupouy-Camet J, Bougnoux ME, Lavareda de Souza S, Thulliez P, Dommergues M, Mandelbrot L, Ancelle T, Tourte-Schaeffer C, Benarous R (1992) Comparative value of polymerase chain reaction and conventional biological tests for the prenatal diagnosis of congenital toxoplasmosis. Ann Biol Clin 50:315-319
52. Forestier F, Hohlfeld P, Sole Y, Daffos F (1998) Prenatal diagnosis of congenital toxoplasmosis by PCR: extended experience. Prenat Diag 18:405-415
53. Grover CM, Thulliez P, Remington JS, Boothroyd J (1990) Rapid prenatal diagnosis of congenital *Toxoplasma* infection by using polymerase chain reaction and amniotic fluid. J Clin Microbiol 28:2297-2301
54. Pelloux H, Weiss J, Simon J, Muet F, Fricker-Hidalgo H, Goullier-Fleuret A, Ambroise-Thomas P (1996) A new set of primers for the detection of *Toxoplasma gondii* in amniotic fluid using polymerase chain reaction. FEMS Microbiol Lett 138:11-15
55. Guy EC, Pelloux H, Lappalainen M, Aspöck H, Hassl A, Melby KK, Holberg-Pettersen M, Petersen E, Simon J, Ambroise-Thomas P (1996) Interlaboratory comparison of polymerase chain reaction for the detection of *Toxoplasma gondii* DNA added to samples of amniotic fluid. Eur J Clin Microbiol Infect Dis 15:836-839
56. Pelloux H, Brun E, Vernet G, Marcillat S, Jolivet M, Guergour D, Fricker-Hidalgo H, Goullier-Fleuret A, Ambroise-Thomas P (1998) Determination of anti-*Toxoplasma gondii* immunoglobulin G avidity: adaptation to the Vidas system (bioMérieux). Diag Microbiol Infect Dis 32:69-73
57. Riss JM, Carboni ME, Franck JY, Mary CJ, Dumon H, Ridings B (1995) Toxoplasmose oculaire: intérêt de l'immunoblot pour la mise en évidence d'une synthèse intra-oculaire d'anticorps. Path Biol 43:772-778
58. Rothova A (1993) Ocular involvement in toxoplasmosis. Brit J Ophthalmol 77:371-377
59. Fricker-Hidalgo H, Pelloux H, Racinet C, Grefenstette I, Bost-Bru C, Goullier-Fleuret A, Ambroise-Thomas P (1998) Detection of *Toxoplasma gondii* in 94 placentae from infected women by polymerase chain reaction, *in vivo*, and *in vitro* cultures. Placenta 19:545-549

1.7. Drugs effective against *Toxoplasma gondii*. Present status and future perspective

F. Derouin

Introduction

Several aspects of the biology and life cycle of *Toxoplasma gondii* are important limiting factors for the evaluation of drugs for the treatment of congenital toxoplasmosis: *(i) T. gondii* is an obligate intracellular parasite which multiplies within a parasitophorous vacuole or a cyst; *(ii)* two distinct parasitic stages i.e. tachyzoites and bradyzoites are present during the course of infection; *(iii)* parasites can invade different organs, mainly brain, striated muscles, lungs, eyes and placenta in case of maternal contamination.

Thus, an ideal drug would be effective, and preferentially parasiticidal, against the different parasitic stages, and would penetrate into cysts and be well distributed in the main sites of infection. In the context of congenital toxoplasmosis, such requirements would also include a good penetration and concentration in the placenta, a transplacental passage and a total lack of fetal toxicity and teratogenic effect.

Presently, there is no drug that fulfils these criteria. For many drugs with known activity against *T. gondii*, informations are dramatically lacking on the precise mode of action, tissue distribution, transplacental passage and safety in pregnant women. Indeed, *in vitro* and *in vivo* animal models have been extensively used to explore these different aspects but the relevance of results obtained in animal models of congenital toxoplasmosis and of chrorioretinitis are questionable, due to the marked differences between the mode of infection and pharmacokinetics of drugs in humans and in animals.

On the other hand, the emergence of cerebral toxoplasmosis as a severe infectious complication in immunocompromised patients has resulted in a better knowledge of the clinical efficacy, limits and tolerance of anti-*Toxoplasma* drugs and also markedly stimulated the search for new active compounds.

In this paper a broad overview of anti-*Toxoplasma* drugs is presented, focusing on their mode of action and activity *in vitro* and in animal model. The interest and limitations of each drug will be discussed in the context of their prescription for treatment of congenital toxoplasmosis.

Inhibitors of folate biosynthesis

In the protozoan *Toxoplasma gondii*, folate compounds are essential factors for several parasitic metabolisms including nucleosides biosynthesis and thereby nucleic acid formation. Unlike mammalian cells, *T. gondii* does not possess a carrier system to uptake preformed folate and must synthesize them *de novo*. Dihydropteroate synthase (DHPS) is one of the enzymes responsible for this synthesis, while dihydrofolate reductase (DHFR) maintains the folate at a reduced state.

Since DHPS is absent in mammalian cells it represents a unique drug target with a potentially high therapeutic index. By contrast, DHRF is represented in both mammalian and protozoa, and the therapeutic index of DHFR inhibitors is limited by the potential toxicity of these drugs on mammalian cells. This represents the main drawback of this family of drugs which may induce a folate deficiency, possibly responsible for severe hematological side effects and embryopathy.

Dihydrofolate inhibitors

Pyrimethamine

This 2.4-diamino pyrimidine is known to be active against *T. gondii* for 50 years [1]. *In vitro*, pyrimethamine is inhibitory for tachyzoite growth for concentrations ≥ 0.05 mg/L and its parasiticidal effect can readily be evidenced, with marked alterations of nucleic and cell division of treated parasites [2-4]. This high inhibitory activity was also confirmed using purified DHFR, pyrimethamine being approximately 1.000 fold more active against the parasite than the human enzyme [5, 6]. However, pyrimethamine was found not effective on intracystic parasites in an *ex-vivo* model [7].

In murine models of acute toxoplasmosis, oral administration of pyrimethamine is protective but the effect on parasitic burdens in infected tissue is only observed 6 days after initiation of treatment, probably corresponding to a delayed accumulation of pyrimethamine in tissues. After cessation of therapy, relapses are constantly observed, as pyrimethamine does not eradicate tissue cysts [1, 8].

Pyrimethamine is almost insoluble in water and is administered orally; the only available form for intravenous use is in combination with sulfadoxine (Fansidar). When administered orally, pyrimethamine is well absorbed but several pharmacokinetics studies performed in adults revealed important individual variations of serum drug levels [9-12]. The peak value is observed at 4 hours and the mean half-life of elimination is estimated at 95 ± 30 hours [13]. In patients treated for toxoplasmic encephalitis, pyrimethamine was found to diffuse into cerebrospinal fluid (CSF), with a serum/CSF ratio ranging form 0.13 to 0.26 [11] and to penetrate in brain tissue, with a higher concentration than in serum after 24 hours of treatment [14].

A shorter serum half-life was noted in infants treated for congenital toxoplasmosis, especially in those receiving phenobarbital [15]. Serum levels in infants treated daily with 1mg/kg were at 1.3 ± 0.5mg/L, and 0.7 ± 0.26 in those treated on alternate days. As in adults, CSF levels ranged for 10 to 25% of serum levels.

Pyrimethamine can cross the placental barrier and diffuse in fetal blood; in pregnant women treated with 25mg/20kg twice monthly, fetal/maternal ratio of serum pyrimethamine was 0.66 ± 0.22 [16]. These results are in agreement with those obtained experimentally in monkeys where pyrimethamine was found to accumulate in the brain with concentrations being 3 to 4 time higher than in serum [17]. Such individual variations is in favor of the monitoring of pyrimethamine levels in order to assess efficacy of therapy. From *in vitro* experiments, a concentration of ≥ 0.5mg/L could be considered sufficient as this concentration is completely inhibitory for *T. gondii* and cytopathic for the parasite in tissue culture [2, 3, 18, 19], especially when combined with sulfadiazine [9].

Since pyrimethamine has been found teratogenic in animals, its use during pregnancy is a concern. Although there is no unequivocal documentation of pyrimethamine-associated birth defects at the dose levels used for malaria prophylaxis, pyrimethamine is contraindicated during the first trimester of pregnancy.

Trimethoprim

This 2-4-diamino-5-(3'4'5'-trimethoxybenzyl)-pyrimidine is inhibitory for *T. gondii* tachyzoite for concentrations ≥ 2mg/L, i.e. a concentration 100 times higher than pyrimethamine in the same culture conditions [3]; this lower efficacy was also confirmed in an assay performed on purified DHFR [5].

In animal models, several studies showed that the administration of trimethoprim alone was not protective [20, 21]. Because of this limited efficacy, trimethoprim is not used alone but is administered in combination with sulfamethoxazole (see below).

Pharmacokinetic data show that trimethoprim is readily absorbed, and produce peak levels of 1.2-2.1mg/L within 1 hour after administration of 160 mg [22]; its half-life is estimated at 7.5 hours. Trimethoprim is widely distributed in tissues and CSF levels are about 40% of serum levels. In aqueous humor, trimethoprim levels are 10 to 50% of serum levels [23, 24].

Trimethoprim readily crosses the placental barrier and is detectable in serum and fetal tissues [25, 26]. However, the teratogenicity and potential toxicity of trimethoprim is not clearly defined.

Other DHFR inhibitors

Pyrimethamine and trimethoprime have a high degree of binding selectivity for *T. gondii* DHFR vs. mammalian DHFR; they are not very potent and are not fully effective when used as single agents.

Several other very potent DHFR inhibitors which have been initially developed as anti-cancer agents are also highly inhibitory for *T. gondii*, such as trimetrexate and piritrexim [5]; however, the high affinity of these compounds to mammalian DHFR is responsible for untoward side effects, mainly myelosuppression.

Epiroprim is a 2.4-diaminobenzylpyrimidine that is structurally related to trimethoprim. It is inhibitory for *T. gondii in vitro* and effective in the treatment of experimental toxoplasmosis when administered orally at a high dosage [27, 28].

PS-15, a novel biguanide, was also found partially effective in an immunosupressed rat model of acute toxoplasmosis [27].

DHPS inhibitors: sulfonamides

As for DHFR inhibitors, the activity of sulfonamides and sulfone was demonstrated more than 50 years ago in murine models of infection [1]. *In vitro* studies performed in tissue cultures or on purified DHPS showed that sulfonamides exhibited a broad range of inhibitory potency [2, 3]. In both studies sulfamethoxazole was found to be the most potent of the sulfonamides tested (IC50 estimated at 1.1mg/L in tissue culture and 0.7mg/L on purified DHPS) whereas sulfadoxine was a poor *Toxoplasma* DHPS inhibitor (IC50 > 30mg/L). Sulfadiazine is one of the most effective compounds, with an IC50 estimated at 2.5mg/L in tissue culture and 2.7mg/L on purified DHPS [29, 2]. This marked inhibitory effect was not associated with morphological alterations of the parasite in tissue culture [29, 4]. In animal models of acute infection, sulfadiazine and sulfamethoxazole administered alone at a high dosage are protective but relapses are constantly observed after cessation of therapy [8].

Sulfonamides are usually administered orally, although sulfadiazine and sulfamethoxazole in combination with trimethoprime are available for intravenous administration. Most of the sulfonamides are absorbed rapidly and variably bind to proteins (bound drug are inactive) producing serum peak levels that range between 30 and 100mg/L. According to their excretion rate, sulfonamides are classified into short or medium acting and long acting sulfonamides. Sulfadiazine and sulfamethoxazole are belonging to the first category, with half-life of 17 and 11 hours, respectively. In contrast, sulfadoxine is characterized by a much slower excretion rate, and half-life of 100-230 hours [13].

Sulfonamides are well distributed through the body and into CSF: the serum/CSF ratio is inversely related to the degree of protein binding and range between 20 and 80%. Little information is available of intraocular penetration; with sulfamethoxazole. Drug concentrations in aqueous humor are comprised between 10 and 40% of those in serum [23, 24]. Sulfonamides readily cross the placenta and are present in the fetal blood and amniotic fluid [25, 26].

Dapsone (4-4 diaminodiphenyl sulfone) is highly effective against *T. gondii* [30]. *In vitro*, a significant inhibition of *Toxoplasma* growth is obtained for concentrations ≥ 0.5mg/L and the IC50 is estimated at 0.55mg/L. This excellent *in vitro* activity was confirmed in murine models of acute toxoplasmosis [1, 30]. Despite of this, the use of dapsone in human and especially during pregnancy is limited by its potential hematological toxicity and risks of hemolytic anemia in patients with G6PDH deficiency.

Drug combinations

Antifolate chemotherapy of toxoplasmosis relies on the combination of folate analogs to inhibit DHFR and a sulfonamide, since the remarkable synergy between these two families of drug has been evidenced *in vitro* and *in vivo* for a variety of drug combinations.

Pyrimethamine + sulfadiazine is considered as the most effective drug combination as it combines two potent DHFR inhibitor and sulfonamide. This combination proved remarkably efficient in the treatment of severe form of toxoplasmosis, both in experimental models and in humans [8, 9, 31] but is ineffective on the cyst form of the parasite [7, 32]. Because of their different half-lives, these two drugs have to be administered separately, once a day for pyrimethamine and 2 or 3 times a day for sulfadiazine, whose half-life is much shorter than that of pyrimethamine. The need for repeated administration of sulfadiazine and the lack of parenteral formulation of pyrimethamine is the main disadvantage of this drug combination although the short half-life of sulfadiazine can be considered as an advantage in the management of untoward side effects in case of sulfonamide intolerance.

Pyrimethamine + sulfadoxine (Fansidar) combines two long half-life drugs at a ratio of 1/20. This drug combination is synergistic *in vitro* [2, 3] and effective in murine models of acute toxoplasmosis [33]. It can be administered orally or parentally and offers a major advantage for long-term treatment since oral administration can be spaced weekly. On the other hand, Fansidar formulation is not suitable for treatment of toxoplasmosis for which a daily dose of 1 to 2mg/kg of pyrimethamine is needed; such treatment would imply the co-administration of 20 to 40mg/kg/day of sulfadoxine which is too high dosage and rate of administration for this long-term sulfonamide.

Due to the unknown teratogenic potential of pyrimethamine, Fansidar is not recommended in pregnant women (at least during the first trimester of pregnancy). In children, long-term administration of Fansidar is well tolerated when concomitantly administered with folinic acid [34].

As for Fansidar, trimethoprim + sulfamethoxazole (cotrimoxazole) is combining two drugs with comparable half-life and is available for oral or parenteral route of administration. Initially, cotrimoxazole was developed as an antibacterial drug and the respective ratio of the two compounds (trimethoprim: 1, sulfamethoxazole: 5) was chosen in order to provide in tissues (mainly lung) the optimum synergistic ratio against bacteria (i.e. 1/20). Several *in vitro* and *in vivo* studies suggest that this ratio may not be optimal on *T. gondii*, due to the poor efficacy of trimethoprim, comparatively to pyrimethamine [21, 35]. Experimental data showed that sulfamethoxazole accounts for most of the anti-*Toxoplasma* activity of the combination and that an increase of dosage of trimethoprim may allow a reduction of the dosage of sulfamethoxazole without loss of prophylactic activity [35]. This would explain why high dosage of cotrimoxazole is needed to cure experimental acute infections in mice [33] and is ineffective on parasitic brain cysts [32]. However, administration of cotrimoxazole in pregnant mice infected with *T. gondii* indicated a better in utero control of congenital toxoplasmosis by cotrimoxazole than by spiramycin [36]. In humans the efficacy of cotrimoxazole has been established for the prophylaxis of *Pneumocystis carinii* and *T. gondii* infections in patients with AIDS, and its wide spread use has resulted in a marked reduction of incidence of cerebral toxoplasmosis [37]. A randomized and a retrospective study also showed that the combination of trimethoprim 10mg/kg/day and sulfamethoxazole 50mg/kg/day was as effective as the standard pyrimethamine + sulfadiazine regimen for the treatment of toxoplasmic encephalitis and was better tolerated [38, 39].

Whether cotrimoxazole can be safely used during pregnancy is subject of debate. On one hand, trimethoprim is not recommended during pregnancy because of its potential teratogenicity when administered at high dosage in animal; on the other hand, cotrimoxazole has been extensively used for years in humans and no study could clearly establish a relationship between administration of cotrimoxazole during pregnancy and fetal toxicity or birth defects [40].

Other combinations of folate inhibitors have been evaluated *in vitro* and *in vivo* showing a synergistic effect which was comfirmed for pyrimethamine + dapsone, PS15 (a new biguanide) + dapsone, and epiroprim + sulfadiazine or + dapsone [27, 28, 41].

Antibiotics

Macrolides, azalides, lincosamides, synergistin, ketolides (MALSK)

Several members of this important family of antibiotics are active against *T. gondii*. This was first demonstrated experimentally in mice [33], then *in vitro* against tachyzoites. Most MALSK inhibit the growth of *T. gondii* tachyzoites but their effect is only observed with prolonged incubation with the drug, reflecting the delayed mode of action of these drugs on the parasite. Their inhibitory effect is progressively increasing with the concentration of the drug into the culture, so that 50% inhibitory concentrations of MALSK range between 0.8 and 15mg/L whereas a complete inhibition of parasitic growth is only observed for high concentration of drug, i.e. 40 to 100mg/L [42, 43]. This observation as well as the fact that no major alterations are seen on treated parasites is suggesting a parasitostatic effect of these drugs.

The mode of action of MALSK on *T. gondii* remains poorly understood. By analogy to that observed in bacterias, one hypothesis is an inhibition of protein synthesis [44, 45] but the site of action and fixation in the parasite has not been demonstrated. Recently, the demonstration of a vestigial procaryotic organelle in *T. gondii* in which a protein synthesis can be conducted, offers a possible explanation for the activity of these antibiotic on eucaryotic organisms [46, 47].

In murine models of acute toxoplasmosis, macrolides are only partially protective even when administered at very high dosages [48].

Spiramycin

Spiramycin was the first macrolide used for treatment of toxoplasmosis in humans. This 16-C macrolide is inhibitory for *T. gondii in vitro* for concentrations ≥ 1mg/L and the IC50 is estimated at 12mg/L [42]. Such a concentration is usually not achieved in serum but may be reached in some tissues such as lung, liver and placenta where spiramycin remarkably concentrates [49]. Transplacental transfer of spiramycin is partial, yielding to low fetal concentrations; in a model of congenital toxoplasmosis in rhesus monkeys, concentrations of spiramycin in neonatal tissues, mainly liver and spleen, were found to be higher than in the serum but were still >10 times lower than those found in the mother [50, 51]; no spiramycin was found in the fetal brain.

Azithromycin

Azithromycin is a 15-membered ring azalide whose activity against *T. gondii* has been clearly evidenced *in vitro* against tachyzoites: the IC50 is estimated at 1.2mg/mL, and a 90% inhibition is obtained at 40mg/L [43]. Indeed, such concentrations are not obtained in serum but may be reached in several tissues (mainly lungs and liver), where azithromycin highly concentrates [52, 53] and is maintained at high levels due the remarkably long half-life of this drug (40 hours). In an experimental model of acute toxoplasmosis, azithromycin concentrations in the brain were almost tenfold higher than the serum concentration after treatment with 200mg/kg/day for 10 days [48]. In humans concentrations ≥ 3mg/L may be obtained in brain tissue within 48 hours after administration of a single 500mg oral dose, whereas it was at very low level in CSF and aqueous humor [54, 55]. One study performed in pregnant women treated with 500mg once daily for 3 days also showed that azithromycin concentrates well in the placental (mean 2.1mg/L for 14 samples) whereas serum level in the mother and cord blood remained very low (i.e. < 0.1mg/L) [56]. In preclinical studies, azithromycin was found to have a teratogenic effect in rat treated with 10 to 200mg/kg for 6 to 15 days and fetal tissue concentrations were found to be higher than in maternal plasma or amniotic fluid [57]; no data is available in humans.

Azithromycin is also characterized by its activity against intracystic bradyzoites. In an *ex-vivo* experiment the incubation of *T. gondii* cyst for 4-6 days with a high concentration of azithromycin (100mg/L) resulted in a marked reduction of the viability and infectivity of intracystic parasites [7]. However, this potential anti-cystic effect was not confirmed in animal model as long term administration of azithromycin to chronically infected mice failed to reduce the mean number of brain cysts [58]. In models of acute toxoplasmosis, azithromycin was also found effective [59] but with a limited effect on brain infection, whereas parasites are cleared from blood and lung of infected mice [60].

Clarithromycin

Clarithromycin is a 6-O-methyl derivative of erythromycin whose activity against *T. gondii* has been demonstrated *in vitro* and *in vivo* [43, 61, 62]. As for other macrolides, a high concentration of the drug or of its 14-OH metabolite is needed to obtain a marked inhibition *in vitro* (IC50: 0.8mg/L, maximum inhibition at 40mg/L) or a significant protection in animal [60, 61]. No information is available on the activity of clarithomycin on cysts *in vitro* or *in vivo*.

Like other macrolides of the "new generation", clarithomycin is characterized by its good diffusion and concentration in various tissues, but information of brain, placental and fetal concentrations are lacking. Of possible interest in the context of congenital toxoplasmosis, is the ocular penetration of clarithromycin, although the concentrations that are achieved in the aqueous humor or vitreous humor do not exceed 0.5mg/L [63].

Roxithromycin

Roxithromycin, an ether oxime derivative of erythromycin, also showed promising activity against *T. gondii*. Its *in vitro* and *in vivo* characteristics and mode of action on *T. gondii* are comparable to those observed with azithromycin or clarithromycin, with an IC50 estimated at 2mg/L; in murine models of acute toxoplasmosis, a significant protection is obtained after treatment with high dosage of roxithromycin [48, 64-66].

Besides its excellent tolerance in humans, roxithromycin has a long elimination half-life (11 hours) and produces a peak serum concentration of 11mg/L within 1.5 hours after oral administration of 300mg. High intracellular and tissue concentrations are also achieved [67] and one study showed that *Toxoplasma* inhibitory concentrations may be achieved in human brain tissue [68].

Clindamycin

Clindamycin is a lincosamide which is usually presented as water soluble hydrochloride or phosphate salts and can be administered orally or parenterally. *In vitro*, clindamycin is highly potent against *T. gondii* but its activity is also characterized by a long lag period between drug administration and effect [42, 69]. Nanomolar drug concentrations blocks parasite replication, but only 2-3 days after treatment, which is a remarkably long delay considering that the tachyzoites undergo 8 generations in this time. Kinetic studies revealed that the drug effects are only observed in the second infectious cycle of the parasite [70]. In one study, the IC50 has been estimated at about 0.001 mg/L and a parasiticidal effect was reported for concentrations ≥ 0.006mg/L [69]. *In vivo*, administration of clindamycin alone is poorly protective in a model of acute toxoplasmosis [8] but has been found efficient in a rabbit model of ocular toxoplasmosis [71].

In humans, clindamycin has a short half-life (3-5 hours), and thus has to be administered 3 to 4 times a day. It is readily absorbed and a peak value of 2.5mg/L is obtained within 1 hour after an oral administration of 150mg. Clindamycin poorly diffuses to CSF but the concentrations that are found inhibitory for *T. gondii in vitro* are achievable in CSF [72] as well as in cord blood [73] and placental tissue [74]. Clindamycin is considered non toxic or teratogenic for the fetus.

Other MALSK

More recently, two ketolides (a new family of derivative of 14-membered ring macrolides) were found active *in vitro* and *in vivo* against *T. gondii*. [75].

Combination of MALSK with other drugs

Due to the moderate activity of MALSK alone on *T. gondii*, the efficacy of their combination with other anti-parasitic drugs has been evaluated experimentally. *In vitro*, a simple additive effect was observed when azithromycin, roxithromycin or clarithromycin were combined with sulfadiazine or pyrimethamine [43, 76]. By contrast, several *in vivo* studies demonstrated a remarkable synergy for the combination of several macrolides (azithromycin, clarithromycin, roxithromycin) and ketolides with other anti-*Toxoplasma* drugs like pyrimethamine, sulfadiazine, minocycline or atovaquone [60-62, 66, 77]. This synergy was especially evidenced with the combination of azithromycin and pyrimethamine. Combination regimen consistently resulted in a marked reduction of the parasitic burdens in blood, lung and brain, compared to those in mice treated with any of the agents alone, and remain negative as long as 30 days after cessation of treatment [60]. One probable hypothesis to explain this synergy is the complementary pharmacokinetics of the compounds on tissue infection.

Minocycline

The efficacy of tetracycline antibiotics on *T. gondii* has been demonstrated for many years especially for oxytetracycline and chlortetracycline [1]. In the seventies' a new generation of tetracycline derivatives were synthetized, including minocycline and doxycycline; both compounds were found effective against *T. gondii*, *in vitro* and *in vivo* [62, 78]. Minocycline was considered as a promising agent for treatment of toxoplasmic encephalitis, due to its high liposolubility which favours CSF diffusion and brain penetration [79], and its synergistic activity when used in combination with a macrolide such as clarithomycin [62].

In addition, it has been found effective for treatment of ocular toxoplasmosis in a rabbit model [80].

However, despite of this activity against *T. gondii* and its good diffusion through the placenta, minocycline is not recommended in the context of congenital toxoplasmosis since it is responsible, as other tetracyclines, of adverse effects on fetal dentition. In addition, pregnant women receiving tetracyclines are particularly vulnerable to certain toxic effects including fatty necrosis of the liver and pancreatitis.

Other antibiotics

Rifabutin-Rifapentin

These rifamycin derivatives were developed for their remarkable activity against *Mycobacteria*. *In vitro* and *in vivo*, rifabutin and rifapentin were found to be active against *T. gondii* [81-83]; a synergistic activity was noted for the combination of rifabutin + atovaquone or clindamycin [83, 84]. Presently, no data are available on the efficacy of rifabutin in human toxoplasmosis.

Fluoroquinolones

Recent data suggest that several members of this important family of antibiotic are active against *T. gondii*, possibly through a unique mechanism of action on the apicoplast [46]. In animal models of acute toxoplasmosis, trovafloxacin was found to be the most effective fluoroquinolone [85]; a synergistic activity was also observed when this drug was combined with several anti-*T. gondii* drugs [86]. Because of their large diffusion and excellent tissue concentration, fluoroquinolones are promising drugs for treatment of toxoplasmosis. Whether they have a place in therapy of congenital toxoplasmosis remain to be determined since their teratogenic potential is still under debate [87].

Atovaquone

Among the drugs that could be considered as an alternative to the use of folate inhibitors and macrolides in the treatment of toxoplasmosis, atovaquone appears as a possible candidate. This broad spectrum anti-parasitic drug is active against *T. gondii* by inhibition of mitochondrial electron transport processes, competing with the biological electron carrier ubiquinone [88]. In vitro, a complete inhibition of the growth of *T. gondii* tachyzoites can be observed at very low concentrations and the IC50 has been estimated at 0.02mg/L) [89-91]; however, individual variations of the IC50 were observed for different strains or *T. gondii* [89]. Of major interest is the activity of atovaquone on cysts; *in vitro* treatment of cysts isolated from brain of chronically infected mice resulted in loss of viability and infectivity of intracystic parasites [7, 90]. This effect was confirmed *in vivo* as prolonged oral treatment of chronically infected mice progressively reduced the mean number of brain cysts comparatively to untreated mice [90, 92, 93]. In addition, the cysts recovered from treated mice presented morphological abnormalities with an increase of lysed or degenerated intracystic bradyzoites [94]. In murine models of acute toxoplasmosis, administration of atovaquone alone resulted in a significant protection of infected mice which correlates with a marked reduction of parasitic burdens in tissues [91]. However, striking variations in the activity of atovaquone against different strains of *T. gondii* was noted [90, 93], suggesting a possible natural resistance of some strains or the rapid selection of drug resistant mutants.

Several drug combinations including atovaquone have been assessed experimentally [83, 91, 95]. *In vitro*, an additive effect was observed when atovaquone was combined with a macrolide, or a sulfonamide, but a significant antagonistic effect was noted between atovaquone and pyrimethamine [91]. However, *in vivo*, the combination of atovaquone with pyrimethamine, macrolides and sulfonamides was more efficient than each drug administered alone, but none of these combinations can be considered as efficient as the reference pyrimethamine-sulfadiazine therapy.

The chemical and pharmacokinetic characteristics of atovaquone have also restricted its clinical use for treatment of toxoplasmosis. Atovaquone is almost insoluble in water and is only available for oral administration. Several clinical and experimental studies have shown that the pharmaceutical formulation of atovaquone is a determinant factor for the bioavailability and therapeutic efficacy [96]. Presently, the administration of the micronized form together with food is recommended since it improves intestinal absorption, and provides seric concentrations that are largely superior to those which are inhibitory for *T. gondii*. At the recommended dosages, atovaquone was also found well tolerated in adults, infants and children [97, 98]; no data are available on transplancental transfer and fetal tissue distribution of atovaquone.

Other drugs

The activity of several drugs effective against Apicomplexan parasites have been examined on *T. gondii*. Among the antimalarial drugs, quinine, chloroquine, melfoquine and primaquine have no effect on *T. gondii* whereas cycloguanyl and artemisin derivatives are inhibitory *in vitro* [99, 100]. *In vivo*, arteether is also effective in mice for treatment of acute toxoplasmosis [101] but the use of this drug in humans might be restricted by its potential neurotoxicity [102].

Recently, a study also showed that 2', 3'-dideoxyinosine (ddI), a nucleoside analog which probably interacts with the purine pathway of *T. gondii*, was inhibitory for tachyzoite growth *in vitro* and induced a significant reduction in the number of cysts in the brain tissue of treated mice [103, 104].

Future directions

From this review, we can outline several complementary orientations for anti-*T. gondii* drug research.

1 – Improvement of our knowledge on the pharmacokinetics of the presently available drugs (cotrimoxazole, atovaquone, macrolides): this would be highly relevant for clinical practice, since information are still lacking on the transplancental passage, fetal diffusion and ocular penetration for most of the currently used compounds.

2 – Development of new compounds belonging to families of drugs that are recognized to be effective against *T. gondii*. This experimental approach has already been developed for DHFR inhibitors, in the objective to identify new compounds with high activity on the parasite and low toxicity on mammalian cells [105]. It should be extended for other drug families, taking advantage of new research tools such as combinatorial chemistry [106] and molecular modeling methods [107] which are particularly time-saving for drug screening activities.

3 – Identification of new drug targets. In this field, a remarkable insight in pharmacological research is the recent demonstration in *T. gondii* of unique biochemical pathways and parasitic structure i.e the apicosplast, that may represent highly specific drug targets. The function of the apicoplast is still not clearly defined but several drugs, including antibiotics such as macrolides and fluoroquinolones can inhibit its DNA replication. Another study indicates that this organelle is responsible for a fatty acid biosynthesis which can be specifically inhibited [108]. The presence of vestigial plant structures within *T. gondii* also offers the opportunity to inhibit the replication of the parasite by blocking plant metabolic pathways such as shikimate synthaze [109] or microtubule synthesis [110, 111]. These new orientations for drug targeting are certainly very promising for the future but a delay of at least several years is to be expected before these new drugs may be proposed in human therapeutics.

References

1. Eyles DE (1956) Newer knowledge of the chemotherapy of toxoplasmosis. N Y Acad Sci 64:252-267
2. Derouin F, Chastang C (1988) Enzyme immunoassay to assess effect of antimicrobial agents on *Toxoplasma gondii* in tissue culture. Antimicrob Ag Chemother 32:303-307
3. Derouin F, Chastang C (1989) In vitro effects of folate inhibitors on *Toxoplasma gondii*. Antimicrob Ag Chemother 33:1753-1759
4. Sheffield HG, Melton M (1975) effect of pyrimethamine and sulfadiazine on the fine structure and multiplication of *Toxoplasma gondii* in cell cultures. J Parasitol 61:704-712
5. Kovacs JA, Allegra CJ, Chabner BA, Swan JC, Drake J, Lunde M, Parrillo JE, Massur H (1987) Potent effect of trimetrexate, a lipid-soluble antifolate, on *Toxoplasma gondii*. J Infect Dis 155:1027-1032
6. Kovacs JA, Allegra CJ, Beaver J, Boarman D, Lewis M, Parrillo JE, Chabner B, Massur H (1989) Characterization of de novo folate synthesis in *Pneumocystis carinii and Toxoplasma gondii*: Potential for screening therapeutic agents. J Infect Dis 160:312-320
7. Huskinson-Mark J, Araujo FG, Remington JS (1991) Evaluation of the effect of drugs on the cyst form of *Toxoplasma gondii*. J Infect Dis 164:170-177
8. Piketty C, Derouin F, Rouveix B, Pocidalo JJ (1990) In vivo assessment of antimicrobial agents on *Toxoplasma gondii* by quantification of parasite in blood, lungs and brain of infected mice. Antimicrob Ag Chemother 34:1467-1472
9. Derouin F, Gerard L, Farinotti R, Maslo C, Leport C (1998) Determination of the inhibitory effect on *Toxoplasma* growth in the serum of AIDS patients during acute therapy for toxoplasmic encephalitis J Acquir Imm Defic Syndr Hum Retrovir 19:50-54
10. Jacobson JM, Davidian M, Rainey PM, Hafner R, Raasch RH, Luft BJ (1996) Pyrimethamine pharmacokinetics in human immunodeficiency virus-positive patients seropositive for *Toxoplasma gondii*. Antimicrob Ag Chemother 40:1360-1365
11. Weiss JM, Harris C, Berger M, Tanowitz HB, Wittner M (1988) Pyrimethamine concentrations in serum and cerebrospinal fluid during treatment of acute *Toxoplasma* encephalitis in patients with AIDS. J Infect Dis 157:580-583
12. Winstanley P, Khoo S, Szawandt S, Edwards G, Wilkins E, Tija J, Coker R, McKane W, Beecking N, Watkin S, Breckenridge A (1995) Marked variation in pyrimethamine disposition in AIDS patients treated for cerebral toxoplasmosis. J Antimicrob Chemother 36:435-439
13. Weidekamm E, Plozza-Nottebrock H, Forgo I, Duback UC (1982) Plasma concentrations of pyrimethamine and sulfadoxine and evaluation of pharmacokinetic data by computerized curve fitting. Bull W H Organ 60:115-122
14. Leport C, Meulemans A, Robine D, Dameron G, Vildé JL (1992) Levels of pyrimethamine in serum and penetration into brain tissue in humans. AIDS 6:1040-1041
15. McLeod R, Mack D, Foss R, Boyer K, Withers S, Levin S, Hubbell J (1992) Levels of pyrimethamine in sera and cerebrospinal and ventricular fluids from infants treated for congenital toxoplasmosis. Antimicrob Ag Chemother 36:1040-1048

16. Trenque T, Marx C, Quereux C, Leroux B, Dupouy D, Dorangeon PH, Choisy H, Pinon JM (1998) Human maternofoetal distribution of pyrimethamine-sulphadoxine. Br J Clin Pharmacol 45:179-180

17. Schoondermark-Van De Ven E, Galama J, Vree T, Camps W, Baars I, Eskes T, Meuwissen J, Melchers W (1995) Study of treatment of congenital *Toxoplasma gondii* infection in rhesus monkeys with pyrimethamine and sulfadiazine. Antimicrob Ag Chemother 39: 137-144

18. Harris C, Salgo MP, Tanowitz HB, Wittner M (1988) In vitro assessment of antimicrobial agents on *Toxoplasma gondii*. J Infect Dis 157:14-22

19. Mack DG, Mc Leod R (1984) New micromethod to study the effect of antimicrobial agents on *Toxoplasma gondii*: comparison of sulfadoxine and sulfadiazine individually or in combination with pyrimethamine and the study of clindamycin, metronidazole and cyclosporin A. Antimicrob Ag Chemother 26:26-30

20. Grossman PL, Remington JS (1979) The effect of trimethoprim and sulfamethoxazole on *Toxoplasma gondii* in vitro and in vivo. Am J Trop Med Hyg 28: 445-455

21. Vischer WA (1973) Comparative study of the efficacy of some sulfanilamide derivatives in clinical use against acute toxoplasmosis in the mouse. Zbl Bakt Hyg I Abt Orig A223:398-40

22. Andreasen F, Elsbourg L, Husted S, Thomsen O (1978) Pharmacokinetics of sulfadiazine and trimethoprim in man. Europ J Clin Pharmacol 14:57-67

23. Pohjanpelto PEJ, Sarmela TJ, Raines T (1974) Penetration of trimethoprim and sulphamethoxazole into the aqueous humor. Brit J Ophthal 58:606-608

24. Salmon JD, Fowle ASE, Bye A (1975) Concentrations of trimethoprim and sulphamethoxazole in aqueous humor and plasma from regimens of co-trimoxazole in man. J Antimicrob Chemother 1:205-211

25. Prokopczyk J, Raczynski A, Troszynski M, Wankowicz B, Wenzel E (1979) Sulfame-thoxazole concentration in the homogenate of the human embryo. Probl Med Wieku Rozwoj 9:132-133

26. Reid DW, Caille G, Kaufmann NR (1975) Maternal and transplacental kinetics of trimethoprim and sulfamethoxazole, separately and in combination. Can Med Assoc J 112:67-72

27. Brun-Pascaud M, Chau F, Garry L, Jacobus D, Derouin F, Girard PM (1996) Combination of PS-15, epriprim, or pyrimethamine with dapsone in prophylaxis of *Toxoplasma gondii* and *Pneumocystis carinii* dual infection in a rat model. Antimicrob Ag Chemother 40:2067-2070

28. Martinez A, Allegra CJ, Kovacs JA (1996) Efficacy of epriprim (Ro11-8958). A new dihydrofolate reductase inhibiteur, in the treatment of acute *Toxoplasma* infection in mice. Am J Trop Med Hyg 54:249-252

29. Allegra CJ, Boarman D, Kovacs JA, Morrison P, Beaver J, Chabner BA, Massur H (1990) Interaction of sulfonamide and sulfone compounds with *Toxoplasma gondii* dihydropteroate synthase. J Clin Invest 85:371-379

30. Derouin F, Piketty C, Chastang C, Chau F, Rouveix B, Pocidalo JJ (1991) Anti-*Toxoplasma* effects of dapsone alone and combined with pyrimethamine. Antimicrob Ag Chemother 35:252-255

31. Leport C, Raffi F, Matheron S, Katlama C, Regnier B, Saimot AG, Marche C, Vedrenne C, Vildé JL. (1988) Treatment of central nervous system toxoplasmosis with pyrimethamine/sulfadiazine combination in 35 patients with the acquired immunodeficiency syndrome. Am J Med 84:94-100

32. Nguyen BT, Stadtsbaeder S (1983) Comparative effects of cotrimoxazole (trimethoprim-sulfamethoxazole), pyrimethamine-sulfadiazine and spiramycin during avirulent infection with *Toxoplasma gondii* (Beverley strain) in mice. Br J Pharmac 79:923-928

33. Garin JP, Paillard B (1984) Toxoplasmose expérimentale de la souris. Activité comparée de : Clindamycine, Midécamycine, Josamycine, Spiramycine, Pyriméthamine-Sulfa-doxine, et Triméthoprime-Sulfaméthoxazole. Ann Pédiat 31:841-845

34. Villena I, Aubert D, Leroux B, Dupouy D, Talmud M, Chelma C, Trenque T, Schmit G, Quereux C, Guenounou M, Pluot M, Bonhomme A, Pinon JM (1998) Pyrimethamine-sulfadoxine treatment of congenital toxoplasmosis: follow-up of 78 cases between 1980 and 1997. Scan J Infect Dis 30:295-300

35. Brun-Pascaud M, Chau F, Garry L, Farinotti R, Derouin F, Girard PM (1996) Altered trimethoprim-sulfamethoxazole ratios for prophylaxis and treatment of *Toxoplasma gondii* and Pneumocystis carinii dual infections in rat model. J Acqu Imm Defic Syndr Hum Retrovir 13:201-207

36. Nguyen BT, Stadtsbaeder (1985) comparative effects of cotrimoxazole (trimethoprim-sulfa-methoxazole) and spiramycin in pregnant mice infected with *Toxoplasma gondii* (Beverley strain). Br J Pharmac 85:713-716

37. Bélanger F, Derouin F, Grangeot-Kéros L, Meyer L and the HEMOCO-SEROCO Group (1999) Incidence and risk factors of toxoplasmosis in a cohort of HIV-infected patients: 1988-1996. Clin Infect Dis 28:575-581

38. Torre D, Casari S, Speranza F, Donisi A, Gregis G, Poggio A, Ranieri S, Orani A, Angarano G, Chiodo F, Fiori G, Carosi G (1998) Randomized trial of trimethoprim-sulfamethoxazole versus pyrimethamine-sulfadiazine for therapy of toxoplasmic encephalitis in patients with AIDS. Antimicrob Ag Chemother 42:1346-1349

39. Torre D, Speranza F, Martegani R, Zeroli C, Banfi M, Airoldi M (1998) A retrospective study of treatment of cerebral toxoplasmosis in AIDS patients with trimethoprim-sulphamethoxazole. J Infect 37:15-18
40. Jacqz-Aigrain E. (personal communication)
41. Chang HR, Arsenisevic D, Comte R, Polak AM, Then RL, Pechère JC (1994) Activity of epiroprim (Ro-11-8958), a dihydrofolate reductase inhibitor, alone and in combination with dapsone against *Toxoplasma gondii*. Antimicrob Ag Chemother 38:1803-1807
42. Derouin F, Nalpas J, Chastang C (1988) Mesure in vitro de l'effet inhibiteur de macrolides lincosamides et synergestines sur la croissance de *Toxoplasma gondii*. Path Biol 36:1204-1210
43. Derouin F, Chastang C (1990) Activity in vitro against *Toxoplasma gondii* of azithromycin and clarithromycin alone and with pyrimethamine. J Antimicrob Chemother 25: 708-711
44. Blais J, Garneau V, Chamberland S (1993) Inhibition of *Toxoplasma gondii* synthesis by azithromycin. Antimicrob Ag Chemother 37:1701-1703
45. Blais J, Tardif C, Chamberland S (1993) Effect of clindamycin on intracellular replication, protein synthesis, and infectivity of *Toxoplasma gondii*. Antimicrob Ag Chemother 37:2571-2577
46. Fichera ME, Roos DS (1997) A plastid organelle as a drug target in apicomplexan parasites. Nature 390:407-409
47. Soldati D (1999) The apicoplast as a potential therapeutic target in *Toxoplasma* and other apicomplexan parasites. Parasitol Tod 15:57
48. Araujo FG, Shepard RM, Remington JS (1991) In vivo activity of the macrolide antibiotics azithromycin, roxithromycin and spiramycin against *Toxoplasma gondii*. Eur J Clin Microbiol Infect Dis 10:519-524
49. Forestier F, Daffos F, Rainault M, Desnottes, Gaschard JC (1987) Suivi thérapeutique foetomaternel de la spiramycine en cours de grossesse. Arch Fr Pediatr 44:539-544
50. Schoondermark-Van De Ven E, Galama EJ, Camps W, Vree T, Russel F, Meuwissen J, Melchers W (1994) Pharmacokinetics of spiramycin in the rhesus monkeys : transplacental passage and distribution in tissue in the fetus. Antimicrob Ag Chemother 38:1922-1929
51. Schoondermark-Van De Ven E, Melchers W, Camps W, Eskes T, Meuwissen J, Galama J (1994) Effectiveness of spiramycin for the treatment of congenital *Toxoplasma gondii* infection in rhesus monkeys. Antimicrob Ag Chemother 38:1930-1936
52. Bergogne-Berezin E (1995) Azithromycine: pharmacologie tissulaire. Path Biol 43: 498-504
53. Girard AE, Girard D, English AR, Gootz TD, Cimochowski CR, Faiella JA, Haskell SL, Retsema JA (1987) Pharmacokinetic and in vivo studies with azithromycin (CP-62,993), a new macrolide with an extended half-life and excellent tissue distribution. Antimicrob Ag Chemother 31:1948-1954
54. Jaruratanasirikul S, Hortiwakul R, Tantisarasart T, Phuenpathom N, Tussanasunthorn-wrong S (1996) Distribution of azithromycin into brain tissue, cerebrospinal fluid, and aqueous humor of the eye. Antimicrob Ag Chemother 40:825-826
55. Tabbara KF, Al-Kharashi SA, Al-Mansouri SM, Al-Omar OM, Cooper H, El-Asrar AM, Foulds G (1998) Ocular levels of azithromycin. Arch Ophthalmol 116:1625-1628
56. Stray-Pedersern B (1996) Azithromycin levels in placental tissue amniotic fluid and blood. 36th Interscience Conference on antimicrobial Agents and Chemotherapy, New orleans, Sept. 15-18th abstract A 68
57. Stadnicki SW, Kessedjian MJ, Stadler J, Tachibana M (1996) Preclinical reproductive and teratology studies with azithromycin. Pharmacom 51:85-95
58. Dumas JL, Chang HR, Mermillod B, Piguet PF, Comte R, Pechere JC (1994) Evaluation of the efficacy of prolonged administration of azithromycin in a murine model of chronic toxoplasmosis. J Antimicrob Chemother 34:111-118
59. Araujo FG, Guptill DR, Remington JS (1988) Azithromycin, a macrolide antibiotic with potent activity against *Toxoplasma gondii*. Antimicrob Ag Chemother 32:755-757
60. Derouin F, Almadany R, Chau F, Rouveix B, Pocidalo JJ (1992) Synergistic activity of azithromycin and pyrimethamine or sulfadiazine in acute experimental toxoplasmosis. Antimicrob Ag Chemother 36:997-1001
61. Araujo FG, Prokocimer P, Lin T, Remington JS (1992) Activity of clarithromycin alone or in combination with other drugs for treatment of murine toxoplasmosis. Antimicrob Ag Chemother 36:2454-2457
62. Derouin F, Caroff B, Chau F, Prokocimer, Pocidalo JJ (1992) Synergistic activity of clarithromycin and minocycline in an animal model of acute experimental toxoplasmosis. Antimicrob Ag Chemother 36:2852-2855
63. Al-Sibai MB, Alkaff AS, Raines D, Alyazigi A (1998) Ocular penetration of oral clarithromycin in humans. J Ocul Pharmacol Therap 14:575-583
64. Brun-Pascaud M, Chau F, Derouin F, Girard PM (1994) Experimental evaluation of combined prophylaxis against murine pneumocystosis and toxoplasmosis. J Infect Dis 170:653-658
65. Chang HR, Pechere JCF (1987) Effect of roxithromycin on acute toxoplasmosis in mice. Antimicrob Ag Chemother 31:1147-1149

66. Romand S, Bryskier A, Moutot M, Derouin F (1995) In vitro and in vivo activities of roxithromycin in combination with pyrimethamine or sulphadiazine against *Toxoplasma gondii*. J Antimicrob Chemother 35:821-832
67. Lassman HB, Puri SK, Ho I, Sabo R, Mezzino MJ (1988) Pharmacokinetics of roxithromycin (RU 965). J. Clin Pharmacol 28:141-152
68. Manuel C, Dellamonica P, Rosset MJ, Safran C, Pirot D, Audegond L (1988) Penetration of roxithromycin into brain tissue. 28th Interscience Conference on antimicrobial Agents and Chemotherapy, Los Angeles, 1988, abstract 1224
69. Pfefferkorn ER, Nothnagel RF, Borotz SE (1992) Parasiticidal effect of clindamycin on *Toxoplasma gondii* grown in cultured cells and selection of a drug-resistant mutant. Antimicrob Ag Chemother 36:1091-1096
70. Fichera ME, Bhopale MK, Roos DS (1995) In vitro assays elucidate peculiar kinetics of clindamycin action against *Toxoplasma gondii*. Antimicrob Ag Chemother 39:1530-1537
71. Tabbara KF, Nozik RA, O'Connor GR (1974) Clindamycin effects on experimental ocular toxoplasmosis in the rabbit. Arch Ophth 92:244-247
72. Gatti G, Malena M, Casazza R, Borin M, Bassetti M, Cruciani M (1998) Penetration of clindamycin and its metabolite N-demethylclindamycin into cerebrospinal fluid following intravenous infusion of clindamycin phosphate in patients with AIDS. Antimicrob Ag Chemother 42:3014-3017
73. Weinstein AJ, Gibbs RS, Gallagher M (1976) Placental transfer of clindamycin and gentamicin in term pregnancy. Am J Obstet Gynecol 124:688-691
74. Philipson A, Sabath LD, Charles D (1973) Transplacental passage of erythromycin and clindamycin. N Engl J Med 288:1219-1221
75. Araujo FG, Khan AA, Slifer TL, Bryskier A, Remington JS (1997) The ketolide antibiotics HMR 3647 and HMR 3004 are active against *Toxoplasma gondii* in vitro and in murine models of infection. Antimicrob Ag Chemother 41:2137-2140
76. Cantin L, Chamberlands S (1993) In vitro evaluation of the activities of Azithromycin alone and combined with Pyrimethamine against *Toxoplasma gondii*. Antimicrob Ag Chemother 37:1993-1996
77. Araujo FG, Khan AA, Bryskier A, Remington JS (1998) Use of ketolides in combination with other drugs to treat experimental toxoplasmosis. J Antimicrob Chemother 42:665-667
78. Chang HR, Comte R, Pechère JC (1990) In vitro and in vivo activity of doxycycline against *Toxoplasma gondii*. Antimicrob Ag Chemother 34:775-780
79. Macdonald H, Kelly RG, Allen ES, Noble JF, Kanegis LA (1973) Pharmacokinetic studies on minocycline in man. Clin Pharmacol 14:852-861
80. Rollins DF, Tabbara KF, Ghosheh R, Nokik RA (1982) Minocycline in experimental ocular toxoplasmosis in the rabbit. Am J Ophth 93:361-365
81. Araujo FG, Slifer T, Remington JS (1994) Rifabutin is active in murine models of toxoplasmosis. Antimicrob Ag Chemother 38:570-575
82. Araujo FG, Khan AA, Remington JS (1996) Rifapentin is active in vitro and in vivo against *Toxoplasma gondii*. Antimicrob Ag Chemother 40:1335-1337
83. Romand S, Della Bruna C, Farinotti R, Derouin F (1996) In vitro and in vivo effects of rifabutin alone or combined with atovaquone against *Toxoplasma gondii*. Antimicrob Ag Chemother 40:2015-2020
84. Araujo FG, Suzuki Y, Remington JS (1996) Use of rifabutin in combination with atovaquone, clindamycin, pyrimethamine, or sulfadiazine for treatment of toxoplasmic encephalitis in mice. Eur J Clin Microbiol Infect Dis 15:394-397
85. Khan AA, Slifer T, Araujo FG, Remington JS (1996) Trovafloxacin is active against *Toxoplasma gondii*. Antimicrob Ag Chemother 40:1855-1859
86. Khan AA, Slifer T, Araujo FG, Polzer RJ, Remington JS (1997) Activity of trovafloxacin in combination with other drugs for treatment of acute murine toxoplasmosis. Antimicrob Ag Chemother 41:893-897
87. Loebstein R, Addis A, Ho E, Andreou R, Sage S, Donnenfeld AE, Schick B, Bonati M, Moretti M, Lalkin A, Pastuzak A, Koren G (1998) Pregnancy outcome following gestational exposure to fluoroquinolones: a multicenter prospective controlled study. Antimicrob Ag Chemother 42:1336-1339
88. Hudson AT (1993) Atovaquone - A novel broad-spectrum anti-infective drug. Parasitol Tod 9:66-68
89. Araujo FG, Huskinson J, Remington JS (1991) Remarkable in vitro and in vivo activities of the hydroxynaphthoquinone 566C80 against tachyzoites and tissue cysts of *Toxoplasma gondii*. Antimicrob Ag Chemother 35:293-299
90. Araujo FG, Huskinson-Mark J, Gutterigde WE, Remington JS (1992) In vitro and in vivo activities of the hydroxynaphthoquinone 566C80 against the cyst form of *Toxoplasma gondii*. Antimicrob Ag Chemother 36:326-330
91. Romand S, Pudney M, Derouin F (1993) In vitro and in vivo activities of the hydroxynaphthoquinone atovaquone alone or combined with pyrimethamine, sulfadiazine, clarithromycin, or minocycline against *Toxoplasma gondii*. Antimicrobial Age Chemother 37:2371-2378

92. Gormley PD, Pavesio CE, Minnasian D, Lightman S (1998) Effects of drug therapy on *Toxoplasma* cysts in an animal model of acute and chronic disease. Invest Ophthalmol Vis Sci 39:1171-1175

93. Sordet F, Aumjaud Y, Fessi H, Derouin F (1998) Assessment of the activity of atovaquone-loaded nanocapsules in the treatment of acute and chronic murine toxoplasmosis. Parasite 5:223-229

94. Ferguson DJP, Huskinson-Mark J, Araujo FG, Remington JS (1994) An ultrastructural study of the effect of treatment with atovaquone in brains of mice chronically infected with the ME49 strain of *Toxoplasma gondii*. Int J Exp Path 75:111-116

95. Araujo F, Lin T, Remington JS (1993) The activity of atovaquone (566C809) in murine toxoplasmosis is markedly augmented when used in combination with pyrimethamine or sulfadiazine. J Infect Dis 167:494-497

96. Torres RA, Weinberg W, Stansell, Leoung G, Kovacs J, Rogers M, Scott J and the Atovaquone/Toxoplasmic Encephalitis Study Group (1997) Atovaquone for salvage treatment and suppression of toxoplasmic encephalitis in patients with AIDS. Clin Infect Dis 24:422-429

97. Freeman CD, Klutman NE, Lamp KC, Dall LH, Strayer AH (1998) Relative bioavailability of atovaquone suspension when administered with an enteral nutrition supplement. Ann Pharmacother 32:1004-1007

98. Hugues W, Dorenbaum A, Yogev R, Beauchamps B, Xu J, McNamara J, Moye J, Purdue L, Van Dyke R, Rogers M, Sadler B (1998) Phase I safety and pharmacokinetics study of micronized atovaquone in human immunodeficiency virus-infected infants and children. Antimicrob Ag Chemother 42:1315-1318

99. Holfels E, McAuley J, Mack D, Milhous WK, McLeod R (1994) In vitro effects of artemisinin ether, cycloguanyl hydrochloride (alone and in combination with sulfadiazine), quinine sulfate, mefloquine, primaquine phosphate, trifluoperazine hydrochloride, and verapamil on *Toxoplasma gondii*. Antimicrob Ag Chemother 38:1392-1396

100. Yang KE, Krug EC, Berens RL (1990) Inhibition of growth of *Toxoplasma gondii* by Qinghaosu and derivative. Antimicrob Ag Chemother 34:1961-1965

101. Chang HR, Pechère JC (1988) Arteether, a qinghaosu derivative in toxoplasmosis Trans Roy Soc Trop Med Hyg 82:867

102. Brewer TG, Grate SJ, Peggins JO, Weina PJ, Petras JM, Levine BS, Heiffer MH, Schuster BG (1994) Fatal neurotoxicity of arteether and artemether. Am J Trop Med Hyg 51:251-259

103. Sarciron ME, Lawton P, Saccharin C, Petavy AF, Peyron F (1997) Effects of 2', 3'-dideoxynosine on *Toxoplasma gondii* cysts in mice. Antimicrob Ag Chemother 41:1531-1536

104. Sarciron ME, Lawton P, Petavy AF, Peyron F (1998) Alterations of *Toxoplasma gondii* induced by 2', 3'-dideoxyinosine in vitro. J Parasitol 84:1055-1059

105. Gangjee A, Elzein E, Queener SF, McGuire JJ (1998) Synthesis and biological activities of tricyclic conformationally restricted tetrahydropyrido annulated furo (2,3-d) pyrimidines as inhibitors of dihydrofolate reductases. J Med Chem 41:1409-1416

106. Gutteridge WE (1997) Designer drugs: pipe-dreams or realities. Parasitology, 114:S145-S151

107. Gozalbes R, Galvez J, Garcia-Domenech R, Derouin F (1999) Molecular search of new active drugs against *Toxoplasma gondii*. SAR and QSAR Environ. Res. 10:47-60

108. Waller RF, Keeling PJ, Donald RGK, Striepen B, Handman E, Lang-Unnasch N, Cowman AF, Besra GS, Roos DS (1998) Nuclear-encoded proteins target to the plastid in *Toxoplasma gondii* and *Plasmodium falciparum*. Proc Natl Acad Sci 95:12352-12357

109. Roberts F, Roberts CW, Johnson JJ, Kyle DE, Krell T, Coggins JR, Coombs GH, Milhous WK, Tzipori S, Ferguson DJP, Chakrabarti D, McLeod R (1998) Evidence for the shikimate pathway in apicomplexa parasites. Nature 393:801-805

110. Estes R, Vogel N, Mack D, McLeod R (1998) Paclitaxel arrests growth of intracellular *Toxoplasma gondii*. Antimicrob Ag Chemother 42:2036-2040

111. Stokkermans TJK, Schwartzman JD, Keenan K, Morrissette NS, Tilney LG, Roos DS (1996) Inhibition of *Toxoplasma gondii* replication by dinitroaniline herbicides. Exp Parasitol 84:355-370

2.1. Clinical aspects of infection during pregnancy

F. JACQUEMARD

Infection in the Pregnant Woman

Primary infection acquired during pregnancy is asymptomatic in about 60% of cases [1]. When present, signs and symptoms are often so slight that they escape the memory of the majority of patients. The most commonly recognized clinical manifestations are mild and non-specific: fatigue, malaise, low grade fever, myalgia and lymphadenopathy. Lymphadenopathy may be localized (the most characteristic sign is a single lymph node enlargement of the posterior cervical region), or it may involve multiple areas (cervical, suboccipital, supraclavicular, axillary and inguinal), including retroperitoneal and mesenteric nodes. Lymphadenopathy can be tender for a few days and is unattached to overlying skin; in some patients it may persist for as long as 6 months but without tendency towards suppuration.

Some other signs are less common: hepatitis, exanthem, polymyositis, dermatomyositis and chorioretinitis have been observed in immunocompetent persons [2].

When enlarged nodes are present, concomittant serological results usually suggest a recent infection: tests for specific IgG and IgM are positive. When the patient is sampled too early after the onset of the lymphadenopathy, the tests can be negative. The diagnosis of recent toxoplasmosis must not be excluded and the study of a later sample, 10 or 15 days after the previous one, should confirm the diagnosis.

Finally, because of their low frequency and their lack of specificity clinical features of acquired infections are not useful for diagnosis but for dating. When the serology of a pregnant woman suggests a recent infection, it is of special interest to search symptoms by retrospective questioning about the time of their onset, which may be a reliable indication of the time of infection. Identification of all primary infections occuring in a given population of pregnant women requires consequently a systematic serological screening.

Clinical manifestations of fetal infection

The infection of the placenta is a prerequisite for congenital transmission. The placenta is infected during the maternal parasitaemic phase which results almost exclusively from a primary infection acquired after conception and very rarely from a reactivation of an infection prior to pregnancy. Then the placenta acts as a source of parasites which are transmitted to the fetus almost immediately after maternal infection, or with a delay of several weeks or longer [2].

Incidence

Table 1. Different clinical forms at birth of 133 infected neonates (most of them diagnosed during pregnancy), according to the date of maternal infection. The majority of neonates suffer from subclinical or mild infection. This is the result of prenatal diagnosis, prenatal treatment of infected foetuses, identification of the most severe forms and eventually medical abortion according to the French law

Date of maternal infection *	N°	Clinical forms							
		Subclinical		Mild		Severe densities		Intracranial	
		N°	%	N°	%	N°	%	N°	%
< 6	1	1	-	-	-	-	-	-	-
6-16	16	10	62,5	6	37,5	-		4	25
17-23	60	37	61,7	23	38,3	-		21	35
24-36	56	40	71,4	15	26,8	1		12	21
all weeks	133	88	66,3	44	33	1	0,7	37	27,8

* weeks of amenorrhea

Clinical aspects during pregnancy

The severity of infection in the fetus depends on the gestational age at the time of transmission of parasites and the manifestations vary according to both following patterns:

1) if transplacental transmission occurs early, that is if the mother has acquired infection early, and if there has been a short delay before the parasites spread from the placenta to the fetus, a progressive disease will occur. This may result in fetal death *in utero* and spontaneous abortion, or in delivery of a live child with signs of central nervous system involvement including hydrocephalus, meningoencephalitis, intracranial calcifications and chorioretinitis. Signs of generalized infection may also be present including hepatosplenomegaly, jaundice, rash, anemia and thrombocytopenia, myocarditis, pericarditis, pleural effusion.

2) If transmission to the foetus occurs later, either because of late acquisition of infection by the mother or because of delayed spreading of parasites

from the placenta to the foetus, the congenital infection will be sublicinal at birth but may evolve months or years after birth and results in eye lesions (chorioretinitis whose prognosis depends of the involvement of the macular area). Some neonates can also present very high protein content in the cerebrospinal fuid.

Early pregnancy maternal infection is rarely transmitted, but it results in severe fetal infection; inversely, late maternal infection is frequently transmitted but it generally results in mild or sublinical fetal infection. As a consequence, approximately 85% of live infants with congenital infection appear normal at birth [2].

Consequences of fetal infection can be evaluated by ultrasound examinations repeatedly performed during pregnancy. In the largest series of 148 fetal infections diagnosed among 2030 infected mothers, Daffos et al [3] reported the following frequencies of ultrasound findings according to the time of maternal infection:

– before 16 weeks: 31/52 fetuses (60%) and 48% had cerebral ventricular dilatation;

– maternal infection between 17 and 23 weeks: 16/63 foetuses (25%) and 12% had cerebral ventricular dilatation but no case was identified among mothers with seroconversion after the 22nd week;

– after 24 weeks: 1/33 fetuses without ventricular dilatation.

The most characteristic alteration is the extensive necrosis of the brain parenchyma because of vascular involment by lesions [2]. Necrotic brain tissue may later calcify and become visible on ultrasound. According to our experience, brain necrosis lesions are always found when infection has been contracted by the mother during the ten first weeks of gestation and has been transmitted to the fetus. Hydrocephalus is characteristically due to peri-acqueductal involment.

Obstruction of the acqueduct of Sylvius leads to the rapid enlargement of the third and lateral ventricules, usually progressive during a short period (one or two weeks). Obstruction of the forarnen of Monro can lead to unilateral hydrocephalus.

Ultrasonographic evidence of this necrosis can be delayed in the second part of pregnancy, sometimes to the end of pregnancy, if at the beginning there was no brain necrosis around the acqueduct of Sylvius.

In a series of 33 cases of medical termination of pregnancy published in 1989 [4], findings at the fetal autopsy were as follows:

Table 2. Results of fetal autopsy according to the term of maternal infection (weeks of amenorrhea)

	Periconceptional n = 2	6-16 S n = 22	17-20 S n = 9
Brain necrosis	2	22	9
Hydrocephalus	2	12	5
Ascitis	-	4	1
Splenomegaly	-	3	1

Ultrasonographic signs

Brain abnormalities are the most common signs which can be seen in case of symptomatic fetal infection, especially when infection has occured during the first half of pregnancy. Repetition of ultrasound scans is mandatory during pregnancy. When the result of prenatal diagnosis has been proved to be negative, the risk of delayed transplacental passage is low but ultrasound scan must be performed each month, to look for the appearance of slight signs of fetal infection. When these signs are present, repetition of amniocentesis should be discussed. When the fetus is infected, ultrasound scans must be performed every two weeks.

Cerebral ventricular dilatation, usually bilateral and symmetrical, is the most common and characteristic sign; it occurs first in the occipital region before involving the entire lateral ventricles. Its evolution may be very rapid over a period of a few days and it is associated with a poor prognosis. Cerebral ventricular dilatations can be present at the time of prenatal diagnosis or appear shortly thereafter in case of infections of the first half of pregnancy and then repetitive and careful ultrasound examinations must be performed even if the ultrasound scan show no evidence of abnormality at the date of amniocentesis (Figs. 1-4). The absence of cerebral ventricular dilatation is not always a good prognosis factor, as major brain lesions can be seen without involment of the acqueduct of Sylvius region.

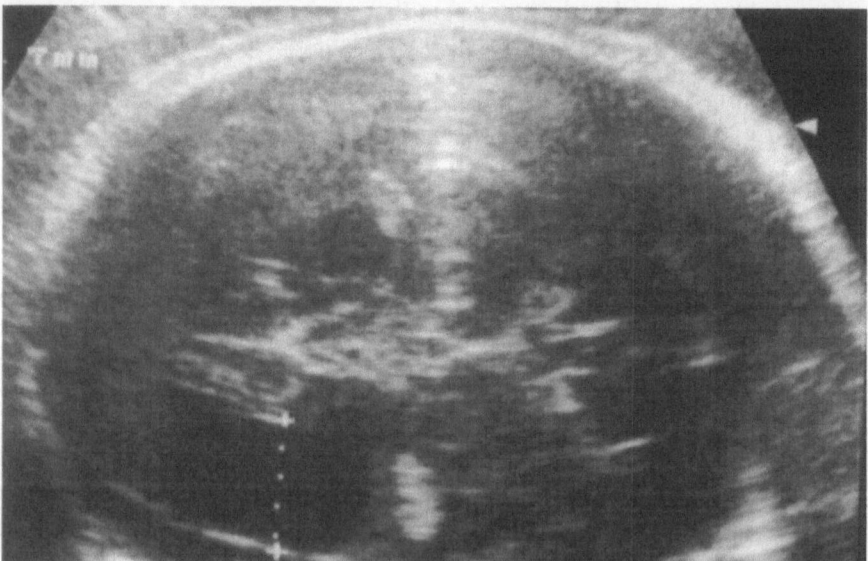

Fig. 1. Cerebral ventricular dilatation at 26 weeks of gestation. Transabdominal ultrasound with axial plane. Maternal infection between 15 and 20 weeks of gestation. Amniocentesis at 22 weeks of gestation: positive. For *Toxoplasma* Ultrasound examination without any abnormality. Appearance at 26 weeks of gestation of mild hydrocephalus

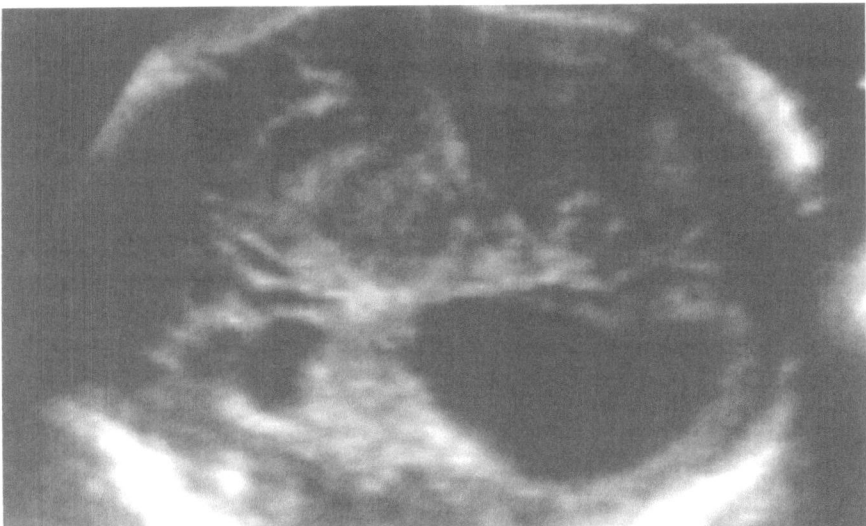

Fig. 2. Cerebral ventricular dilatation at 32 weeks of gestation. Transabdominal ultrasound with axial plane. Maternal infection between 12 and 18 weeks of gestation. Amniocentesis at 24 weeks of gestation: positive. Ultrasound examination without any abnormality. Maternal treatment with pyrimethamine and sulfadiazine. Appearance at 30 weeks of gestation of mild hydrocephalus with rapid evolution

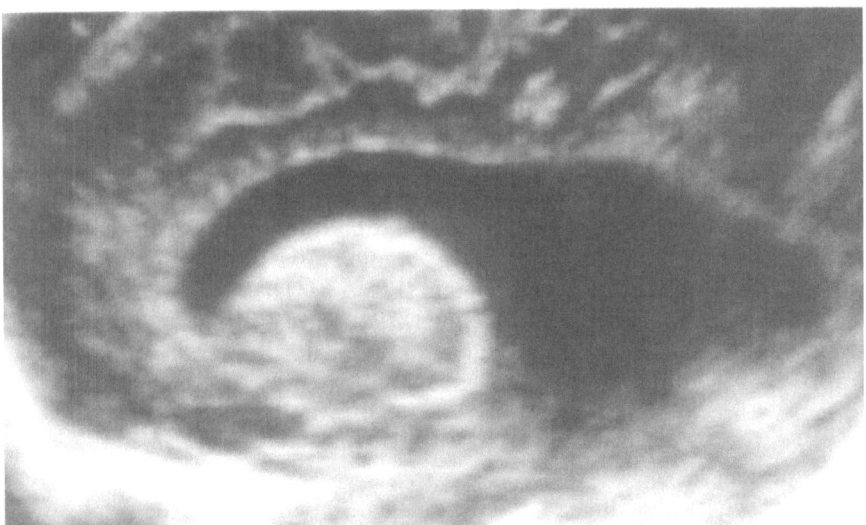

Fig. 3. Hydrocephalus at 32 weeks of gestation. Transvaginal ultrasound with trans-fontanellar sagittal plane. Maternal infection between 12 and 16 weeks of gestation. Amniocentesis at 22 weeks of gestation: negative. Ultrasound examination without any abnormality. Appearance at 32 weeks of gestation of multiple intracranial densities and mild hydrocephalus . Second amniocentesis: positive

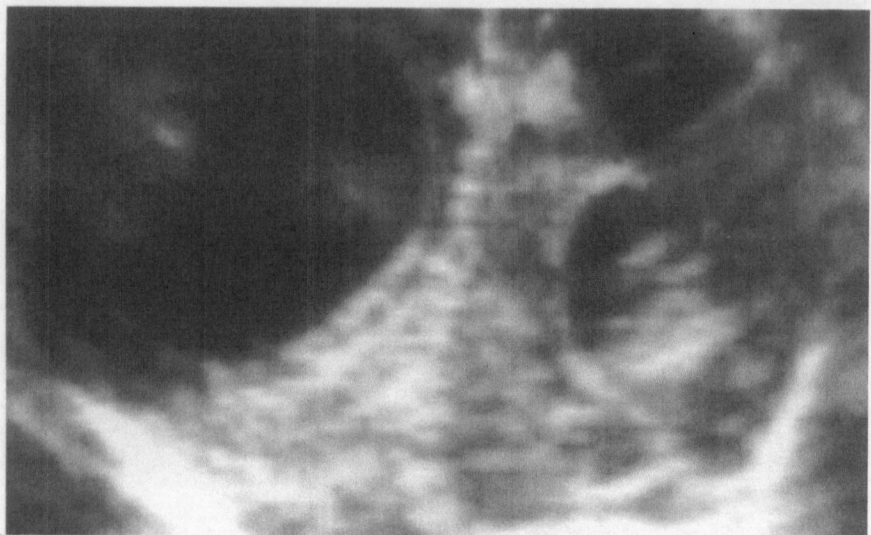

Fig. 4. Hydrocephalus at 32 weeks of gestation. Transvaginal ultrasound with trans-fonta-nellar coronal plane. Same fetus as previous (asymmetric cerebral ventricular dilatation)

Intracranial densities (i.d.) correspond to intracranial calcifications obser-ved after birth; they are often poorly calcified at the time of prenatal diagno-sis and less frequently observed than ventricular dilatation [4, 5]. There is usually a discrepancy between the number of i.d. that can be observed during the pregnancy and after birth, probably because the ultrasound identification of these densities is difficult. Ultrasound examination of the fetal brain must be systematically done not only in the axial plane but also in the coronal, sagittal and parasagittal (oblique) planes through the anterior fotnanelle, which can be accessed and subsequently used as an acoustic window. If the fetus is in a vertex presentation, imaging the fetal brain with high frequency transvaginal probes results in high-quality images. Improvement of the qua-lity of the ultrasound probes and standardization of the planes and sections lead to more accurate diagnosis of intracranial densities during pregnancy and offer comparable images as those obtained after birth by high frequency probes through the anterior fontanelle. (Fig. 5-8). These densities cannot be seen with magnetic resonance imaging (MRI). After birth, computed tomop-graphy (CT) allows accurate neuroanatomic localization and count of intra-cranial calcifications.

Hyperechogenic fetal bowel is also an ultrasonographic marker of fetal infection (toxoplasmosis as well as CMV). This sign can be encountered in two situations:

– evidence at the time of amniocentesis of hyperechogenic fetal bowel leads to the practice of prenatal diagnosis not only for toxoplasmosis but also CMV fetal infection, cystic fibrosis, fetal karyotyping, and amniotic digestive enzyme assays;

– appearance during the follow-up of a presumed non-infected fetus (pre-natal diagnosis already performed and negative) of hyperechogenic bowel:

this situation can be a marker of fetal infection and a second amniocentesis should be discussed.

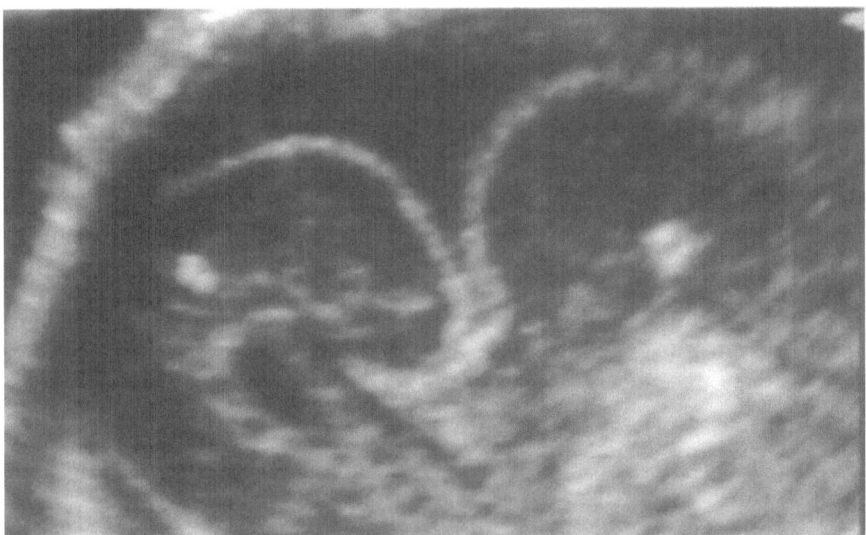

Fig. 5. Intracranial densities at 26 weeks of gestation. Transvaginal ultrasound with transfontanellar oblique plane (parasagittal). Maternal infection between 14 and 18 weeks of gestation. Amniocentesis at 23 weeks of gestation: diagnosis of fetal infection. Ultrasound examination without any abnormality. Appearance at 26 weeks of gestation of multiple intracranial densities

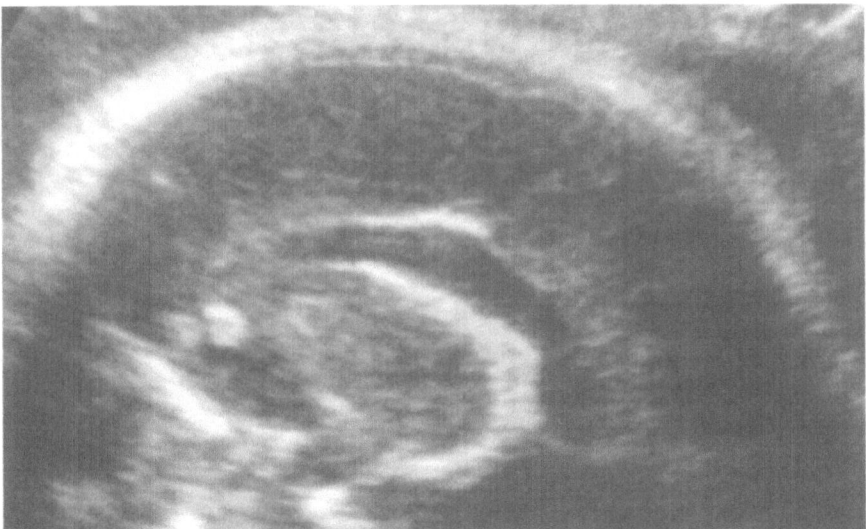

Fig. 6. Intracranial densities at 32 weeks of gestation. Transvaginal ultrasound with transfontanellar sagittal plane. Maternal infection between 12 and 16 weeks of gestation. Amniocentesis at 22 weeks of gestation: negative. Ultrasound examination without any abnormality. Appearance at 32 weeks of gestation of multiple intracranial densities and mild hydrocephalus. Second amniocentesis: positive

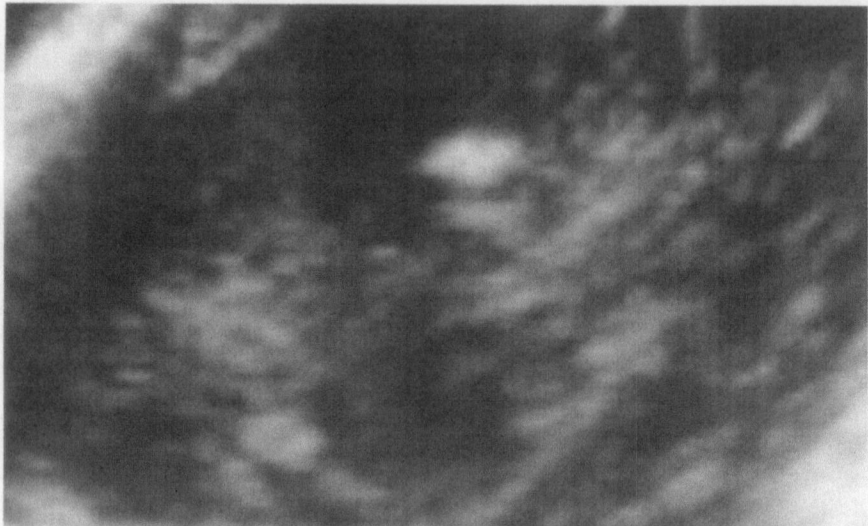

Fig. 7. Intracranial densities at 32 weeks of gestation. Transvaginal ultrasound with trans-fontanellar oblique plane (same foetus as previous)

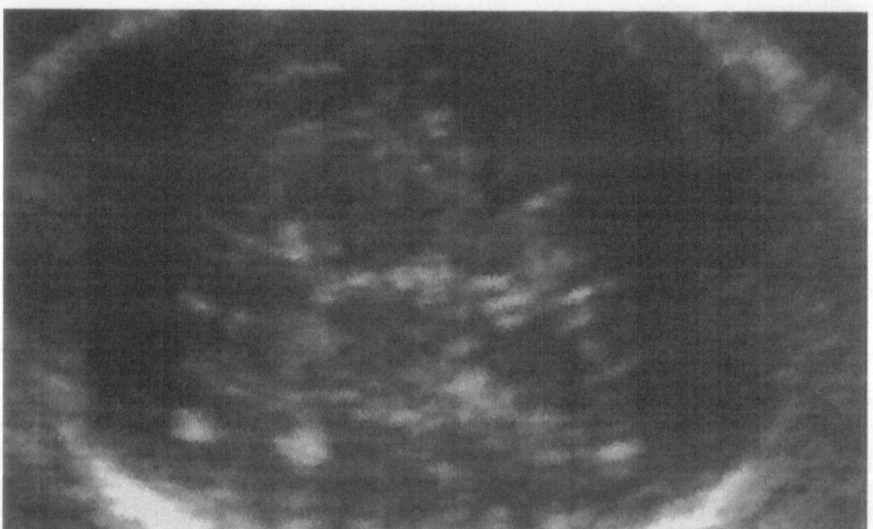

Fig. 8. Intracranial densities at 31 weeks of gestation. Transabdominal ultrasound with axial plane. Maternal infection between 13 and 22 weeks of gestation. Amniocentesis at 26 weeks of gestation: positive. Maternal treatment with pyrimethamine and sulfadiazine. Ultrasound examination without any abnormality at this moment. Appearance at 31 weeks of gestation of multiple intracranial densities

Other ultrasonographic signs correspond to placental inflammation, hepatic involvement and effusions, showing that fetal toxoplasmosis is a multisystemic disease. Some of them may be transient.

Placenta is often enlarged with a "frosted glass" aspect. Enlargement of the liver and liver densities are often observed when the fetus presents liver enzyme elevation on fetal blood sampling (when it was performed previously for prenatal diagnosis). Ascitis, pleural effusion, pericardic effusion must also be searched for.

Ultrasound monitoring is not sufficient for a definite diagnosis of fetal infection because signs are not pathognomonic of *Toxoplasma* infection. Their appearance can be observed later regarding the date of transmission and above all, most infected fetuses (those infected in the second half of pregnancy) are not severely damaged and cannot be identified.

Forming a prognosis

Most of the fetuses infected during the ten first weeks of pregnancy have a poor neurological prognosis due to the presence of hydrocephalus and brain necrosis. Ocular lesions are usually associated. Few of these fetuses can have a good prognosis after treatment with pyrimethamine and sulfadiazine but in most of the cases, early fetal infection leads to the appearance (sometimes late during the course of pregnancy) of hydrocephalus. Fifty per cent of the fetuses infected before 16 weeks will develop hydrocephalus, and the prognosis remains uncertain for the others. When the pregnancy continues, careful examinations of the fetal brain must be performed frequently, and the parents must know that the neurological prognosis, and moreover the ocular prognosis, remain uncertain. The prognosis of intracranial densities is difficult to establish during pregnancy. The presence of few intracranial calcifications seems not correlated with neurological sequelae although the responsibility for convulsive seizures during childhood and adolescence has been discussed, whithout certainty. When there are many intracranial densities involving all the parts of the brain, the neurological prognosis is more difficult to establish, but possibly poor, especially in case of intection during the first half of pregnancy. The presence of intracranial densities is well correlated with the presence of chorioretinitis at birth, as shown in Table 3.

Table 3. Correlations between the presence of intracranial densities and chorioretinitis at birth (133 infected neonates)

Intracranial densities	Presence n = 37	Absence n = 96
Associated chorioretinitis	9 24,3%	7 17,3%
No chorioretinitis	28 75,7%	89 92,7%

In utero MRI of the brain can be proposed in case of congenital toxoplasmosis when there is a doubt concerning the brain development. Intracranial densities cannot be demonstrated in this way, but normal development of brain gyri and cell migration can be assessed. We recently observed localised and severe impairment of the gyri after early fetal infection (during the first trimester of pregnancy).

Other ultrasound signs (placenta enlarged, hepatomegaly, splenomegaly) indicate a generalized disease, often associated with neurologic and ocular diseases.

References

1. Daffos F, Forestier F, Capella-Pavlovsky M et al (1988) Prenatal management of 746 pregnancies at risk for toxoplasmosis. N Engl J Med 318:271-275
2. Remington JS, McLeod R, Desmonts G (1995) Toxoplasmosis. *In:* Klein JO, Remington JS (eds). Infections diseases of the fetus and newborn infant. WB Saunders, Philadelphia, pp. 140-267
3. Daffos F, Mirlesse V, Hohlfeld P, Jacquemard F, Thulliez P, Forestier F (1994) Toxoplasmosis in pregnancy. Lancet 344:541
4. Hohlfeld P, Daffos F, Thulliez P, Autrant C, Couvreur J, MacAleese J, Descombey D, Forestier F (1989) Fetal toxoplasmosis: outcome of pregnancy and infant follow-up after *in utero* treatment. J Pediatr 115 (5.1):765-769
5. Hohlfeld P, MacAleese J, Capella-Pavlovsky M et al (1991) Fetal toxoplasmosis: ultrasonographic signs. Ultrasound Obstet Gynecol 1:241-244

2.2. Diagnosis in the pregnant woman

U. GROSS, H. PELLOUX

The pregnant woman

Introduction

In most countries, screening programs for toxoplasmosis during pregnancy do not exist, so far. Reasons for that are economi, discussion of epidemiological importance of prenatal infection and uncertainty of serological interpretations in several cases. However, the existing screening systems in Austria and France indicate that medical advantages arising from such programs seem to justify those additional costs for the healths systems [1, 2].

Serological screening is useful for (i) identification of women at risk in order to prevent later infection by educating them to obey relevant protective behavior and measures, and (ii) for identification of pregnant women with primary infection in order to offer them early therapy. It thus would be desirable if the immune status of a woman is known before or early during pregnancy. Several methods are available which finally allow to diagnose the stage of infection.

Indirect diagnosis

Animal studies indicate that parasitemia is present for only a very limited time following acute infection [3]. Therefore and since the parasite thereafter is predominantely localized within the brain, diagnosis of primary infection during pregnancy has mainly to rely on serological methods to detect *Toxoplasma*-specific antibodies.

Conventional serological methods

The Sabin Feldman dye test (DT) is considered as a reference test and is based on the observation that viable tachyzoites can be stained with alkaline methylene blue, whereas specific antibodies in human sera lyse the parasite in the presence of external complement [4]. The titer is defined as the serum dilution at which half of the parasites are killed by the activation of the complement system through formation of antigen-antibody complexes. When titers are compared with an international standard reference serum, results can be expressed in international units (IU) per milliliter of serum. This test, which detects IgG1, IgG3 and IgM antibodies directed against surface antigens of the parasite, is positive within 7-10 days after infection. Since positive results usually persist at low levels throughout life, monitoring past infections before pregnancy can be achieved by the DT.

Direct Agglutination (DA) of formalin-fixed tachyzoites by IgG antibodies in human serum samples that were treated with mercaptoethanol has been shown to be a useful screening test during pregnancy. However, it has to be noted that early infection can be missed when still only IgM antibodies are present. When differently fixed tachyzoites are used in the differential agglutination test (HS/AC test), diagnosis can be improved since AC antigens detect acute-phase-specific IgG antibodies against *Toxoplasma gondii* [5].

Finally, tests like the ELISA, ISAGA, immunofluorescence assay (IFA) and immunoblot can be used to differentiate between IgG, IgM, IgA, and IgE antibodies against *Toxoplasma gondii* [6-12]. Depending on the assay, care has to be taken to avoid false-positive IgM results, which might occur in sera that contain either antinuclear antibodies or that are positive for the rheumatoid factor [13].

Immunoglobulins

Understanding the kinetics and specificity of antibodies is important for the correct interpretation of test results. However, a great variability in the amount and kinetics of the development of *Toxoplasma gondii*-specific antibodies exists among pregnant women [14]. The immunological variation depends on parasite factors (i. e. parasite strain, parasite stage; cyst versus sporozoite, inoculum size) and the immune competence of the host. In addition, the sensitivity and specificity of a test system largely depends on the parasite antigen that is used for detection of antibodies and on the type of antibody that is looked for. Likewise, when different tests are compared with each other, a great individual variation in the peak amounts of antibodies results [14]. All these factors that contribute to the result of a serological test makes it impossible to give a defined and generalized comment. Therefore, although some general hints are given, one always has to keep in mind that in individual cases the kinetics of antibody rise and decrease varies considerably, and therefore, it is usually impossible to estimate the precise time of infection based on the results that were obtained from a single serum sample. It is mandatory to test at least two sequentially obtained samples in parallel. In order to properly diagnose active infection, these samples should be drawn at least with an interval of 2 weeks. However, especially in those tests which are performed with fourfold dilutions (i.e. DT), acute infection cannot be excluded when titers in these two serum samples do not differ significantly.

IgG. Specific IgG antibodies always develop after primary infection in immunocompetent patients [14]. It has been shown that titers in the dye test usually rise more rapidly – generally within 4 weeks after infection – than those measured in the agglutination test or IFA [13, 15]. However, although the peak of IgG production usually is reached within 4 to 8 weeks, based on the factors listed above, the ranges until the peak is reached has been shown for the dye test to vary between 2 to 21 weeks and for other IgG-specific tests even 4 to 36 weeks [14]. IgG antibodies usually persist lifelong at low levels and thus are useful for monitoring previous infection especially when serum samples are investigated before pregnancy. High avidity of IgG antibodies in contrast to antibodies with low avidity seems to be a useful tool to exclude acute infection [16-19]. However, those serum samples, which demonstrate IgG antibodies of low avidity have to be further investigated in order to confirm acute toxoplasmosis.

IgM. Specific IgM antibodies usually develop rapidly within 1-2 weeks after infection and reach their peak within 1-4 weeks, although the variation in reaching the peak test-dependently varies between 1-18 weeks [14]. Persistence of IgM antibodies for more than 6 months – and sometimes even for years – has been shown by most commercially available ELISA and ISAGA test systems [14, 20]. Although in contrast to ELISA, the IFA has the shortest persistence of positivity in most cases [20], the presence of IgM does not necessarily confirm a very recent infection.

IgA. Specific IgA antibodies usually start to develop a little later than IgM antibodies and reach their peak between 3 to 4 weeks after infection. However, this time period varies considerably among individual pregnant women in a range of 2-21 weeks [14]. Since most IgA-specific tests seem to be less sensitive than IgM tests [14], long persistence does not occur as often as for IgM antibodies and IgA usually disappear between 4 to 7 month [8, 15]. However, one has to note that the absence of IgA does not necessarily exclude recent infection [15].

IgE. Only a few laboratories have included evaluation of specific IgE antibodies by either the ELISA or the ISAGA technique in their program of diagnosis of *Toxoplasma* infection. Although these tests have a limited sensitivity, the presence of specific IgE antibodies may correlate with acute infection [21]. They start to develop earlier than IgA and follow the kinetics of IgM. However, in contrast to these two immunoglobulin classes, specific IgE antibodies seem not to persist for more than 3 to 5 months [9, 22].

Direct diagnosis

As mentioned before, direct diagnosis of acute toxoplasmosis during pregnancy usually is of limited value. In most cases, EDTA blood from the women is analysed for the presence or absence of the parasite, its nucleic acids or its antigen products when the results from serology are uncertain or indicate acute infection. For direct diagnosis from amniotic fluid please refer to Chapter 2.2. Although inoculation of clinical specimen in cell cultures or mice (not suitable for untreated EDTA blood) is also useful for demonstration of vitality of the parasite, PCR has become the most common direct diagnostical method to date [23, 24]. In general, PCR results should always be judged with care and together with serological data. Several investigators analysed the presence of circulating antigen(s) during infection [25-27]. However, their very low sensitivity make methods for the detection of circulating antigen unuseful for routine diagnosis of active *Toxoplasma* infection during pregnancy.

Screening protocols

Unfortunately, no standardized screening protocols for toxoplasmosis during pregnancy exist within Europe. Indeed, differences are present between and even within countries and include the frequency of sampling, the methods that are used and the interpretation. Therefore, protocols will be presented (i) from France and Austria, where screening is mandatory, and (ii) from Germany, where no mandatory screening program exists to date.

Screening in France and Austria

In France, screening was established by an official text from the government in 1978. Serological investigations of serum samples have to be performed monthly as soon as the pregnancy is recognized. It is necessary to use two quantitative techniques for both IgG and IgM antibodies. The fact that screening is made on a monthly basis allows a better detection of seroconversions, the worst case being a toxoplasmic contamination occuring the day after blood has been drawn: in this case, the seroconversion will be detected one month later the earliest. However, the interpretation of serology can be difficult at the time of the first sampling when no previous results are available. This is often the case when serology is not performed before pregnancy, but in the third month of pregnancy, just before the legal dead-line to declare it to the social insurance system. The decisional scheme of such protocol is summarized in Fig. 2, Stage 1.

In Austria, screening is performed on a trimestrial basis [1]. While this type of protocol is less expensive, and less aggressive for women than the one performed in France, detection of seroconversion may not be as quick as in a monthly protocol and thus can lead to a delay before treatment is installed.

Screening in Germany

In Germany, where screening is not mandatory, the German Society of Hygiene and Microbiology (DGHM) has recently suggested a sequential screening protocol [20] (Fig. 2, Stage 2). According to this protocol and to keep the costs low, it is sufficient to use IgG tests for screening since highly acute infections (IgG-negative, IgM-positive) are rare and will be diagnosed at the latest when a control serum sample is analysed 2 to 3 months later. IgG-negative patients should be all screened 2 to 3 months. In case of a positive IgG result, the same serum sample has to be tested for the presence of specific IgM antibodies. In reality, most laboratories simultaneously also determine IgM antibodies at the first stage. High IgM antibody titers indicate active or acute

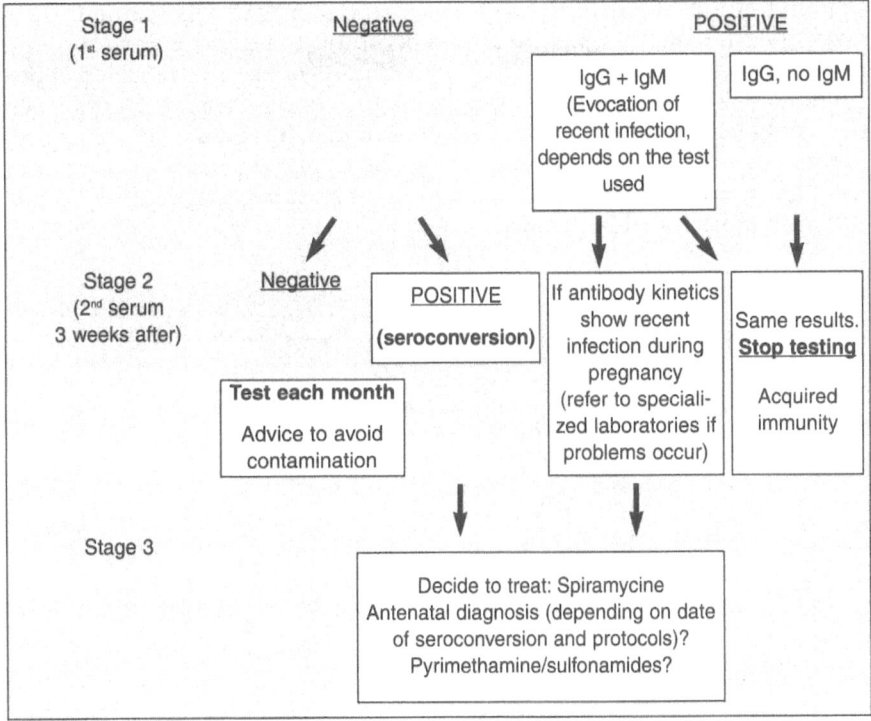

Fig. 1. Screening protocol in France

infection, which finally should be confirmed or excluded in specialized laboratories. The suspected diagnosis must be approved by a control serum sample which should be drawn 2 to 3 weeks later.

It is suggested that each non-specialized laboratory can perform screening tests (DA, IFA, CFT, IgG-ELISA, IgG-ISAGA), and IgM tests. In contrast, tests for the determination of IgA and IgE antibodies, DT, IgG avidity, use of recombinant antigens, and methods for direct diagnosis (for example, PCR) should only be performed in specialized laboratories.

Interpretation of results

Background

Even if the sensitivity and specificity of serological methods used for diagnosis of acquired toxoplasmosis have been improved during the last years, the interpretation of the results in pregnant women is often difficult and presents numerous traps [14, 28-30]. As outlined before, it is quite impossible to give a general interpretation since the different kits available on the market are not identical and test results are influenced by several parasite and host factors [5, 31, 32]. Thus, each person who is involved in diagnosis, should be aware of all the characteristics of the tests he/she uses. Furthermore, for a given test, the interpretation of results is obviously highly dependent on the number of sera available, and the dates of these related to the duration of pregnancy [14, 20, 33]. However, it is possible to define some patterns of results, that could lead to a clear interpretation. But, in daily routine, one must keep in mind that all patterns of results are possible, and that their interpretation must be very careful, and always based on at least two consecutively drawn serum samples tested in parallel.

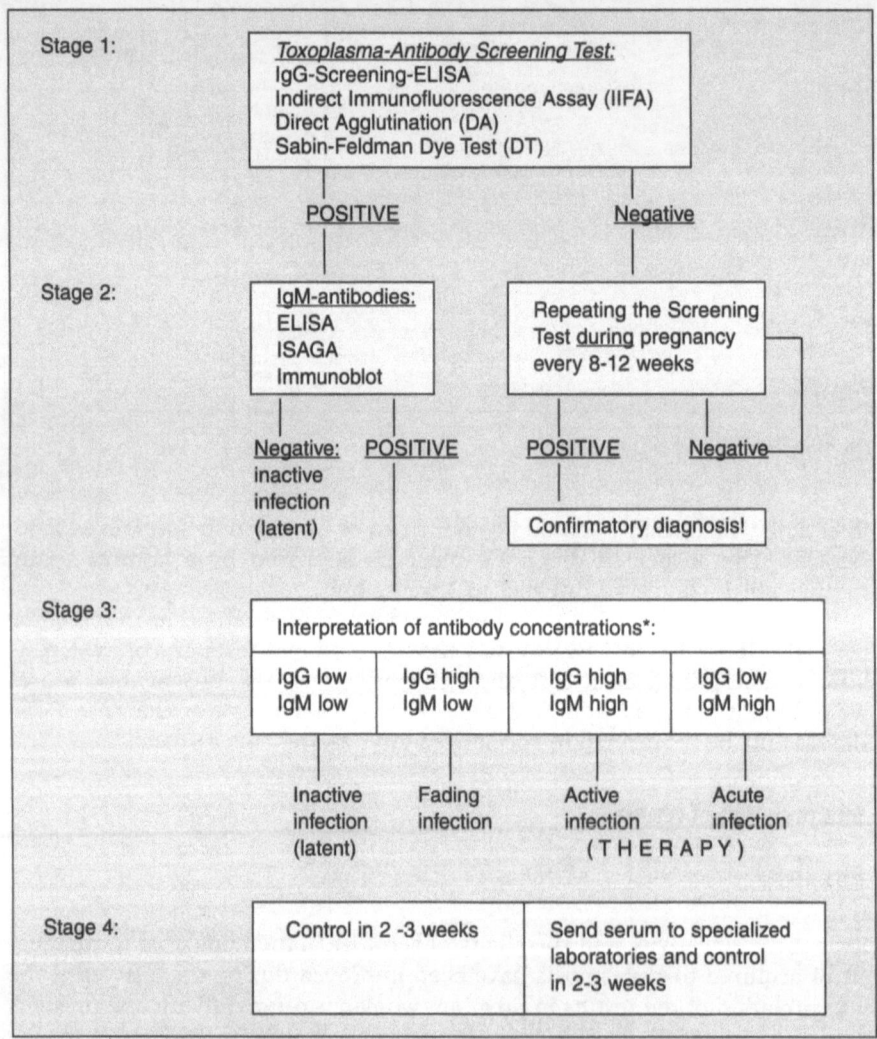

* Depending on the test that is used and the internal standards, each laboratory has to define its own criteria on an individual basis for high and low IgG and IgM values.

Figure 2. Suggestion for a screening protocol in Germany [34]

Negative and then positive

The easiest situation is when at least 2 consecutive samples are available (for instance during monthly screening). If the first one is negative, and the second one is positive, this allows (if technical problems are excluded and if the woman is not immunocompromised or has not received immunoglobulins) to affirm a seroconversion. Then, the problem is to judge as precisely as possible the date of infection taking into account the interval between the two serum samples and the kinetics of the serological methods used. One has to note that the appearance of non-specific IgM antibodies, which are not associated with *Toxoplasma* infection, could eventually hinder correct diagnosis.

IgG alone

Since IgM is usually present during acute infection, the presence of only IgG antibodies at stable levels in two consecutively drawn serum samples, at least 2 weeks apart, allows to diagnose that the infection occurred long time ago and that the woman has immunity against *Toxoplasma gondii*. However, this interpretation must also take into account the date of the beginning of pregnancy.

Presence of IgM and/or IgA antibodies

The presence of IgM and/or IgA antibodies is often the reason why a non specialized laboratory refers serum samples to a specialized one. The presence of such isotypes can be the first sign of a seroconversion, if alone, but is more often associated with IgG. In this case, the interpretation of the presence of IgM and/or IgA is difficult because of the persistance of these immunoglobulins for eventually a long time (up to several years for IgM) [14, 28, 35]. Thus, interpretation must be based on the association of techniques (such as IgG avidity) and on the comparison with the results of other sequential serum samples [16, 17, 19]. Finally, specialized laboratories should always be consulted in cases where diagnosis is uncertain.

Interpretation of antibody kinetics and titers

Here again, it is of paramount importance for the person who performs diagnosis to accurately know the characteristics of the test kits in use. Knowing the kinetics of antibodies is of main importance in the case of serological results that are unclear and difficult to interprete on one or two serum samples [36]. In such a case, the use of kinetic curves allows to extrapolate the probable date of seroconversion. However, such results must be interpreted carefully, since individual variations may occur which may lead to erroneous results [14].

How to decide whether to treat or not

In case of seroconversion during early pregnancy, treatment with spiramycin is used by some because of its absence of adverse effects (intolerance in the mother has been described very rarely). Other drugs, such as pyrimethamine-sulfadiazine or pyrimethamine-sulfadoxine can be used later during pregnancy and/or after antenatal diagnosis.

There is certainly no seroconversion: what to do? If serological tests remain negative during a regular screening (monthly, trimestrial, or other), advices to avoid infection must be given or repeated. Treatment is not necessary when repeatedly drawn serum samples remain negative.

Seroconversion is certain: what to do? If seronconversion is certain, treatment must be immediately initiated. Then, depending on the gestational age at conversion, antenatal diagnosis should be performed.

Seroconversion is uncertain: what to do? If seroconversion is uncertain but the techniques were performed in a non-specialized laboratory, serum samples should be referred to a reference laboratory in order to perform other techniques (i. e. such as IgG avidity or/and serologic methods using different antigens compared to the techniques used first). However, if seroconversion cannot be confirmed or excluded, it is necessary to obtain additional serum samples in order to more precisely analyse the kinetic curves of the antibodies. In some cases it might remain difficult to definitely confirm the presence or absence of a primary infection.

Conclusion

In congenital toxoplasmosis, demonstration of seroconversion of the mother is the first step of the medical management of the mother *and* the fetus. Thus, diagnosis during pregnancy is of paramount importance. Since to date the only way to affirm primary *Toxoplasma gondii* infection of the mother is based on serological methods, the responsibility of the diagnosis relies on the medical microbiologist who has the obligation to accurately assess the value and limits of the techniques he or she is using. Finally, interdisciplinary management between the gynecologist and the microbiologist should lead to clarify whether primary infection is present or not in order to decide on treatment of the pregnant woman.

References

1. Aspöck H, Pollack A (1992) Prevention of prenatal toxoplasmosis by serological screening of pregnant women in Austria. Scand J Infect Dis 84:32-38
2. Coradello H, Thalhammer O (1984) Toxoplasmosis screening of pregnant women in Austria. Z Geburtsh u Perinat 188:197-200
3. Derouin F, Garin YJ (1991) *Toxoplasma gondii:* blood and tissue kinetics during acute and chronic infections in mice. Exp Parasitol 73:460-468
4. Sabin AB, Feldman HA (1949) Dyes as microchemical indicators of a new immunity phenomenon affecting a protozoan parasite (*Toxoplasma*). Science 108:660-663

5. Dannemann BR, Vaughan WC, Thulliez P, Remington JS (1990) Differential agglutination test for diagnosis of recently acquired infection with *Toxoplasma gondii*. J Clin Microbiol 28:1928-1933

6. Decoster A, Caron A, Darcy F, Capron A (1988) IgA antibodies against P30 as markers of congenital and acute toxoplasmosis. Lancet i:1104-1107

7. Foudrinier F, Marx-Chemla C, Aubert D, Bonhomme A, Pinon JM (1995) Value of specific immunoglobulin A detection by two immunocapture assays in the diagnosis of toxoplasmosis. Eur J Clin Microbiol Infect Dis 14:585-590

8. Groß U, Roos T, Appoldt D, Heesemann J (1992) Improved serological diagnosis of *Toxoplasma gondii* infection by detection of immunoglobulin A (IgA) and IgM antibodies against P30 by using the immunoblot technique. J Clin Microbiol 30:1436-1441

9. Groß U, Keksel O, Dardé ML (1997) IgE antibodies as markers for activity of *Toxoplasma gondii* infection. Clin Diagn Lab Immunol 4:247-251

10. Paul M, Goullier-Fleuret A, Pelloux H, Ambroise-Thomas P (1996) The importance of the detection of anti-IgA antibodies in acquired toxoplasmosis. Acta Parasitol 4:227-233

11. Pinon JM, Chemla C, Villena I, Foudrinier F, Aubert D, Puygauthier-Toubas D, Leroux B, Dupouy D, Quereux C, Talmud M, Trenque T, Potron G, Pluot M, Remy G, Bonhomme A (1996) Early neonatal diagnosis of congenital toxoplasmosis: value of comparative enzyme-linked immunofiltration assay immunological profiles and anti-*Toxoplasma gondii* immunoglobulin M (IgM) or IgA immunocapture and implications for postnatal therapeutic strategies. J Clin Microbiol 34:579-583

12. Roos T, Martius J, Groß U, Schrod L (1993) Systematic serologic screening for toxoplasmosis in pregnancy. Obstet Gynecol 81:243-250

13. Remington JS, Desmonts G (1990) Toxoplasmosis. In: Remington JS, Klein JO (eds) Infectious diseases of the fetus and newborn infant. WB Saunders, Philadelphia, pp 89-195

14. Jenum PA, Stray-Pedersen B (1998) Development of specific immunoglobulins G, M, and A following primary *Toxoplasma gondii* infection in pregnant women. J Clin Microbiol 36:2907-2913

15. Bessières MH, Roques C, Berrebi A, Barre V, Cazaux M, Séguéla JP (1992) IgA antibody response during acquired and congenital toxoplasmosis. J Clin Pathol 45:605-608

16. Cozon GJN, Ferrandiz J, Nebhi H, Wallon M, Peyron F (1998) Estimation of the avidity of immunoglobulin G for routine diagnosis of chronic *Toxoplasma gondii* infection in pregnant women. Eur J Clin Microbiol Infect Dis 17:32-36

17. Hedman K, Lappalainen M, Seppâla I, Mäkelä O (1989) Recent primary *Toxoplasma* infection indicated by a low avidity of specific IgG. J Inf Dis 159:736-740

18. Jenum P, Stray-Pedersen B, Gundersen AG (1997) Improved diagnosis of primary *Toxoplasma gondii* infection in early pregnancy by determination of antitoxoplasma immunoglobulin G avidity. J Clin Microbiol 35:1972-1977

19. Pelloux H, Brun E, Vernet G, Marcillat S, Jolivet M, Guergour D, Fricker-Hidalgo H, Goullier-Fleuret A, Ambroise-Thomas P (1998) Determination of anti-*Toxoplasma gondii* immunoglobulin G avidity: adaptation to the Vidas system (bioMérieux). Diag Microbiol Infect Dis 32:69-73

20. Gorgievski-Hrisoho M, Germann D, Matter L (1996) Diagnostic implications of kinetics of immunoglobulin M and A antibody responses to *Toxoplasma gondii*. J Clin Microbiol 34:1506-1511

21. Wong SY, Hadju MP, Ramirez R, Thulliez P, McLeod R, Remington JS (1993) Role of specific immunoglobulin E in diagnosis of acute *Toxoplasma* infection and toxoplasmosis. J Clin Microbiol 31:2952-2959

22. Pinon JM, Toubas D, Marx C, Mougeot G, Bonnin A, Bonhomme A, Villaume M, Foudrinier F, Lepan H (1990) Detection of specific immunoglobulin E in patients with toxoplasmosis. J Clin Microbiol 28:1739-1743

23. Groß U, Roggenkamp A, Janitschke K, Heesemann J (1992) Improved sensitivity of the polymerase chain reaction for detection of *Toxoplasma gondii* in biological and human clinical specimen. Eur J Clin Microbiol Infect Dis 11:33-39

24. Grover CM, Thulliez P, Remington JS, Boothroyd JC (1990) Rapid prenatal diagnosis of congenital *Toxoplasma* infection by using polymerase chain reaction. J Clin Microbiol 28:2297-2301

25. Candolfi E, Derouin F, Kien T (1987) Detection of circulating antigens in immunocompromised patients during reactivation of chronic toxoplasmosis. Eur J Clin Microbiol Infect Dis 6:44-48

26. Hafid J, Tran Man Sung R, Raberin H, Akono ZY, Pozzetto B, Jana M (1995) Detection of circulating antigens of *Toxoplasma gondii* in human infection. Am J Trop Med Hyg 52:336-339

27. von Knapen F, Panggabean SO (1977) Detection of circulating antigen during acute infections with *Toxoplasma* gondii by enzyme-linked immunosorbent assay. J Clin Microbiol 6:545-547

28. Liesenfield O, Press C, Montoya JG, Gill R, Isaac-Renton JL, Hedman K, Remington JS (1997) False-positive results in immunoglobulin M (IgM) *Toxoplasma* antibody tests and importance of confirmatory testing : the Platelia Toxo IgM test. J Clin Microbiol 35:174-178

29. Pelloux H, Fricker-Hidalgo H, Goullier-Fleuret A, Ambroise-Thomas P (1997) Detection of anti-*Toxoplasma* immunoglobulin M in pregnant women. 35:2187

30. Wong SY, Remington JS (1994) Toxoplasmosis in pregnancy. Clin Infect Dis 18:853-862
31. De Champs C, Pelloux H, Cambon M, Fricker-Hidalgo H, Goullier-Fleuret A, Ambroise-Thomas P (1997) Evaluation of the second generation IMx toxo IgG antibody assay for detection of antibodies to *Toxoplasma gondii* in human sera. J Clin Lab Anal 11:214-219
32. Petithory JC, Ambroise-Thomas P, De Loye J, Pelloux H, Goullier-Fleuret A, Milgram M, Buffard C, Garin JP (1996) Serodiagnosis of toxoplasmosis: a comparative study of a series of control sera using various currently available tests and expression of the results in international units. WHO Bull 74:291-298
33. Candolfi E, Kien T (1990) Les nouvelles données de l'interprétation de la sérologie de la toxoplasmose par l'évaluation comparée d'anciennes et de nouvelles techniques sérologiques. Spectra Biol 90:55-62
34. Janitschke K, Kimmig P, Seitz HM, Frosch M, Groß U, Hlobil H, Reiter-Owona I (1998) MIQ - Parasitosen. Gustav Fischer Verlag, Stuttgart
35. Pelloux H, Ciapa P, Goullier-Fleuret A, Ambroise-Thomas P (1993) Evaluation du système Vidas pour le sérodiagnostic de la toxoplasmose. Ann Biol Clin 50:875-878
36. Lebech M, Joynson DHM, Seitz HM, Thulliez P, Gilbert RE, Dutton GN, Ovlisen B, Petersen E (1996) Classification system and case definitions of *Toxoplasma gondii* infection in immunocompetent pregnant women and their congenitally infected offspring. Eur J Clin Microbiol Infect Dis 15:799-805

2.3. Laboratory diagnosis of fetal toxoplasmosis

S. Romand, P. Thulliez

Introduction

Since 1985, prenatal diagnosis of congenital toxoplasmosis can be reliably performed in women with suspected or confirmed *Toxoplasma* infection acquired during pregnancy [1]. Availability of this recent diagnostic procedure has profoundly changed the management of congenital infection before birth and more specifically algorithms of decisions regarding prenatal treatment or medical terminations of pregnancy which were previously based mostly on the sole basis of maternal infection. Therefore, termination of pregnancy for maternal infection with *Toxoplasma gondii* has now become unusual thanks to prenatal diagnosis along with the possibility to treat infected fetus in utero via mother with the combination regimen of pyrimethamine (PYR) and sulfadiazine (SDZ) [2]. These major advances in the field of diagnosis and therapy has allowed to shift indications of medical termination of pregnancy for toxoplasmosis almost exclusively for cases with severe lesions detected by ultrasonography.

Since initial studies of prenatal diagnosis, diagnostic procedures have been deeply modified after the introduction of the polymerase chain reaction (PCR) at the begining of the 90's, which led to being abandonned progressively several of the previously developed techniques.

Indications of prenatal diagnosis

Prenatal diagnosis should be recommended to all women with proven or highly suspected *Toxoplasma* primary infection during pregnancy. Thus, given the limited but significant risk of fetal loss associated with cordocentesis or amiocentesis, such indication should be restricted only to documented and appropriate cases. For several authors, prenatal diagnosis may not be suitable for periconceptional infections or maternal infections acquired before the 7th or the 8th week of amenorrhea (WA), since in these cases the risk of fetal loss following amniocentesis (around 0.5%) is equivalent or higher than the risk of congenital toxoplasmosis [3]. On the other hand, in case of late maternal infection beyond 34 gestational week, or for those occurring a few days before expected delivery, the estimated risk of fetal infection is so high (80%)

that a presumptive curative treatment combining PYR plus SDZ without prenatal diagnosis has been recommended by some authors [4, 5].

Prenatal diagnosis from 1985 to 1990

Before the development of PCR techniques, prenatal diagnostic techniques
were based upon demonstration of specific and non specific signs of fetal
infection with *T. gondii*. These investigations included amniocentesis along
with cordocentesis for fetal blood sampling. Amniocentesis was designed for
isolation of *T. gondii* by mouse inoculation and cell culture, whereas both specific and non specific tests were performed on fetal blood.

Isolation of Toxoplasma gondii

Isolation of *T. gondii* from fetal blood or amniotic fluid constitutes proof of
fetal infection. From 20 WA, 1.5 to 4ml of fetal blood (FB) and 10 to 30ml of
amniotic fluid (AF) are sampled for analysis. Pellet of amniotic fluid and
whole blood clot are injected intraperitoneally or subcutaneously into mice.
After 3 to 6 weeks, inoculated mice that develop a specific anti-*Toxoplasma*
antibody response are sacrificed and examined for the presence of brain
cysts. Sensitivity of isolation of *T. gondii* either from fetal blood or amniotic
fluid was similar and ranged from 49 to 72% [1, 3, 4, 6-8]. Isolation of *T. gondii* from tissue culture of amniotic fluid was subsequently developed and allowed to obtain more rapid results within 4 days [9]. However, this method
revealed frequently less sensitive than mouse inoculation [8-10].

Non specific tests on fetal blood

Non specific tests comprise detection of eosinophilia, thrombocytopenia and
elevation of hepatic enzymes (γ-glutamyl-transpeptidase and lactate des-
hydrogenase). These non specific signs are only indicative of congenital toxoplasmosis and are not predictive of the severity of foetal lesions. However,
demonstration of these abnormalities was useful to make a therapeutic decision before infection was confirmed by specific tests or isolation of *T. gondii*
[11].

Specific tests on fetal blood

Specific tests include detection of anti-*Toxoplasma* IgM by immunocapture
ISAGA combined with isolation of *Toxoplasma* by mouse inoculation [12].
Due to immaturity of the fetal immune system, cordocentesis was not per-
formed before 20 WA to detect a specific antibody response. Sensitivity of
IgM detection in fetal blood for prenatal diagnosis ranged from 21 to 57% and
seemed to increase with gestational age at the time of puncture [3, 10].
Detection of specific IgA in combination with IgM also appeared as a valuable
marker for diagnosis of fetal infection [5, 13-15].

Combination of techniques

When combined together, conventional techniques yielded high sensitivity (92%) and negative predictive value (99%) and were thus reliable to demonstrate a fetal infection [3, 5, 6]. However, major drawbacks were associated with these procedures, i.e. time consuming procedures to demonstrate the purity of the fetal blood, a significant risk of fetal loss associated with fetal blood sampling and a long delay (3 to 6 weeks) before obtaining a definitive diagnosis after mouse inoculation [1, 6, 16].

Prenatal diagnosis with the use of polymerase chain reaction (PCR) test

From the early 90's, the development of PCR techniques applied on AF represented a major breakthrough for a more accurate, safe and rapid result of prenatal diagnosis.

In addition PCR test may be prescribed from the 18 WA as opposed to conventional methods which could not be performed before 20 WA [3].

Current recommendations for an accurate prenatal diagnosis of congenital toxoplasmosis are summarized in Table 1.

Table 1. Recommendations for prenatal diagnosis of congenital toxoplasmosis

Indications	Maternal primary *Toxoplasma* infection during pregnancy
Amniocentesis	• > 18th week of pregnancy • > 4 weeks after maternal infection • AF sample = 10 to 20 ml
Technique	• PCR on amniotic fluid + • mouse inoculation of amniotic fluid
PCR	• Target: B1 repeated sequence • DNA extraction • Monitoring of sensitivity (internal control) • Prevention of contamination (Uracyl-DNA-glycosylase)
Delay of result	• PCR = 24 hours • Mouse inoculation = 3 to 6 weeks

Background

Following initial promising results in experimental studies [17], Grover et al [8] first reported on the accuracy and usefulness of PCR for direct detection of *T. gondii* DNA in amniotic fluid. In this study, PCR targeting the repeated B1 sequence gene of *T. gondii* was more sensitive than mouse inoculation or tissue culture and detected *T. gondii* in 8 of 10 AF samples of cases with proven congenital infection. Other promising results were obtained with PCR detection of several DNA targets of *T. gondii*, including the single copy gene of surface protein P30 [18, 19] or a one-hundred fold repeated sequence of 18s ribosomal DNA [20]. For the first time, a simple method of prenatal diagnosis based on AF analysis allowed to obtain reliable results within a short delay (24 hours). Moreover, fetal blood sampling, which carries a higher risk of fetal loss [21] than amniocentesis, could be no longer necessary. However, in these initial studies, sporadic false positive reactions occurred and optimal sensitivity was not achieved. Although most laboratories now use the B1 protein gene as the most relevant and reliable target in routine practice [22], the PCR technique, because of its widespread use is far from being standardized and its sensitivity and specificity may vary greatly between laboratories. Thus, the diagnostic value of PCR on AF largely depends on the experience and technical ability within each laboratory.

Specificity of prenatal diagnosis with PCR

Important variations in specificity of PCR between different laboratories were identified in two recent interlaboratory comparison studies of artificial AF samples without *T. gondii* or containing known amounts of *T. gondii* DNA or whole tachyzoites [22, 23]. All laboratories were known to perform PCR methods with a high level of sensitivity. Nevertheless, in each study, 2 of 5 and 4 of 15 evaluated laboratories found one or more control samples to be falsely positive. These serious dicrepancies could be related to the choice of relevant primers but also with specific in-house developed procedures of the reaction which may differ in many ways. However, no particular PCR protocol could be clearly related with a higher risk of false positive results although laboratories using nested PCR seemed to have a higher rate of false positive tests. Nevertheless, it must be emphasized that in 5 of 6 false positive results, uracyl-DNA-glycosylase was not used to prevent carry-over contamination of samples. These investigations also highlighted contamination risks associated with handling steps. Other false positive results have been reported by some authors using different PCR protocols. Thus, Dupouy-Camet et al [7] using P30 gene targeted PCR obtained 2 positive PCR results in 34 non infected infants. In more recent clinical reports by Pratlong et al [5] and Jenum et al [24], the specificity of prenatal diagnosis using B1 targeted PCR was only of 94% and 97%, respectively. On the other hand, Hohlfeld et al [3] also using B1-PCR reported no case of false positive result in 339 consecutive AF samples from women infected during pregnancy, since all 37 positive prenatal diagnoses were confirmed either by conventional methods or by subsequent autopsy findings or serological postnatal follow-up.

Since a decision making process currently relies almost exclusively on the result of PCR analysis on AF, it is of utmost importance that specificity and positive predictive value of prenatal diagnosis using PCR has to be optimized in order to prevent any unnecessary and potentially toxic treatment or termination of pregnancy. Thus, given the important rate of false positive results found in some laboratories, some authors strongly recommend that PCR should not be used alone for prenatal diagnosis of congenital infection [22]. In this view, mice inoculation with AF is still retained as a confirmatory method to overcome some possible important variations in quality of testing with PCR. Besides, this latter method allows isolation and preservation of *T. gondii* strains. However, PCR on AF has proved to be far more sensitive than any other diagnostic test and in a number of cases, a positive PCR can be the only method to demonstrate a fetal infection in otherwise asymptomatic children.

Sensitivity of prenatal diagnosis with PCR

Differences in sensitivity in relation with the techniques used

Initial clinical studies with PCR have reported a rather low sensitivity of PCR. In 1990, Dupouy-Camet et al [7] determined that sensitivity of P30 targeted PCR was similar to that of cell culture and mouse inoculation of AF (70%). Thus, in this study and in other first reports PCR appeared only as an additional test to confirm or improve the performances of prenatal diagnosis but could not be considered as a complete alternative to other conventional methods.

However, further data have demonstrated the reliability and higher sensitivity of PCR compared with conventional methods. In 1994, Hohlfeld et al [3] reported a significant advance in B1-PCR reliability with the addition of an internal positive control to avoid false negative reactions, and the use of a specific decontamination step with uracyl-DNA-glycosylase to prevent carry-over contamination. In their series of 339 consecutive AF samples for prenatal diagnosis, Hohlfeld et al [3] identified 37 fetal infections in 38 infants with congenital toxoplasmosis diagnosed antenatally or at birth, including 3 cases for which PCR was the only positive test. In this report, PCR sensitivity was evaluated at 97.4% (and negative predictive value at 99.7%) as compared with an overall sensitivity of parasitologic tests ranging from 64% to 72%.

Finally, these results have demonstrated that a reliable PCR test performed on AF could fully replace other conventional prenatal diagnostic methods. However, in order to achieve optimal sensitivity of prenatal diagnosis it might be advisable to continue to use mouse inoculation since the semi-quantitative PCR testing has shown that when parasite burden was low, inoculation could still be positive [3]. In our experience, some rare discrepancies between isolation of *T. gondii* by mouse inoculation of AF and a negative PCR test have been observed. Such discrepancies might be explained by both a small parasite burden and the difference of processed volumes: a pellet of 10 ml of AF is usually inoculated into mice whereas 1.5 is required for PCR. Yet, our group ceased using tissue culture, except when the AF sample contained a high proportion of blood which may inhibit the reaction [25].

Nevertheless, significant variations in sensitivity between investigators have also been demonstrated by Pelloux et al [22] using artificial AF samples spiked with tachyzoites of *T. gondii*. Among 15 European laboratories involved in prenatal diagnosis, 9 were able to detect a single parasite whereas 2 found no *Toxoplasma* in any of the 8 positive aliquots. Again, no clear link with specific technical procedures was found to explain such important dicrepancies. In a large screening program involving more than 35.000 pregnant women in Norway, Jenum et al [26] performed prenatal diagnosis with a nested PCR in 6 women. Nevertheless, the nested PCR method used in this study detected only 2/6 fetal infections (sensitivity = 33%), as compared with other conventional methods. This rather low sensitivity may be explained by the PCR technique used but also by the fact that amniocentesis was performed as soon as maternal infection was identified regardless of delay between estimated maternal infection and amniocentesis. Moreover, contrasting with current recommendations, amniocentesis was performed from 12 WA in some cases, although reliability of PCR before 18 WA has not been evaluated [3]. Thus, in order to avoid false negative results due to the delay of parasite transfer from placenta to the fetus, it is recommended to perform prenatal diagnosis from 18 WA and at least 4 weeks after the estimated date of maternal infection [3].

Differences in sensitivity in relation with the selection of cases

In a number of cases, differences between investigators in the PCR sensitivity are likely to be explained not only by lack of technical standard but also by major differences in selection and definition of cases of congenital infection. So far, in most studies, performances of PCR have been assessed comparatively to conventional prenatal diagnostic methods, without taking into account the definitive status of infants with a negative prenatal diagnosis, which can be determined only after birth and during subsequent long-term follow-up of the child. Therefore, the sensitivity and negative predictive values of PCR on AF may be overestimated, since a significant number of offsprings are lost to follow-up after birth.

Pratlong et al [5], in a retrospective study involving 286 pregnancies demonstrated congenital infection in 7 of 211 children (3.3%) with negative antenatal diagnosis. All these children had subclinical toxoplasmosis which was diagnosed at birth or during pediatric follow-up. In a first prospective study conducted by Gratzl et al [27] in 49 infants born to mothers with primary *Toxoplasma* infection during pregnancy, both specificity and sensitivity of PCR performed on AF were determined at 100% for the 11 infected and 38 non infected infants who were followed up until 1 year of age.

Furthermore, preliminary data obtained in our centre from an ongoing european multicentre prospective study on congenital toxoplasmosis (EMSCOT) enabled us to reliably estimate the sensitivity and negative predictive values of PCR test as compared with the status of infection in 83 children born to mothers with confirmed seroconversion who have completed a one year follow-up. Although using a similar PCR protocol, our results markedly contrasted with those obtained by Gratzl et al [27] since overall sensitivity and negative predictive value of prenatal diagnosis were estimated at 65% and 75.4%, respectively (Table 2). In our series 14 infants with congenital toxoplasmosis diagnosed after birth had a negative prenatal diagnosis performed with PCR and mouse inoculation. Interestingly, for these 14 cases, the median age of gestation at maternal infection was estimated at 30 weeks.

Therefore, given the high rate of parasite transmission during the third trimester of pregnancy, these results may raise the question of a presumptive curative treatment with PYR plus SDZ in case of maternal infection occurring late during pregnancy, without performing prenatal diagnosis. Such view is supported by several authors [4, 5].

Table 2. Performances of prenatal diagnosis in a cohort of children born to mothers with *Toxoplasma* infection during pregnancy

Amniocentesis (PCR + mouse inoculation)	Children (Nb)		
	Congenital TOXOPLASMOSIS	Infection RULED OUT	Total
Positive	26	0	26
Negative	14	43	57
Total	40	43	83

Sensitivity = 26/40 = 65%; Negative predictive value = 43/57 = 75,4%

Overall, these preliminary results along with other reports show that a negative antenatal diagnosis cannot rule out the possibility of a delayed transmission of parasite following amniocentesis. One case illustrating such delayed transmission has been reported by Hohfeld et al [3]. In this case a late onset of ultrasound abormalities following a negative prenatal diagnosis led to perform a subsequent amniocentesis which eventually allowed to detect the presence of *T. gondii*. Since then, several similar cases have been documented in our centre.

Before the use of PCR for prenatal diagnosis, it was already known that not all cases of congenital toxoplasmosis could be detected prenatally. Of 89 congenital infections, Hohlfeld et al [28] reported 9 cases (10%) with a negative prenatal diagnosis, including one with a severe form. Nevertheless, in spite of a higher sensitivity of PCR, as compared with conventional methods, a significant proportion of cases still cannot be diagnosed antenatally. Hence, in case of a negative result of prenatal diagnosis, obstetricians should be aware to continue treatment with spiramycin, along with a careful ultrasound monitoring throughout pregnancy and a long-term follow-up of child in order to definitively rule out congenital infection.

Conclusion

In countries such as France and Austria where a serological screening program for detection of *Toxoplasma* infection during pregnancy is mandatory, the possibility to perform a safe and accurate prenatal diagnosis is a critical issue.

Direct detection of *Toxoplasma* DNA in amniotic fluid by PCR is currently viewed as the most sensitive, specific, safe and rapid method for diagnosis of fetal infection. As far as a PCR method is considered totally specific of

Toxoplasma infection, it reliably represents a complete alternative to other conventional methods of prenatal diagnosis. Sampling the amniotic fluid only makes the prenatal diagnosis safer and consequently more achievable to physicians and more acceptable to patients.

However, since the risk of amniocentesis is not negligible, this procedure should be offered only to pregnant women with serologically proven or highly suspected primary infection.

Initial enthusiasm engendered by the high performances of the PCR should be tempered by the fact that all congenital infections cannot be identified since a delayed transmission of *Toxoplasma* may occur after the date of amniocentesis.

References

1. Desmonts G, Daffos F, Forestier F, Capella-Pavlovsky M, Thulliez P, Chartier M (1985) Prenatal diagnosis of congenital toxoplasmosis. Lancet 1:500-504
2. Couvreur J, Thulliez P, Daffos F et al (1991) Foetopathie toxoplasmique. Traitement *in utero* par l'association pyrimethamine-sulfamides. Arch Fr Pediatr 48:397-403
3. Hohlfeld P, Daffos F, Costa JM, Thulliez P, Forestier F, Vidaud M (1994) Prenatal diagnosis of congenital toxoplasmosis with a polymerase chain reaction test on amniotic fluid. N Engl J Med 331:695-699
4. Berrebi A, Kobuch WE, Bessières MH et al (1994) Termination of pregnancy for maternal toxoplasmosis. Lancet 344:36-39
5. Pratlong F, Boulot P, Villena I, Issert I, Tamby I, Cazenave J, Dedet JP (1996) Antenatal diagnosis of congenital toxoplasmosis: evaluation of the biological parameters in a cohort of 286 patients. Br J Obst Gyn 103:552-557
6. Daffos F, Forestier F, Capella-Pavlovsky M et al (1988) Prenatal management of 746 pregnancies at risk for congenital toxoplasmosis. N Engl J Med 318:271-275
7. Dupouy-Camet J, Bougnoux ME, Lavareda de Souza S, Thulliez P, Dommergues M, Mandelbrot L, Ancelle T, Tourte-Schaefer C, Benarous R (1992) Comparative value of polymerase chain reaction and conventional biological tests for the prenatal diagnosis of congenital toxoplasmosis. Ann Biol Clin (Paris) 50:315-319
8. Grover CM, Thulliez P, Remington JS, Boothroyd JC (1990) Rapid prenatal diagnosis of congenital *Toxoplasma* infection by using polymerase chain reaction on amniotic fluid. J Clin Microbiol 28:2297-2301
9. Derouin F, Thulliez P, Candolfi E, Daffos F, Forestier F (1988) Early prenatal diagnosis of congenital toxoplasmosis using amniotic fluid samples and tissue culture. Eur J Clin Microbiol Infect Dis 7:423-425
10. Thulliez P (1990) Toxoplasmose congénitale: résultats de 105 diagnostics prénatals positifs (VIII th ICOPA, Paris). Bull Soc Fr Parasitol 8:1001
11. Berrebi A, Cohen-Khallas Y, Bessières MH, Rolland M, Sarramon MF, Fournier A (1992) Valeur prédictive des signes non spécifiques d'infection foetale dans la toxoplasmose congénitale. J Gynecol Obstet Biol Reprod (Paris) 21:791-794
12. Desmonts G, Naot Y, Remington JS (1981) Immunoglobin M-immunosorbent agglutination assay for diagnosis of infectious diseases: diagnosis of acute congenital and acquired *Toxoplasma* infections. J Clin Microbiol 14:486-491
13. Bessières MH, Roques C, Berrebi A, Barre V, Cazaux M, Seguela JP (1992) IgA antibody response during acquired and congenital toxoplasmosis. J Clin Pathol 45:605-608
14. Decoster A, Darcy F, Caron A et al (1992) Anti-P30 IgA antibodies as prenatal markers of congenital *Toxoplasma infection*. Clin Exp Immunol 87:310-315
15. Le Fichoux Y, Marty P, Chan H (1987) Les IgA sériques spécifiques dans le diagnostic de la toxoplasmose. Ann Pediatr 34:375-379
16. Daffos F, Capella-Pavlovsky M, Forestier F (1985) Fetal blood sampling during pregnancy with use of a needle guided by ultrasound: a study of 606 consecutive cases. Am J Obstet Gynecol 153:655-660
17. Burg JL, Grover CM, Pouletty P, Boothroyd JC (1989) Direct and sensitive detection of a pathogenic protozoan, *Toxoplasma gondii* by polymerase chain reaction. J Clin Microbiol 27:1787-1792
18. Dupouy-Camet J, Lavareda de Souza S, Bougnoux ME, Mandelbrot L, Hennequin C, Dommergues M, Benarous R, Tourte-Schaefer C (1990) Preventing congenital toxoplasmosis. Lancet ii: 1017-1018

19. Savva D, Morris JC, Johnson JD, Holliman RE (1990) Polymerase chain reaction for detection of *Toxoplasma gondii*. J Med Microbiol 32:25-31
20. Cazenave J, Forestier F, Bessières MH, Broussin B, Begueret J (1992) Contribution of a new PCR assay to the prenatal diagnosis of congenital toxoplasmosis. Prenat Diag 12:120-128
21. Ghidini A, Sepulveda W, Lockwood CJ, Romero R (1993) Complications of fetal blood sampling. Am J Obstet Gynecol 168:1339-1344
22. Pelloux H, Guy E, Angelici MC, Aspöck H et al (1998) A second european collaborative study on polymerase chain reaction for *Toxoplasma gondii*, involving 15 teams. FEMS Microbiol Letters 165:231-237
23. Guy EC, Pelloux H, Lappalainen M et al (1996) Interlaboratory comparison of polymerase chain reaction for the detection of *Toxoplasma gondii* DNA added to samples of amniotic fluids. Eur J Clin Microbiol Infect Dis 15:836-839
24. Jenum PA, Holberg-Petersen M, Melby KK, Stray-Pedersen B (1998) Diagnosis of congenital *Toxoplasma gondii* infection by polymerase chain reaction (PCR) on amniotic fluid samples. The norwegian experience. Acta Pathol Microbiol Immunol Scand 106:680-686
25. Weiss LM, Udem SA, Salgo M, Tanowitz HB, Wittner M (1991) Sensitive and specific detection of *Toxoplasma* DNA in an experimental murine model: use of *Toxoplasma gondii*-specific cDNA and the polymerase chain reaction. J Infect Dis 163:108-186
26. Jenum PA, Stray-Pedersen B, Melby KK, Kapperud G, Whitelaw A, Eskild A, Eng J (1998) Incidence of *Toxoplasma gondii* infection in 35.940 pregnant women in Norway and pregnancy outcome for infected women. J Clin Microbiol 36:2900-2906
27. Gratzl R, Hayde M, Kohlhauser C, Hermon M, Burda G, Strobl W, Pollak A (1998) Follow-up of infants with congenital toxoplasmosis detected by polymerase chain reaction analysis of amniotic fluid. Eur J Clin Microbiol Infect Dis 17:853-858
28. Hohlfeld P, Daffos F, Thulliez P et al (1989) Fetal toxoplasmosis: outcome of pregnancy and infant follow-up after in utero treatment. J Pediatr 115:765-769

2.4. Effect of treatment of the infected pregnant woman and her foetus

B. Stray-Pedersen and W. Foulon

Introduction

If primary *Toxoplasma* infection is identified in a pregnant woman today, antiparasitic treatment is mandatory. The aim is primarily to prevent the mother-to-foetal transmission and secondly to treat or reduce any damage in an already infected foetus. Whenever foetal infection is diagnosed, two options are considered: pregnancy termination or continuation of pregnancy with antiparasitic treatment of the infected maternal-foetal unit.

Problems in evaluating the benefit of treatment

For 40 years two antiparasitic regimens (spiramycin and/or pyrimethamine-sulphonamides) have been employed in the therapeutic approach. Their effect on preventing vertical transmission and congenital disease has been discussed for years. Admittedly, the efficacy of antenatal treatment has been difficult to evaluate since it depends on factors such as the antenatal screening procedure, the gestational stage of maternal seroconversion and how soon after acquisition the infection is recognised. Another important factor is whether or not fetal infection is diagnosed before the start of treatment [1].

Today prenatal diagnosis may be offered to every newly infected pregnant woman, and it may thus be possible to establish if vertical transmission has occurred before initiation of treatment. Antenatal treatment studies not taking into account fetal infection can only be used to evaluate if treatment is effective on the parasitic infection in the placenta, and on the development of symptoms, signs and complications in infected children.

It should be born in mind that congenital toxoplasmosis exhibits great variation in severity and outcome, and that long term follow-up studies have to be required for proper evaluation of effectiveness. The main problem is however, the lack of randomised placebo controlled trials [2]. Moreover, such treatment studies are not likely to be carried out because it is considered unethical to withhold therapy from an infected foetus [3].

Drugs used in pregnancy

The drugs that have been used in the treatment of pregnant women are spiramycin and pyrimethamine together with sulphonamides (P+S) [4]. The usual regimen, dosage and duration of therapy are given in Table 1.

Table 1. Treatment of *Toxoplasma* infection in pregnant women

Drugs	Pregnant women
Spiramycin	3 g = 9 MIU /day
	or
Pyrimethamine (P)	25 mg /day (First day: double dose)
Sulfadiazine (S)	50-100mg /day (Initially: double dose)
	or
Fansidar	2 tablets/week
	(25 mg pyrimethamine + 500 mg sulphadoxine tablet)

During pyrimethamine therapy
  Folinic acid   5-15 mg twice weekly
  Blood cells counts   (platelet, white cells) every 1-2 weeks

Indications
Pregnant women with primary infection
  • Before conception   No need for treatment
  • Suspected cases   Spiramycin until diagnosis
Proven cases of maternal infection:
  – 1st trimester: Spiramycin continuously
  – 2nd, 3rd trimester: Spiramycin continuously, or P+S
                            (3 weeks), then Spiramycin (3 weeks)

Evidence of foetal infection
(positive amniotic fluid)   Repeated courses until delivery.
                            P+S (3 weeks), then Spiramycin (3-6 weeks)
                            or
                            Fansidar : 2 tablets weekly

Spiramycin

This drug is a macrolide, which is completly safe to use in pregnancy. It concentrates markedly in the tissue, and its concentration in placenta is found to be five times higher than that of the corresponding maternal serum. Transplacental passage has been confirmed with accumulation of the drug in all fetal organs except the brain [5].

In the 1960s' the antenatal treatment program comprised one 3-weeks course of spiramycin or repeated courses at different intervals [6]. However Daffos and colleagues [7] indicated that continuous daily treatment throughout pregnancy was more effective. It is shown that spiramycin slowly reduces the *Toxoplasma* load in the tissue requiring administration for at least three weeks to be effective [8].

Pyrimethamine and sulphonamides

The P+S combination (pyrimethamine usually with sulphadiazine) is the traditional and most successful regime for treating *Toxoplasma* infection. Pyrimethamine crosses the placental barrier and concentrates both in brain and retinal tissue [5]. In addition, the combination has proven to be more effective than spiramycin in treating Toxoplasma placentitis [9].

Since both drugs are folic acids antagonists, the combination may induce reversible bone marrow suppression. Peripheral white cells and platelet counts should be regularly monitored during treatment. It is usual to add folinic acid (not folic acid) 5-15 mg twice weekly to prevent hematologic complications. In humans, pyrimethamine has no known teratogenic effect. An editorial in Lancet [10] stated that pyrimethamine (used as malaria prophylaxis) was safe even in early pregnancy, but folinic acid should be added as a supplement. As a precaution in the first trimester, spiramycin treatment is preferred rather than pyrimethamine [11].

Fansidar (pyrimethamine 25 mg + sulphadoxine 500 mg) has been used especially in France and Switzerland. The advantage is that it can be administered once weekly or twice monthly, which, contributes to a high compliance [12]. The dose of pyrimethamine is, however, much lower than when pyrimethamine is given daily in the P-S combination.

Other drugs

Both spiramycin and P-S suppress the proliferation of parasites, but do not eliminate the tissue cysts. There is a need for initiating trials with new, maybe more effective drugs also in pregnant women, but the possibilities that these drugs are teratogenic or harmful for the foetus have been limiting factors.

Azithromycin and atovaquone are new drugs that have shown activity against tissue cysts in animal studies.

Azithromycin

This new azalide antibiotic has been used successfully in treatment of AIDS patients with cerebral toxoplasmosis [13]. A study of pregnant women who were treated with 500 mg azithromycin once daily for 3 days during the last weeks of pregnancy showed that azithromycin concentration in placental tissue were 10-90 times higher than that in maternal or cord blood [14]. No adverse event was observed in the mothers nor in the new-borns. Today azithromycin is considered as an alternative treatment for chlamydial infection in pregnancy [15], but more studies are needed to evaluate the effect on congenital toxoplasmosis.

Atovaquone

In animal models atovaquone is not teratogenic, has no effect on fertility and induces no chromosomal changes. It has proven effective in the treatment of

cerebral toxoplasmosis in patients with AIDS [16]. There are so far no available data on the use in clinical settings of pregnant women, neither on transplacental transfer nor on fetal tissue distribution (see chapter 4.6). The drug
has been administered in HIV-infected children as a prophylactic against
Pneumocystis carinii, and is regarded as safe.

Clindamycin

This drug is considered to be safe and non toxic for the foetus [17]. It has
been used in ocular toxoplasmosis. It crosses the placental barrier, but no
report exists on the effect in preventing or modifying congenital toxoplasmosis. The drug may be used in women not tolerating the usual drugs.

Treatment regimens in Europe

A questionnaire answered by 14 centres in 11 different European countries
showed that standard therapy in infected pregnant women consisted of spiramycin, while P+S was administered when fetal infection was diagnosed
(Stray-Pedersen unpublished data). Some centres recommended P+S as the
first choice to mothers infected in the third trimester due to the high frequency of mother-to-foetal transmission. P+S alternated always with spiramycin, but different strategies existed about the period of time in the alternating cycle. Usually P+S was administrated daily for 3 weeks, while spiramycin for 3-6 weeks.

If the foetus proved uninfected, two centres stopped the spiramycin treatment, while others continued treatment throughout pregnancy.

Five European centres reported that according to their clinical practice
seroconverting mothers with infected foetuses were offered Fansidar once
weekly or twice monthly [12]. Folinic acid was always added.

In a new recommendation from Italy [18], a single course of P+S is proposed to be given as soon as seroconversion is documented in the mother. In
addition, spiramycin is prescribed at the same time and continued until the
end of pregnancy, whereas P+S is to be stopped after 3-4 weeks. If the foetus
proves to be infected, P+S is recommended to be given in cycles while the spiramycin therapy is given continuously. They base their proposal on the documented efficiency of P+S to attack the parasite in the brain, the faster transplacental passage and the longer half-life of these drugs compared with spiramycin. Continuous administration of spiramycin throughout pregnancy
should prevent the parasite from entering the proliferative stage [19].

Effect of treatment on placental infection

The placenta is a key organ in the mother-to-fetal transmission of *Toxoplasma
gondii*. Demonstration of the parasite in placental tissue means most probably congenital infection[20]. During the acute stage of infection, when mater-

nal parasitaemia occurs, *Toxoplasma* may colonise the placenta which then remains infected for the rest of pregnancy. Thus, if left untreated, the placenta may act as a reservoir, supplying viable organisms to the foetus at any time throughout pregnancy [5]. It has been postulated that the transmission of parasites across the placenta is a delayed process, which gives time for initiating of treatment [21].

In a study of 542 pregnant women, Desmonts and Couvreur [22] reported that parasites were detected less frequently in the placentas of spiramycin-treated mothers (19%) than in untreated mothers (50%). Maternal therapy reduced the placental infection in pregnancy from 25% to 8% in the first trimester, from 54% to 19% in the second trimester and from 65% to 44% in the third trimester, indicating that spiramycin treatment during pregnancy had a great impact on placental infection.

The superior effect of P+S to spiramycin became evident when the two regimens were compared. In a retrospective study of congenitally infected infants from different periods, Couvreur et al [9] detected parasites in (41/46) 89% of placentas of untreated or inadequately treated women, in (89/118) 75% placentas of spiramycin treated women, and in only (10/20) 50% of those of women treated with P+S.

A similar beneficial effect was reported some years later when P+S or Fansidar alternating with spiramycin was given to infected foetuses and compared with those receiving only spiramycin. The parasitological findings of the placentas were significantly reduced from 77% positivity in the spiramycin group to 42% in the pyrimethamine group [23]. In summary, spiramycin seems to reduce the parasitic infection in placenta by 30-60%, while the P+S combination is more effective.

Effect of treatment on maternal-foetal transmission rate

There are few studies comparing the effect of ante/prenatal treatment versus no treatment on the maternal-foetal transmission rate [24] (Table 2). Moreover, no randomised comparisons exist.

The classic studies of Desmont and Couvreur [25] reported a significant reduction in the incidence of congenitally infected infants born to treated (23%) versus untreated (55%) mothers. The conclusion drawn was that spiramycin reduced the risk of fetal toxoplasmosis by 60%. Other studies from Europe [26-28] also report that prenatal treatment has a positive significant effect by lowering the vertical transmission rate. However, only one study [26] take into account the date of maternal seroconversion – a factor which may greatly influence the transmission rate. Thus, erroneous conclusions may be drawn if the gestational age at the time of maternal infection is not controlled for in the compared groups.

Recently, however, two studies have found that treatment (mainly spiramycin) in pregnancy did not reduce the maternal-foetal transmission rate.

Lyon/Copenhagen study [29]

In the period 1988-93, 564 pregnant women with *Toxoplasma* seroconversion from Lyon, France were treated with continuous spiramycin. However, if the maternal seroconversion occurred late (after 32 gestational week) or infection was diagnosed in the foetus, 3 weeks courses of P+S alternating with spiramycin were prescribed. The transmission rate was observed to 24%.

The Lyon group was compared with 135 women from Copenhagen where neonatal screening were performed in the period 1992-95 and the infected mothers identified retrospectively [30]. No treatment was instituted in pregnancy. The fetal transmission rate in this group was 21%. Thus, no significant differences were observed between the treated and untreated pregnant population. It has to be emphasised that two different screening programs were employed in the two cohorts. Admittedly, in Lyon during the same period of time 32 women-not included in the study- did not receive any treatment. They were infected at the end of pregnancy and had a transmission rate that was remarkably higher than the treated group in Lyon [2].

The European multicenter study [31]

In a multicentre study comprising 5 European *Toxoplasma* reference centres (Brussels, Helsinki, Lille, Oslo, Reims), 144 consecutive seroconversions in pregnancy were registered retrospectively. Sixty-four of the women (44%) gave birth to congenitally infected infants. The transmission rate varied between 0% when infection took place before 5th gestational week to 93% when infection occurred at the end of pregnancy (between gestational week 31-35). Prenatal treatment was started as soon as the seroconversion was detected and confirmed. Antiparasitic drugs were administrated to 119 of the infected pregnant women. Eighty-two percent received spiramycin initially. Vertical transmission was observed in 72% (18/25) of the mother-infant pairs who did not receive therapy, and in 39% (46/119) of the mother-infant pairs who were treated prenatally. This difference may seem significant, but when the time of maternal infection was controlled for in the two groups, it was not. The multivariate analysis indicated that neither the administration of antibiotics nor the time lapse between infection and the start of therapy did influence the transmission of infection (p = 0.7 and 0.3, respectively). The only parameter that was found to predict transmission was the time of maternal infection. The earlier the infection took place in pregnancy, the less frequent transmission occurred (p < 0.0001).

In conclusion, these two latter studies may indicate that the fetal infection probably occurs in the majority of cases early after the maternal infection during the maternal parasitemia, and thus the time lag in placenta may not be of a great importance for the transmission rate. If treatment is going to influence the transmission rate, it has to be given very soon after acquisition.

Table 2. Effect of treatment in pregnancy on the maternal-foetal transmission rate

| Investigators | Year | Place | Total number | Therapy | Infected mothers | | Infected infants | |
					Treated	Untreated	Treated mothers	Untreated mothers
Desmonts and Couvreur	1984	Paris	542	S	388	154	22%	52% *
Excler et al	1985	Lyon	134	S	104	30	21%	47% *
Lambotte et al	1976	Liege	129	S	28	110	0%	10% *
Douche et al	1996	France	98	S/P+S	69	29	13%	100% *
Kräubig	1966	Germany		P+S	59	84	5%	17%
Wallon et al	1997	Lyon/Cph		S/P+S	564 (Lyon)	125 (Cph)	24%	21%
Foulon et al	1998	5 European centers	144	S/P+S	119	25	39%	72%

* Significant difference

Effect of treatment on foetal infection

In the 60s' and 70s', Desmonts and Couvreur [25] found that antenatal treatment with spiramycin led to a significant reduction in vertical transmission rate, but no improvement in the clinical outcome of the infected offspring. In fact the percentage of infected infants, which had clinically apparent infection or disease was almost identical in treated and untreated pregnancies (28% vs 32%). The conclusion drawn was that even if antenatal spiramycin treatment reduced the risk of foetal toxoplasmosis, it did not modify the pattern of infection in an already infected foetus.

Maybe this poor efficacy was dose-related, with inadequate foetal blood concentration, which is only half of that in the mother, leading to insufficient fetal tissue levels [1].

In fact, when antenatal treatment with spiramycin was supplemented with P+S, a significant reduction in the number of severely affected babies was observed and a shift to less severe and subclinical forms [7, 32].

The superior effect of P+S treatment was confirmed by Couvreur and colleagues [23] in their study of only infected foetuses (diagnosed *in utero*) and where P+S had significant beneficial effect on the parasitological and serological signs of the evolutive fetopathy observed in the newborn period.

In the Multicentre European Study [31] the effect of prenatal treatment on the development of sequelae up to the age of one year, was analysed in 140 children born of 140 seroconverting mothers. Sequelae were found in 19 children of whom 9 had severe sequelae. These were 7 out of 25 (28%) children born to mothers who did not receive antiparasitic therapy and 12 out of 115 (10%) children to mothers who received therapy. Multivariate analysis showed that the administration of prenatal therapy was predictive for the absence of sequelae (p = 0.026, OR = 0.30, 95% CI = 0.10-0.86). Moreover, in the group which had received antibiotics, a positive correlation on the development of sequelae and the time lapse between infection and the start of antibiotic therapy was seen. The sooner antibiotics were given after the maternal infection, the less frequent sequelae was found in the neonate (p = 0.02). Furthermore, multivariate analysis showed that prenatal treatment reduced the appearance of severe sequelae in the neonate 7 times (p = 0.007, OR = 0.14, 95% CI = 0.03-0.58). Twenty percent of the untreated mothers got children with severe sequelae as compared to only 3.5% of the treated mothers. Most of the women received spiramycin; however, no significant difference in beneficial effect was observed between the two treatment regimens.

In summary, prenatal antiparasitic therapy given to infected mothers during pregnancy greatly reduced the development of sequelae in the infected infants. An early start of treatment after acquisition resulted in a significant reduction of the number of severely affected infants.

Termination of pregnancy

Medical abortion carried out solely on the basis of maternal infection in pregnancy is today unnecessary.

Between 0-21% of women acquiring toxoplasmosis during the first trimester will transmit the infection, and some of the infected foetuses will die (spontaneous abortion, intrauterine death) or be severely affected. If treatment is instituted early, Hohlfeldt and colleagues [32] claim that only 4-8% will be infected, but still 10% of the infected liveborn infants will suffer severe disease. If the mother seroconvert between 12 and 20 gestational week, the risks are 5-23% for congenital infection and 40-64% for clinical signs [31, 33].

Today, infected foetuses may be identified by prenatal diagnosis. In Toulouse, Berrebi at al. [34] investigated 27 infected liveborn infants whose mothers were infected in first (3 cases) or in the second trimester of pregnancy (24 cases). Prenatal diagnosis was performed and antiparasitic treatment was given. In the newborn period 10 of the 27 infected newborns (37%) had one or more clinical signs of congenital toxoplasmosis, but 9 of these 10 infants did not show any symptoms of toxoplasmosis later on. Only 3% of the mothers with proven fetal infection opted for termination. The authors concluded that there was no need to abort infected foetuses if repeated fetal ultrasounds were normal, and antiparasitic treatment were instituted.

Another group in Lyon [35] agrees with the Toulouse group and state that only infected foetuses with abnormal ultrasound are at very high risk of severe disease. In Paris, Daffos et al. [36] however are far less optimistic about the prognosis.

In their recent study of 148 foetal infections diagnosed prenatally, three groups were identified in respect to prognosis. When infection occurred before 16 weeks gestation, 60% of the foetuses (31/52) had ultrasound evidence of infection (eg. ascites, pericarditis, or necrotic brain foci) and 48% had cerebral ventricular dilation. When infection occurred between 17 and 23 weeks, 25% of the foetuses (16/63) had ultrasound signs and only 12% had ventricular dilation. After 24 weeks only 1 of the 33 foetuses had ultrasound signs and none had hydrocephalus. Given the very poor prognosis in early pregnancy, the Paris group accept parental requests for termination when infection occurs before 16 weeks [32, 36]. They claim that at this gestational age there are always large areas of brain necrosis at necropsy. Even in foetuses without ventricular dilation, the group thinks that ventricular dilation will ensue if the pregnancies were to be continued.

The current practice and our recommendation to women infected in early pregnancy is to advise amniocentesis as soon as possible [1, 37]. If the amniotic fluid yields no parasite or *Toxoplasma* antigen, the woman can be reassured that foetal infection is unlikely, and she should be advised to continue her pregnancy with follow up of the newborn infant.

In those few cases where foetal infection is proven in the first or early second trimester (before 16th gestational week), termination may be an option. In addition, if fetal abnormalities are observed on ultrasound, termination on medical indication is discussed with the parents.

Treatment of HIV-infected pregnant women

Several cases of congenital toxoplasmosis have been described among children of mothers co-infected with human immunodeficiency virus (HIV) and

Toxoplasma gondii [13]. Even infections of consecutive pregnancies have been reported [38]. But this is not a common phenomenon, the risk of mother-to child transmission has been observed to be very low in chronically HIV- infected women both in Europe [39] and in USA [40] and only in those who are severely immunocompromised.

The American Academy of Pediatrics [41] recommends today that serologic testing for *Toxoplasma* should be performed on all HIV-infected pregnant women. A seropositive pregnant woman with symptomatic *Toxoplasma* infection and/or severe HIV infection (e.g. CD4 lymphocyte counts < 100 cells/mm) should receive antitoxoplasmic treatment in pregnancy in an attempt to interrupt transmission of *T. gondii* [40]. For those living in high risk areas for *Toxoplasma* infection, this advice may also be appropriate for HIV-uninfected patients who are severely immunocompromised for other reasons (e.g. patients with Hodgkin's lymphoma or systemic lupus erythematosus, who are receiving high-dose steroids) [42].

Summary

For 30 years treatment in pregnancy has been thought to reduce the mother-to-foetal transmission rate; however, no controlled randomised trial has been performed, and in previous studies the date in pregnancy of maternal infection has not been taken into account.

Recent studies have shown that maybe the hypothesis from 1970ies that the placenta acts as a barrier for the parasite and that there is a time lag before infection of the foetus, are not valid in the majority of cases. Prenatal diagnosis indicates that the foetus most likely acquires the infection soon after the maternal acquisition during the maternal parasitemia.

Prenatal antibiotic therapy after primary infection in pregnancy reduces the placental infection, but may have little or no impact on the foetal-maternal transmission rate. However, the crucial point is the outcome of the infected children. Treatment started in pregnancy has shown to reduce significantly sequelae in infected children and in particular severe sequelae at one year of age. The sooner antibiotics have been given after the maternal acquisition in pregnancy, the less frequent sequelae have been observed.

Thus, the proper management of infection in pregnancy today is to start the treatment as soon as possible after seroconversion. This however, necessitates serologic screening of pregnant women, which allows detection of women at risk of infection.

References

1. Stray-Pedersen B (1992) Toxoplasmosis in pregnancy. In: Gilbert GL (ed) Infectious Diseases. Challenges for the 1990's. Bailliere's Clinical Obstetrics and Gynaecology, Bailliere Tindall, London 17:1-107
2. Wallon M (1998) Prévention primaire et secondaire de la toxoplasmose congénitale: evaluation et propositions pour une meilleure efficacité. (Thesis, University of Lyon), pp 1-227

3. Stray-Pedersen B (1992) Treatment of Toxoplasmosis in the Pregnant Mother and Newborn Child. Scand J Infect Dis (Suppl) 84:23-31

4 WHO publication (1988) Report of the WHO consultation on Public Health Aspects of Toxoplasmosis. WHO/CDS/VPH 74:2-14

5 Schoondermark-Van de Ven E, Galama J, Vree T, Camps W, Baars I, Eskes T, Meuwissen J, Melchers W (1995) Study of Treatment of Congenital Toxoplasma gondii Infection in Rhesus Monkeys with Pyrimethamine and Sulfadiazine. Antimicrob Agents Chemother 39:137-144

6. Desmonts G, Couvreur J (1974) Congenital toxoplasmosis. A prospective study of 378 pregnancies. N Eng J of Med 290:1110-1116

7. Daffos F, Forestier F, Capella-Pavlovsky M, Thulliez P, Aufrant C, Valenti D, Cox WL (1988) Prenatal management of 746 pregnancies at risk for congenital toxoplasmosis. N Engl J Med 318:271-275

8. Schoondermark-Van de Ven E, Galama J, Camps W, Vree T, Russel F, Meuwissen J, Melchers W (1994) Pharmacokinetics of Spiramycin in the Rhesus Monkey: Transplacental Passage and Distribution in Tissue in the Fetus. Antimicrob Agents Chemother 38:1922-1929

9. Couvreur J, Desmonts G, Thulliez P (1988) Prophylaxis of congenital toxoplasmosis. Effects of spiramycin on placental infection. J Antimicrob Chemiother 22:193-200

10. Editorial (1983) Pyrimethamine combination in pregnancy. Lancet ii: 1005-1007

11. WHO publication (1990) WHO Model Prescribing Information on Drugs used in Parasitic Diseases. Geneva WHO, pp 53-60

12. Villena I, Aubert D, Leroux B, Dupouy D, Talmud M, Chemla C, Trenque T, Schmit G, Quereux C, Guenounou M, Plutot M, Bonhomme A, Pinon JM (1998) Pyrimethamine-sulfadoxine Treatment of Congenital Toxoplasmosis: Follow-up of 78 Cases Between 1980 and 1997. Scand J Infect Dis 30:295-300

13. Remington JS, McLeod R, Desmonts G (1995) Toxoplasmosis In: Remington JS, Klein JO (eds) Infectious diseases of the fetus and newborn.Vol 4 WB Saunders, Philadelphia, pp 140-267

14. Stray-Pedersen B (1996) Azithromycin Levels in Placental Tissue, Amniotic Fluid and Blood. Interscience Conference on Antimicrobial Agents and Chemotherapy, New Orleans, Sept 15-18, Abstract A68

15. Brockelhurst P, Rooney G (1998) The treatment of chlamydia trachomitis infection in pregnancy. The Cochrane Database of Systematic Reviews 4

16. Kovacs JA (1992) Efficacy of atovaquone in treatment of toxoplasmosis in patients with AIDS. Lancet 340:637-638

17. Briggs GG, Freeman RK, Yaffe SJ (eds) (1998) Drugs in Pregnancy and Lactation. Williams and Wilkins, Baltimore

18. Vergani P, Ghidini A, Ceruti P, Strobelt N, Spelta A, Zapparoli B, Rescaldani R (1998) Congenital toxoplasmosis: efficacy of maternal treatment with spiramycin alone. Am J Reprod Immun 39:335-340

19. Schoondermark-Van de Ven E, Melchers W, Camps W, Eskes T, Meuwissen J, Galama J (1994) Effectiveness of Spiramycin for Treatment of Congenital Toxoplasma gondii Infection in Rhesus Monkeys. Antimicrob Agents Chemother 38:1930-1936

20. Lebeck M, Joynson DHM, Seitz HM, Thulliez P, Gilbert RE, Dutton GN, Oevlisen B, Petersen E (1996) Classification System and Case Definitions of Toxoplasma gondii Infection in Immunocompetent Pregnant Women and Their Congenitally Infected Offspring. Eur J Clin Microbiol Infect Dis 15:799-805

21. Desmonts G, Couvreur J (1974) L'isolement du parasite dans la toxoplasmose congeni-tale. Arch Franç Péd 31:157-166

23. Couvreur J, Thulliez P, Daffos F, Aufrant C, Bompard Y, Gesquiere A, Desmonts G (1993) In utero treatment of toxoplasmic fetopathy with the combination pyrimethamine-sul-fadiazine. Fetal Diagn Ther 8:45-50

24. Eskild A, Oxman A, Magnus P, Björndal A, Bakketeig L (1996) Screening for toxoplas-mosis in pregnancy: what is the evidence of reducing a health problem? J Med Screen 3:88-194

25. Desmonts G, Couvreur J (1984) Toxoplasmose congénitale. Etude prospective de l'issue de la grossesse chez 542 femmes atteintes de toxoplasmose acquise en cours de gesta-tion. Annales de Pédiatrie 31:805-809

26. Excler JL, Piens MA, Maisonneuve H, Pujol E, Garin JP (1985) Dépistage de la toxo-plasmose acquise chez la femme enceinte et de la toxoplasmose congénitale chez le nou-veau-né. Lyon Med 253:3-38
27. Lambotte R, Bassleer J, Beaudouin PH, Senterre J, Lhoist R (1976) Toxoplasmose congé-nitale: evaluation du bénéfice thérapeutique prénatal. J Gynecol Obstet Biol Reprod (Paris) 5:265-269
28. Douche C, Benabdesselam A, Mokhtari F, Le Mer Y (1996) Value of prevention of conge-nital toxoplasmosis. J Fr Ophtalmol 19:330-334
29. Wallon M, Peyron F, Lebech M, Petersen E, Gilbert R, Dunn D (1997) Prenatal treatment and the risk of congenital toxoplasmosis: preliminary findings from two cohort studies. European Society for Pediatric Research, Hungary
30. Lebech M, Andersen O, Christensen NC, Nielsen HE, Hertel J, Peitersen B, Rechnitzer C, Larsen SO, Norgaard-Pedersen B, Petersen E (1999) Feasibility of neonatal screening for *Toxoplasma* infection in the absence of prenatal treatment. Danish Congenital Toxoplasmosis Study Group. Lancet 353:1834-7
31. Foulon W, Villena I, Stray-Pedersen B, Decoster A, Lappalainen M, Pinon M, Jenum PA, Hedman K, Naessens A (1999) Treatment of toxoplasmosis during pregnancy: a multi-center study of impact on fetal transmission and children's sequelae at one year of age. American J Obstet Gynecol 180:410-5
32. Hohlfeld P, Daffos F, Thulliez P, Aufrant C, Couvreur J, MacAleese J, Descombey D, Forestier F (1989) Fetal toxoplasmosis: Outcome of pregnancy and infant follow-up after in utero treatment. J Pediatrics 115:765-769
33. Dunn D, Wallon M, Peyron F, Petersen E, Peckham C, Gilbert R (1999) Mother-to-child transmission of toxoplasmosis: Risk estimates for clinical counselling. Lancet 353:1829-1833
34. Berrebi A, Kobuch WE, Bessieres MH, Bloom MC, Rolland M, Sarramon MF, Roques C, Fournie A (1994) Termination of pregnancy for maternal toxoplasmosis. Lancet 344:36-39
35. Wallon M, Gandilhon F, Peyron F, Mojon M (1994) Toxoplasmosis in pregnancy (letter). Lancet 344:541
36. Daffos F, Mirlesse V, Hohlfeld P, Jacquemard F, Thulliez P, Forestier F (1994) Toxoplasmosis in pregnancy (Letter). Lancet 344:541
37. Jenum PA (1999) Diagnosis and epidemiology of *Toxoplasma gondii* infection among pregnant women in Norway (Thesis, National Institute of Public Health), pp 1-412
38. Mitchell CD, Erlich SS, Mastrucci MT, Hutto SC, Parks W, Scott GB (1990) Congenital toxoplasmosis occurring in infants perinatally infected with human immunodeficiency virus 1. Pediatr Infect Dis J 9:512
39. Dunn D, Newell ML, Gilbert R (1997) Low risk of congenital toxoplasmosis in children infected with human immunodeficiency virus. Ped Infect Dis J 16(1):84
40. Minkoff H, Remington JS, Holman S, Ramirez R, Goodwin S, Landesman S (1997) Vertical transmission of *Toxoplasma* by human immunodeficiency virus-infected women. Am J Obstet Gynecol 176:555-559
41. American Academy of Pediatrics (1998) Antiretroviral Therapy and Medical Management of Pediatric HIV Infection. Pediatrics 102(4S-II):1005-1062
42. Wong S-Y, Remington JS (1994) State-of-the-art clinical article. Clin Inf Dis 18:853-862

3.1. Clinical picture. Neonatal signs and symptoms

M. HAYDE, A. POLLAK

Introduction

Postnatal infection with the protozoan *Toxoplasma gondii* is clinically asymptomatic in up to 90 percent of cases [1]. Since the pathogenicity of the parasite for the immunocompetent individual is limited, the course of infection with *Toxoplasma gondii* is subclinical in most cases, despite the generalized character of the infection with subsequent parasitemia of the host.

While postnatal infection predominantly occurs by oral uptake of viable oocysts, prenatal infection occurs only if pregnancy and primary maternal infection coincide. The parasitemia which follows maternal infection leads to placental infection and placental lesions, resulting in secondary fetal infection via hematogenous propagation.

For the unborn, infection with the parasite can be disastrous. The severity of clinical symptoms increases with the duration of fetal exposure to the parasite. Infection in early pregnancy is usually incompatible with survival of the unborn because of substantial damage of the trophoblast. Thus, overt clinical infection meets more the definition of a fetopathy rather than embryopathy [2]. Fetal infection with *Toxoplasma gondii* can cause either congenital *Toxoplasma* infection or congenital toxoplasmosis.

The term "congenital *Toxoplasma* infection" should be used for an infection which had occured during pregnancy, but without apparent clinical signs and symptoms in the newborn. Diagnosis of fetal infection is done by direct detection of the parasite in amniotic fluid with the polymerase chain reaction, by mice inoculation of amniotic fluid or by tissue culture [3, 4]. Postnatally, congenital *Toxoplasma* infection is confirmed by follow-up-serology, if persisting or increasing titers of *Toxoplasma*-specific antibodies in a clinically healthy child are observed. During antiparasitic treatment of the child specific antibodies may disappear but reappear after cessation of treatment in infected children.

The term "congenital toxoplasmosis" is used, if an infected fetus or child later in life develops symptoms typical for *toxoplasma* infection. In only a small proportion of neonates with congenital toxoplasmosis all three signs of the classic triad, hydrocephalus, intracerebral calcifications and retinochoroiditis (Figs 1-6) first described by Wolf will be observed, in the majority of the cases only one or two of these symptoms are apparent [5].

Ten percent of congenitally infected neonates are showing structural damage at birth (congenital toxoplasmosis), the others are subclinical (congenital *Toxoplasma* infection) [6] but might develop visual impairment or even amaurosis due to retinochoroiditis later in life if not treated appropriately [1, 7].

Children with subclinical infection may also develop other neurologic sequelae. The spectrum ranges from hydro- or microcephalus to psychomotor retardation, seizures and deafness [8].

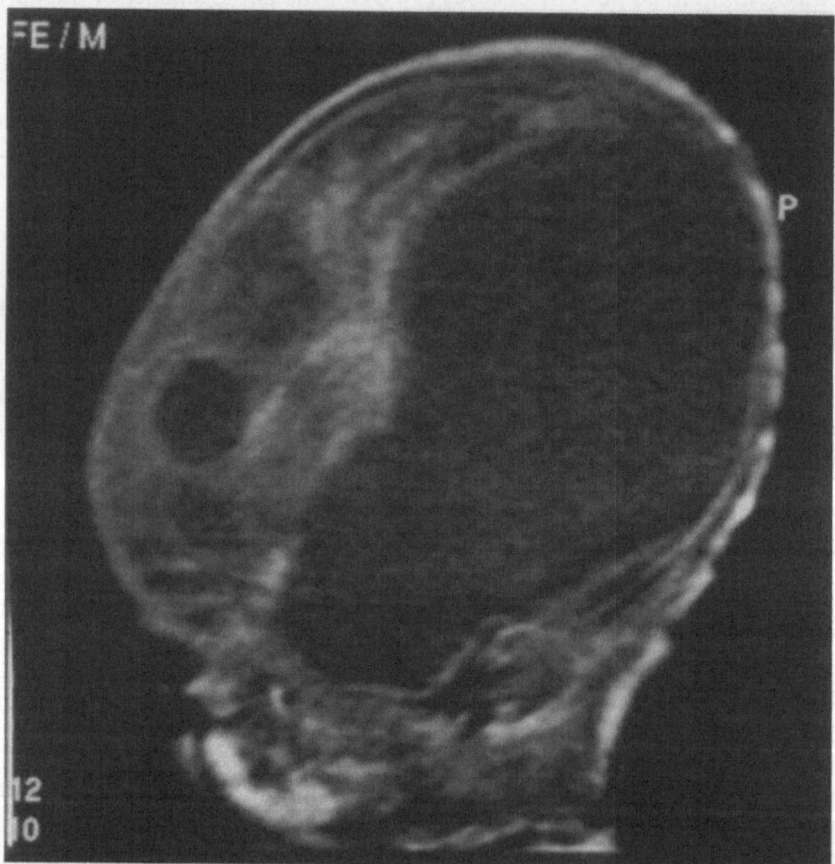

Fig. 1. Magnetic resonance imaging of the brain of a girl, age two days with hydrocaephalus (gestational week 32). Bulbus and orbita are developed only rudimentary (microphthalmus). Ventricular dilatation with parieto-occipital accentuation. Rarification of brain tissue in the temporo-parieto-occipital region. Delayed cortical maturation approximating gestational weeks 24-26

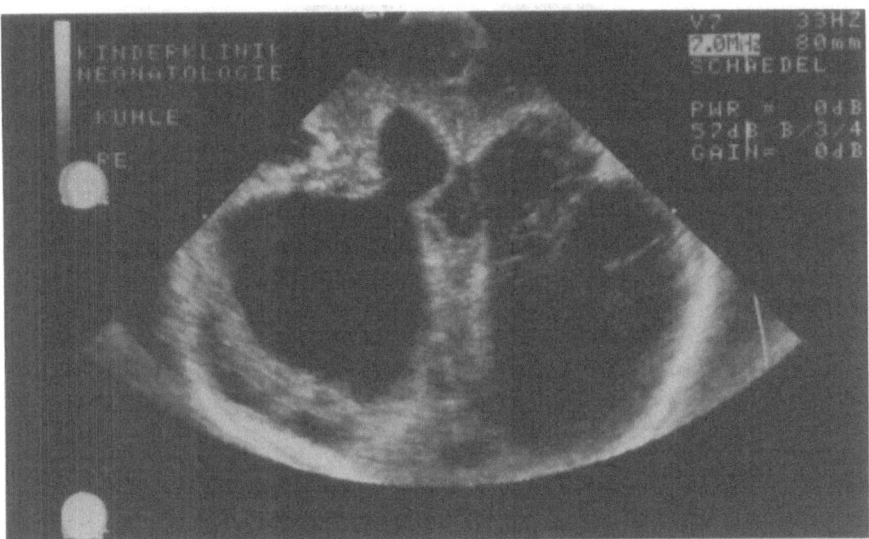

Fig. 2. Brain ultrasonography of a female neonate with intracerebral calcification (*arrow*) and hydrocephalus

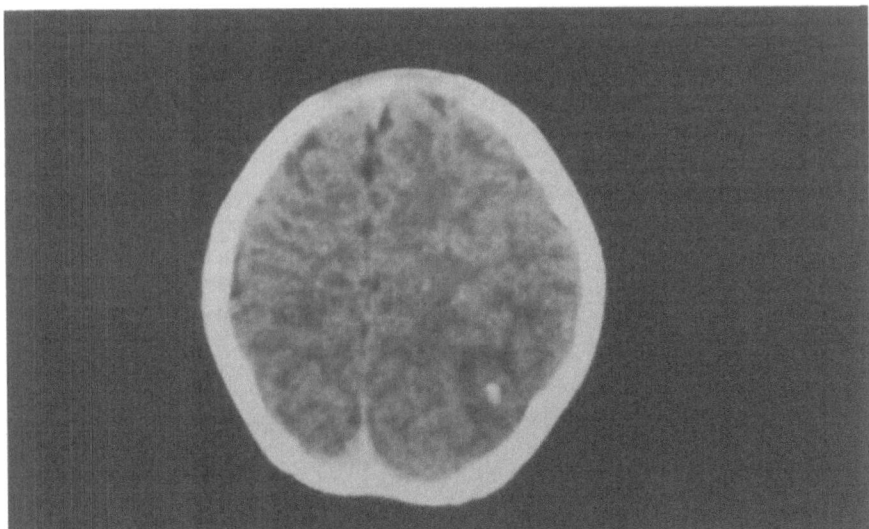

Fig. 3. CT-scan of an infected neonate with intracerebral calcification

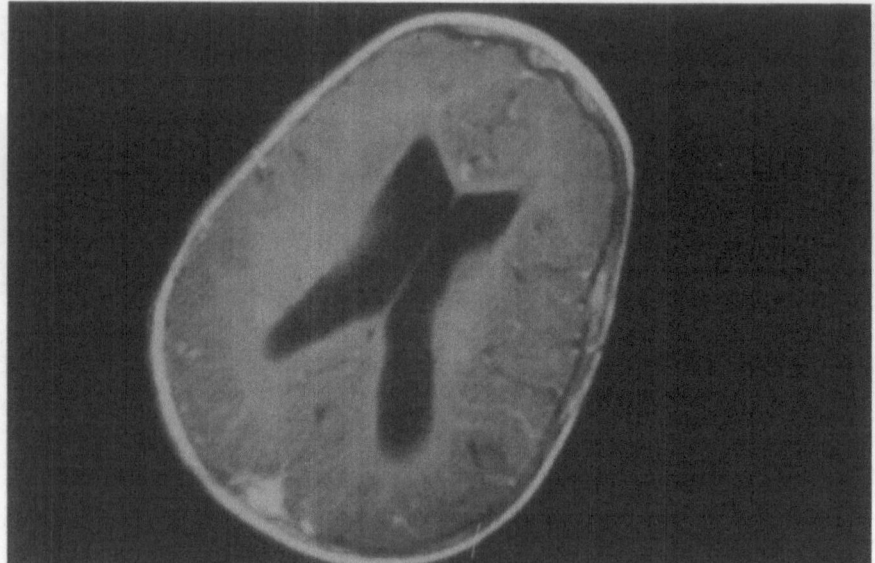

Fig. 4. MRI scan of same neonate (Image 3) showing ventricular dilatation

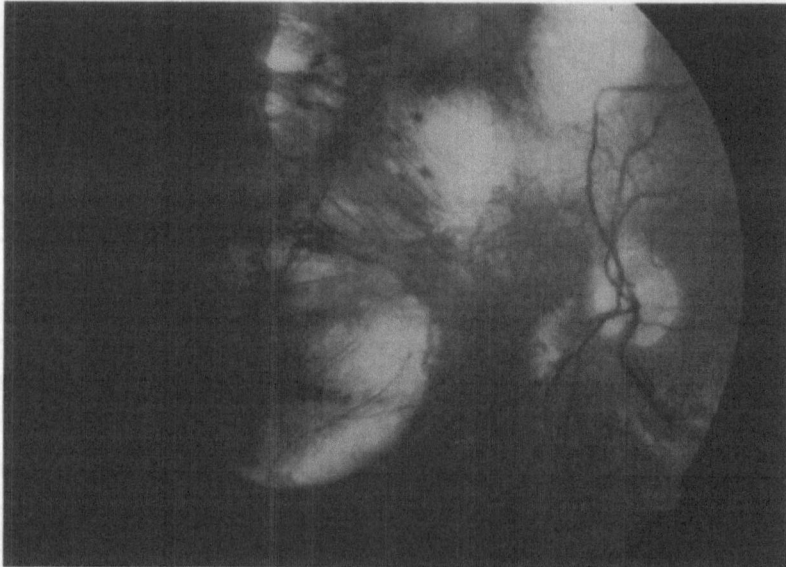

Fig. 5. Ocular fundus with old retinochoroidal lesions in the nasal region between the big vessels. The posterior pole and the macula are free of lesions

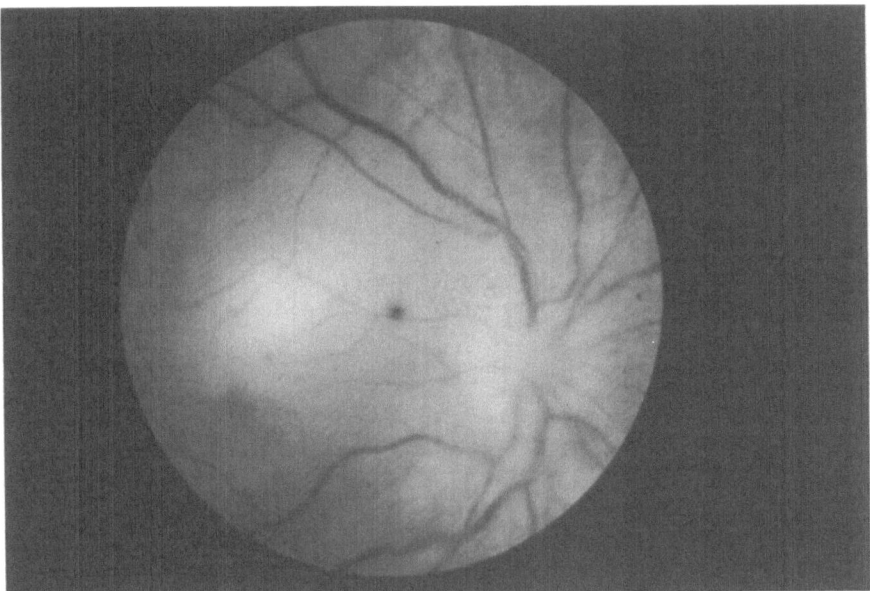

Fig. 6. Ocular fundus of an infected newborn with acute retinochoroiditis

Infection and clinical picture

A strong relationship exists between the timepoint of fetal infection relative to birth (i.e. duration of fetal exposure to the parasite) and the type fetal injury [6]. Other factors, such as length of fetal incubation time (i.e. time difference between maternal and fetal parasitemia), maternal antibody transfer to the fetus, infection dose and strain virulence may also play important roles [9]. As a consequence of the interaction of these factors, the clinical picture of congenital toxoplasmosis varies from asymptomatic to severe manifestation.

Figure 6 is displayed for a better understanding of factors which lead to different clinical manifestations of the fetal disease. The scheme summarizes Thalhammer's hypothesis of sequence of events in which the parasite damages the fetus.

Three clinical entities can be differentiated. They are consecutive stages of the same process occuring in a rather uniform manner. According to the duration of fetal infection one can differentiate: 1) the stage of generalization; 2) the stage of acute encephalitis, and 3) the stage of postencephalitic damage. Until today this model is the basis for categorizing neonatal *Toxoplasma*-associated diseases [10, 11].

The clinical classification into four different neonatal disorders by Remington et al. [1] is based on Thalhammer's observations (Table 1). In Desmonts and Couvreur's clinical classification of the disease [12] similar considerations are applied (Table 2).

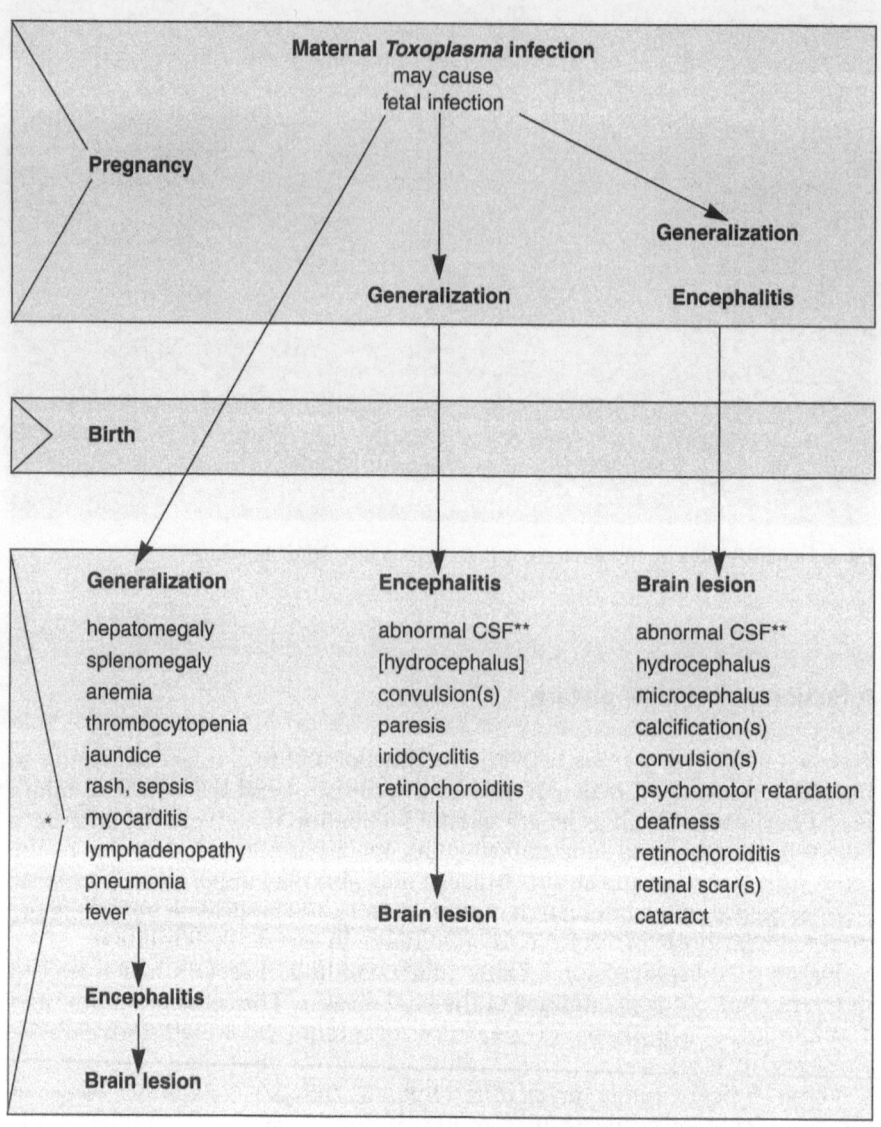

Fig. 6. Scheme of congenital toxoplasmosis. The clinical picture apparent at birth depends
on the stage of the fetal infection relative to the timepoint of birth

Table 1. Four forms of congenital *Toxoplasma* infection [1]

1. Neonatal disease
Severely affected newborn with symptoms of generalized infection, signs referable to CNS always present. Formation of sequelae not mitigated by treatment

2. Disease manifesting during the first months of life
Children are diagnosed to be infected months after birth independently from severity of symptoms (late recognition of disease), but also children in which manifestation of symptoms occurs late, which were normal at birth (delayed onset of disease). Disease with delayed onset may be severe and occurs most often in premature infants; in full-term infants course is usually mild. Signs and symptoms may disappear after treatment

3. Disease manifesting later in life
Sequelae or relapse of a previously undiagnosed infection during infancy, childhood or adolescence. Mostly retinochoroiditis, rarely neurological symptoms (convulsions) or stenosis of aquaeduct (hydrocephalus)

4. Subclinical infection
90 percent of infected children may be clinically normal and just show persistent or even rising IgG-titers. They may suffer no untoward sequelae or may develop retinochorioiditis, deafness, hydrocephaly, psychomotor or mental retardation years later

Table 2. Classification of congenital *Toxoplasma* infection according to clinical signs by Desmonts and Couvreur [12]

1. The child with neurological disorder
Hydrocephalus, microcephalus, microphthalmus with or without retinochoroiditis. Symptoms may be present at birth or may be diagnosed later (diagnosis of hydrocephalus as a sign of postencephalitic cerebral damage after months of normal psychomotor development)

2. The child with severe, generalized illness
Maculopapular exanthema, purpura, pneumonia, severe and prolonged jaundice, hepatosplenomegaly. Uveitis and ventricular enlargement may be be still absent

3. The child with mild disorder and solitary signs of prenatal infection
Hepatosplenomegaly and jaundice with or without thrombocytopenia occur as unspecific symptoms. Their relationship with congenital *Toxoplasma* infection is often established retrospectively after detection of retinochoroidal foci

4. The child with subclinical infection

In comprehensive retrospective studies of infected newborns originating from pregnancies, where infection was not identified and therefore not treated, a variety of symptoms and severe organ manifestations were described [13-16]. The severity of organ damage is probably a function of the timespan of undisturbed action of the parasite on fetal tissues, preferentially on neurological tissue such as brain and eyes.

In the more recent studies, in which antiparasitic treatment was offered to pregnant women, fewer babies were reported to be severely affected. Therefore, an attempt to characterize the clinical picture as completely as possible may lack actuality [17].

Table 3a. Neonates with congenital toxoplasmosis without prenatal treatment. Frequency of occurrence of ocular symptoms at birth in per cent

Reference	Roizen [23]	McAuley [18]	Guerina [19]	Eichenwald [14]	Alford [16]	Koppe [24]
Number of newborns	36	29	5	44	10	5
Retinochoroiditis/retinal scar	56	59	100	66	20	80
Uveitis	–	–	20	–	–	–
Vitritis	–	–	20	–	–	–
Blindness	–	–	40	–	–	–
Microphthalmus	22	24	–	–	–	–

Table 3b. Neonates with congenital toxoplasmosis without prenatal treatment. Frequency of occurrence of neurological symptoms at birth in per cent

Reference	Roizen [23]	McAuley [18]	Guerina [19]	Eichenwald [14]	Alford [16]	Koppe [24]
Number of newborns (n)	36	29	5	44	10	5
Hydrocephalus	44	34	80	–	10	–
Microcephalus	14	17	20	–	–	–
Cerebral atrophy	–	–	80	–	–	–
Intracerebral calcifications	72	66	100	4	–	–
Seizures	17	17	–	18	–	–
Pathological muscular tonus	58	66	–	–	–	–
Abnormal neurologic exam	–	–	–	–	10	–
Abnormal CSF●	59	69	–	84	80	20
Abnormal white matter density	56	59	–	–	–	–

●) Abnormal cerebrospinal fluid: pleocytosis and/or increased protein and/or parasites detected

Table 3c. Neonates with congenital toxoplasmosis without prenatal treatment. Systemic symptoms at birth in per cent

Reference	Roizen [23]	McAuley [18]	Guerina [19]	Eichenwald [14]	Alford [16]
Number of newborns	36	29	5	44	10
Hepatomegaly	50	62	20	77	10
Splenomegaly	56	69	–	90	10
Jaundice	64	76	20	80	10
Rash	14	17	–	25	–
Lymphadenopathy	–	–	–	68	–
Anemia	17	21	–	77	10
Thrombocytopenia	39	48	–	–	10
Eosinophilia	–	–	–	18	–
Abnormal bleeding	–	–	–	18	–
Hypoglycemia	19	24	–	–	–
Hypoxemia	11	14	–	–	–
Hypothermia	–	–	–	20	–
Fever	11	10	–	77	–
Pneumonia	8	10	–	41	–
Vomiting	–	–	–	48	–
Diarrhea	–	–	–	25	–
Neutropenia	3	3	–	–	–
Sepsis	–	48	–	–	–
Respiratory distress	17	21	–	–	–
Petechiae	17	21	–	–	–

In order to describe signs and symptoms of affected newborns with congenital disease more precisely, available data were categorized depending on whether treatment was offered to the mother or not.

In Tables 3a-3c, ocular, neurological and systemic symptoms are listed. More often, individual symptoms of the classic triad (hydrocephalus, intracerebral calcifications and retinochoroiditis) were observed, rarely the complete triad [5, 14].

In Table 3c the frequency of systemic symptoms in newborns from untreated pregnancies is shown. According to Thalhammer (Fig. 1: generalized disease), Remington et al. (Table 1: neonatal disease), Desmonts and Couvreur (Table 2: the child with severe, generalized disease) these symptoms are observed if birth and fetal generalization coincide. Fetal *Toxoplasma* infection might result in prematurity and/or intrauterine growth retardation. In the studies of Mc Auley, Alford and Couvreur prematurity was observed in 38, 50 and 14 per cent, whereas intrauterine growth retardation were seen in 20 and 14 per cent respectively. Children born to treated mothers appear to show more often postencephalitic lesions than symptoms of generalized disease such as those listed in Table 3c.

Table 4a. Fetal outcome data after maternal infection and prenatal treatment

Reference	Hohlfeld [21]	Daffos [22]	Couvreur [25]	Gratzl [3]	Villena [26]
Pregnancies	1270*	746	500	49	676
Not infected	1180 (92,9)**	702 (94,2)	396 (79,2)	38 (77,6)	598 (88,5)
Termination	34 (2,6)	24 (3,2)	0	1 (2,0)	0
Subclinical at birth	44 (3,5)	12 (1,6)	47 (9,4)	7 (14,3)	65 (9,6)
Clinical disease at birth	11 (0,9)	7 (0,9)	56 (11,2)	2 (4,1)	13 (1,9)
Neonatal death	1 (0,1)	1 (0,1)	1 (0,2)	1 (2,0)	0

* absolute numbers; ** (per cent)

Table 4b. Neonates with congenital toxoplasmosis after prenatal treatment. Frequency of occurrence of symptoms and organ manifestations detected at birth in per cent

Reference	Hohlfeld $ [21]	Daffos # [22]	Daffos $ [22]	Couvreur § [25]	Couvreur $ [25]	Gratzl § [3]	Villena $ [26]
Number of newborns	11	5	2	22	34	2	13
Retinochoroiditis/retinal scar	27	–	50	50	44	50	77
Microphthalmus	–	–	–	–	–	–	15
Hydrocephalus	–	20	50	–	3	50	23
Meningoencephalitis	–	–	50	–	–	–	–
Ventricular dilatation	9	–	–	–	–	50	–
Intracerebral calcifications	73	80	50	55	32	–	46
Seizures	–	–	–	–	3	–	–
Pathological muscular tonus	–	–	–	5	3	–	–
Abnormal CSF•	9	–	–	32	15	–	–

#) all women were treated from diagnosis onwards throughout pregnancy with sulfadiazine/pyrimethamine
§) pregnant women were treated with pyrimethamine+sulfonamides and spiramycine
$) pregnant women were treated with spiramycine alone
•) abnormal cerebrospinal fluid: pleocytosis and/or increased protein and/or parasites detected

In Table 4a fetal outcome data from five studies are listed. These data refer to pregnancies where infection was detected and a treatment was subsequently initiated.

In Table 4b frequency of symptoms and signs of organ manifestations after prenatal treatment are listed. Interestingly, the typical symptoms of generalized disease were not described, perhaps as a result of fetal treatment. Neonates treated prenatally, predominantly suffer from intracerebral calcifications, ventricular dilatation and retinal scars of past retinochoroiditis.

References

1. Remington JS, McLeod R, Desmonts G (1995) Toxoplasmosis. In: Remington JS, Klein JO (eds) Infectious diseases of the fetus and newborn infant. 4th edn, Philadelphia, WB Saunders, pp 140-267
2. Thalhammer O (1983) Toxoplasmose und Schwangerschaft. Prophylaxe, Früherkennung und Therapie. Zbl Gynäkol 105:1086-1092
3. Gratzl R, Hayde M, Kohlhauser Ch, Hermon M, Burda G, Strobl W, Pollak A (1998) Follow-up of Infants with Congenital Toxoplasmosis detected by polymerase chain reaction analysis of amniotic fluid. Eur J Clin Microbiol Inf Dis 17:853-858
4. Hayde M, Pollak A, Gratzl R, Hermon M, Trittenwein G, Häusler M, Arzt W, Bernaschek G (1996) Die Bedeutung der Nachsorge von Kindern mit pränataler Toxoplasma-Infektion. Mitt Oesterr Ges Tropenmed Parasitol 18:125-130
5. Wolf A, Cowen D, Paige BH (1939) Toxoplasmic encephalomyelitis. A case of granulomatous encephalomyelitis due to a protozoan. Am J Pathol 15:657-694
6. Desmonts G, Couvreur J (1979) Congenital toxoplasmosis: a prospective study of 542 women who acquired toxoplasmosis during pregnancy. In: Thalhammer O, Baumgarten K, Pollak A (eds), Pathophysiology of congenital disease, Perinatal Medicine 6th European Congress, Georg Thieme, Stuttgart, pp. 51-60
7. Koppe JG, Kloostermann GJ, Roever-Bonnet H, Eckert-Stroink JA, Loewer-Sieger DH, Bruijne JI (1974) Toxoplasmosis and pregnancy, with a long-term follow up of the children. Eur J Obstet Gynaecol Reprod Biol 4:101-110
8. Wilson CB, Remington JS, Stagno S, Reynolds DW (1980) Development of adverse sequeleae in children born with subclinical congenital toxoplasma infection. Pediatrics 66:767-774
9. Thalhammer O (1967) Pränatale Erkrankungen des Menschen. Georg Thieme Verlag, Stuttgart, pp 121-157
10. Thalhammer O (1966) Die angeborene Toxoplasmose. In: Kirchhoff H, Kräubig H (eds). Toxoplasmose. Georg Thieme, Stuttgart, pp. 161-173
11. Raue W (1975) Die Klinik der konnatalen Toxoplasmose. In: Wildführ G, Wildführ W (eds). Toxoplasmose. VWB Gustav Fischer Verlag, Jena, pp. 135-150
12. Desmonts G, Couvreur J (1974) Toxoplasmosis. In: Conn RB (ed) Current diagnosis 7. WB Saunders Company, Philadelphia, pp. 274-297
13. Feldman HA (1958) Toxoplasmosis. Pediatrics 22:559-574
14. Eichenwald HA (1960) A study of congenital toxoplasmosis, with particular emphasis on clinical manifestations, sequelae and therapy. In: Siim JC (ed) Human Toxoplasmosis. Munksgaard, Copenhagen, pp 41-49
15. Couvreur J, Desmonts G (1962) Congenital and maternal toxoplasmosis. Dev Med Child Neurol 4:519-530
16. Alford CA, Stagno S, Reynolds DW (1974) Congenital toxoplasmosis: clinical, laboratory and therapeutical considerations, with special reference to subclinical disease. Bull NY Acad Med 50:160-181
17. Chatterton JMW (1992) Pregnancy. In: HoYen D, Alex WL Joss (eds) Human Toxoplasmosis, Medical Publications, Oxford, New York, Tokyo, pp.144-183
18. McAuley J, Boyer KM, Patel D, Mets M, Swisher C, Roizen N, Wolters C, Stein L, Stein M, Schey W, Remington J, Meier P, Johnson D, Heydeman P, Holfels E, Withers S, Mack D, Brown C, Patton D, McLeod R (1994) Early and Longitudinal Evaluations of Treated Infants and Children and Untreated Historical Patients with Congenital Toxoplasmosis: The Chicago Collaborative Treatment Trial. Clin Inf Dis 18:38-72
19. Guerina NG, Hsu HW, Meissner CH, Maguire JH, Lynfield R, Stechenberg B, Abroms I, Pasternack MS, Hoff R, Eaton RB, Grady GF (1994) Neonatal serologic screening and early treatment for Congenital Toxoplasma gondii infection. N Engl J Med 330:1858-1863

20. Couvreur J, Demonts G, Tournier G, et al (1984) Étude d'une série homogène de 210 cases de toxoplasmose congénitale chez des nourissons agés de 0 a 11 mois et dépistes de facon prospective. Annales de Pediatrie 31:815-819
21. Hohlfeld P, Daffos F, Thulliez Ph, Aufrant C, Couvreur J, MacAleese J, Descombey D, Forestier F (1989) Fetal toxoplasmosis: Outcome of pregnancy and infant follow-up after in utero treatment. J Pediatrics 115:765-769
22. Daffos F, Forestier F, Capella-Pavlovsky M, Thulliez Ph, Aufrant C, Valenti D, Cox WL (1988) Prenatal management of 746 pregnancies at risk for congenital toxoplasmosis. N Engl J Med 318:271-275
23. Roizen N, Swisher CN, Stein MA, Hopkins J, Boyer KM, Holfels E, Mets MB, Stein L, Patel D, Meier P, Withers S, Remington J, Mack D, Heydemann PT, Patton D, McLeod R (1995) Neurologic and developmental outcome in treated congenital toxoplasmosis. Pediatrics 1:11-20
24. Koppe JG, Loewer-Sieger DH, Roever-Bonnet H (1986) Results of 20-Year Follow-up of Congenital Toxoplasmosis. Lancet 1:254-255
25. Couvreur J, Thulliez Ph, Daffos F, Aufrant Ch, Bompard Y, Gesquière A, Desmonts G (1993) In utero Treatment of Toxoplasmic Fetopathy with the Combination Pyrimethamine-Sulfadiazine. Fetal Diagn Ther 8:45-50
26. Villena I, Aubert D, Leroux B, Dupouy D, Talmud M, Chemla C, Trenque T, Schmit G, Quereux C, Guenounou M, Pluot M, Bonhomme A, Pinon JM (1998) Pyrimethamine-sulfadoxine Treatment of Congenital Toxoplasmosis: Follow-up of 78 cases between 1980 and 1997. Scand J Infect Dis 30:295-300

3.2. Ophthalmology in the neonate with congenital toxoplasmosis

A.P. Brézin

Introduction

Congenital infection by *Toxoplasma gondii* is a leading cause of visual impairment in children and the most frequent infectious etiology. Although congenital toxoplasmosis may affect many organs, eye manifestations are the most common. Lesions of retinochoroiditis affect visual function according to their localization relative to the macula and to the optic disc. After the neonatal period, scarred lesions of retinochoroiditis may reactivate or new lesions may appear. Therefore, in cases of congenital toxoplasmosis, even when fundus examination is normal at birth, a careful long-term ophthalmic follow-up is necessary.

Ophthalmic examination: goals and methods

Visual function

Visual function refers to a variety of studies that evaluate visual acuity, binocular interaction, color vision and visual field. Only visual acuity may be assessed in the first year of life. Before 2.5 to 3 years, when children become able to accomplish subjective visual acuity tests, the ability to " fixate and follow " a target is the principal acuity test used to assess central visual function. While at birth no reliable method to assess visual acuity is available, the accuracy of visual acuity testing increases with the age of children. In some children with severe congenital toxoplasmosis, cognitive deficits may prevent in the long term adequate testing of visual acuity.

The impact of chorioretinal lesions on visual acuity is a function of their localization relative to the optic disc and to the macula (Figs. 1-3). Non macular lesions do not affect visual acuity, except in cases of macular dragging, observed in the presence of large necrotic peripheral retinochoroiditis (Fig. 4). When strictly central and extensive, macular lesions are systematically associated with poor visual acuity. In other cases, the impact of macular lesions on visual function depends on the degree of sparing of the fovea, which is the central part of the macula. In their study of the eye manifestations of 94 children with congenital toxoplasmosis, Mets et al. [1] have shown that, in some cases, visual acuity may be significantly better than anticipated from the appearance of the macula in the retinal examination. When macular lesions are present in both eyes, even with similar appearance, asymetrical visual acuities are often observed. Although a central chorioretinal lesion has an impact on visual acuity, the peripheral visual field remains intact.

Eye movement and alignment are assessed during each pediatric ophthalmic examination. Convergent and divergent deviations of the eyes are referred, respectively, as esotropias and exotropias. Children with a loss of central fixation in one eye linked to a macular chorioretinal lesion are at a high risk of strabismus. These deviations are not observed in the immediate neonatal period, but appear secondarily. When bilateral macular lesions are present, sensory deprivation nystagmus may frequently be observed.

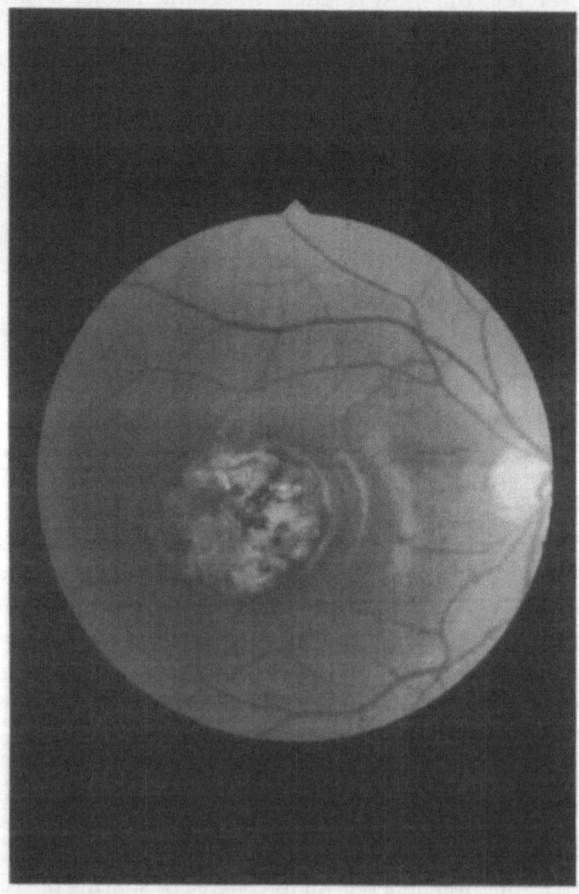

Fig. 1. Central scarred, pigmented and atrophic retinochoroiditis. Visual Acuity < 20/200

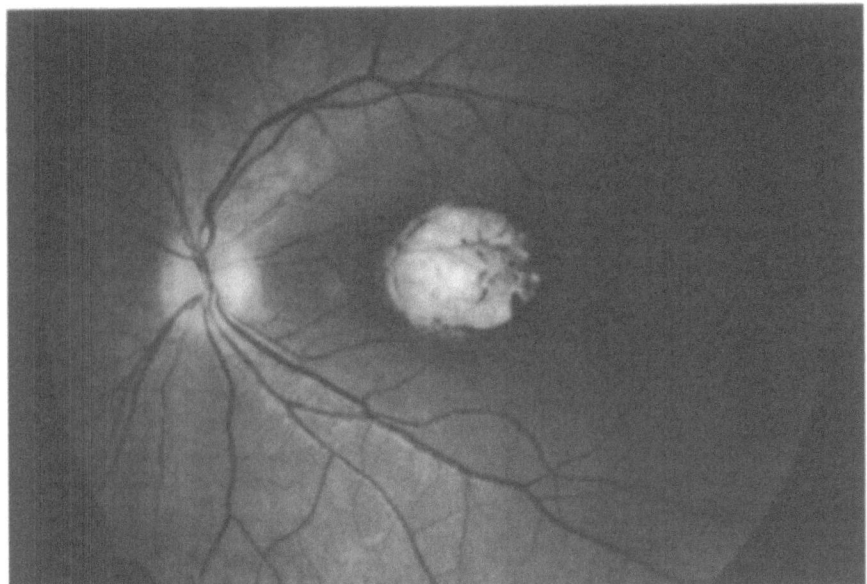

Fig. 2. As in figure 1

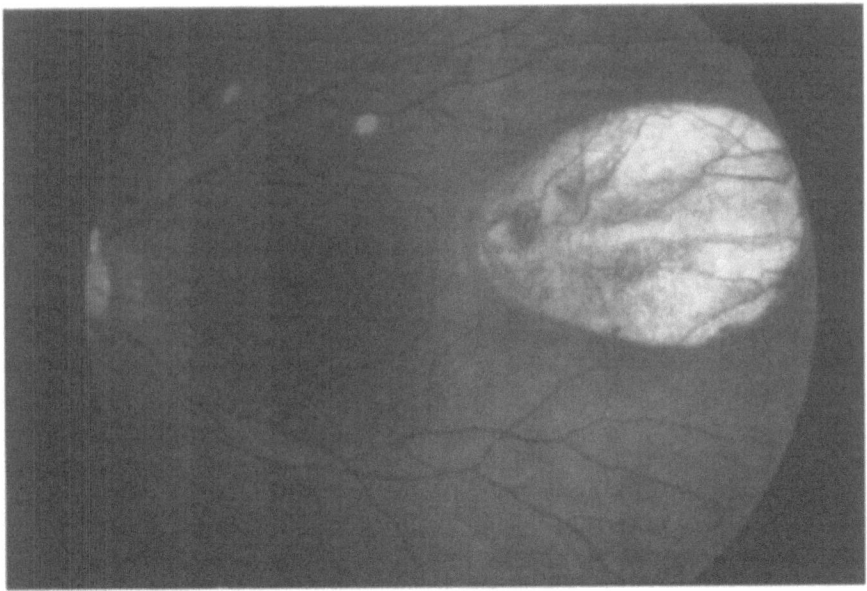

Fig. 3. Extensive, scarred, pigmented and atrophic retinochoroiditis, temporal to the macula. Visual Acuity 20/20

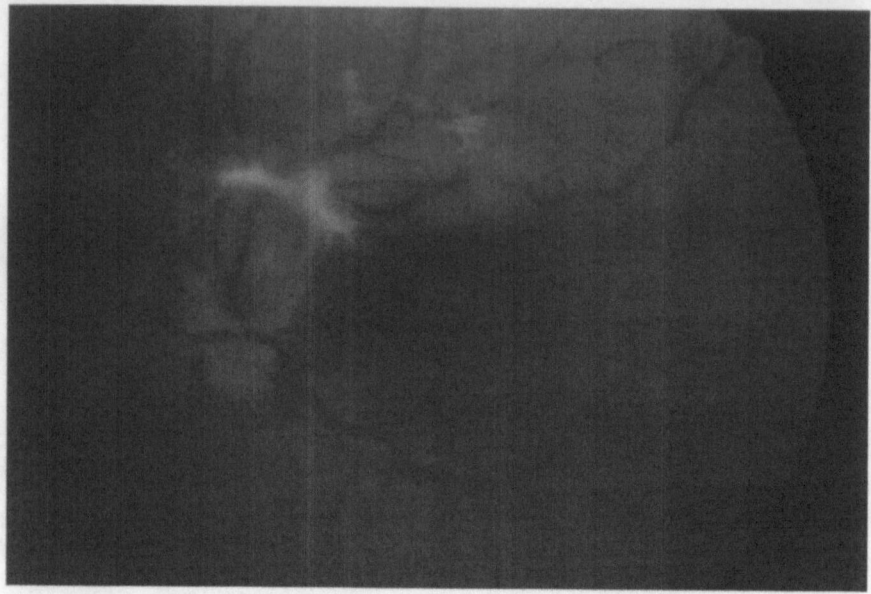

Fig. 4. Macular dragging, secondary to an extensive peripheral toxoplasmic necrosis (not seen on photograph)

Examination of the anterior segment

The slit-lamp is the instrument used for the examination of the anterior segment of the eye (cornea, anterior chamber, iris and lens). Portable slit-lamps are particularly useful to examine uncooperative preverbal children.

The anterior segment is not the primary site of manifestations in ocular toxoplasmosis. However, prolonged severe inflammation of the vitreous may yield, by contiguity, an anterior uveitis and/or secondary cataracts. The most severe cases of congenital toxoplasmosis affect the development of the eye, leading to microphthalmia, microcornea or even phtisis.

Examination of the posterior segment

Pupillary dilatation, usually by 1 percent tropicamide, is necessary for a correct examination of the fundus. Although still widely used in many European practices because of its portability and simplicity, the direct ophthalmoscope should not be used in neonates with congenital toxoplasmosis. Its inadequacies include a field of vision covering only about 8 degrees of the fundus and limitations to visualize the peripheral retina.

The binocular indirect ophthalmoscope, used with a hand-held 28 or 30 Diopters lens, is the instrument of choice to screen for toxoplasmic lesions. Its field of view up to 58° allows a good visualization of the fundus, even in uncooperative, crying children. An eyelid speculum is often necessary.

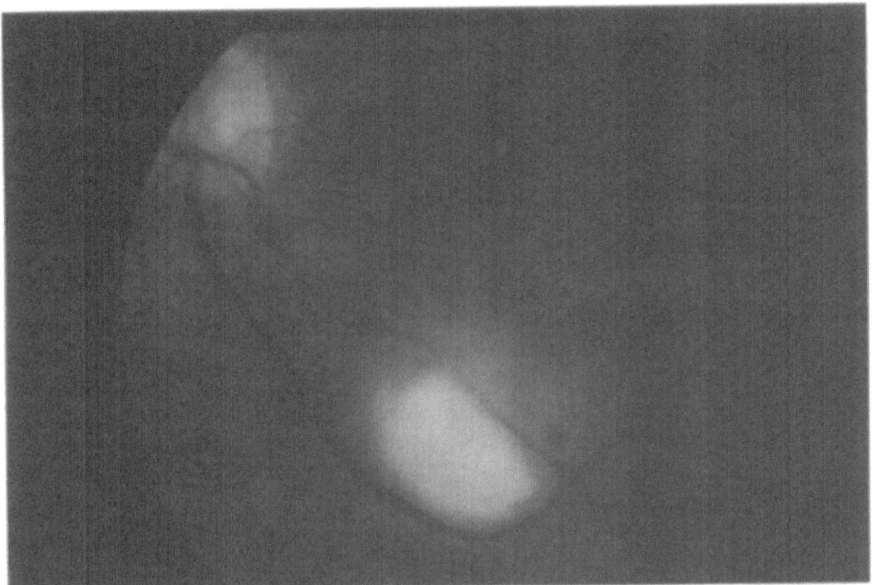

Fig. 5. Active, white, retinochoroiditis, with adjacent vasculitis. A pigmented dot on the supero-temporal edge of the active retinochoroiditis is evocative of an older, scarred lesion

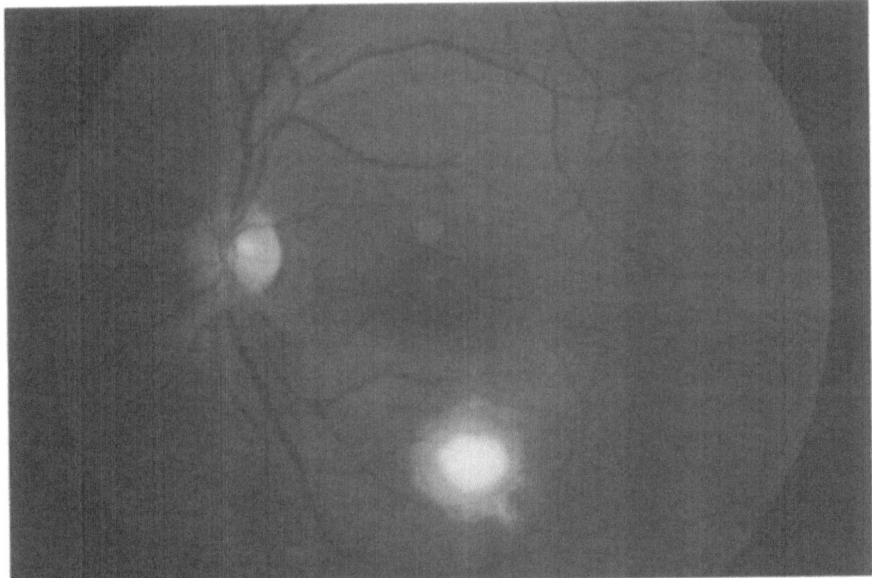

Fig. 6. Active, white, retinochoroiditis. The onset of scarring is seen as a more pigmented ring around the active lesion

Results of fundus examination should be reported on standardized drawings, indicating the size of lesions (the unit is the disc diameter) and their localization in regard to the disc, macula and retinal vessels.

An active retinochoroiditis is characterized by a whitish and edematous area, often with neighboring vasculitis (Figs 5, 6). Scarred lesions are pigmented and/or atrophic scars.

Schedule of ophthalmic examinations

In cases of congenital toxoplasmosis, ophthalmic examinations should not be limited to the neonatal period. Lesions may be absent at birth or may not have been visualized during the first examination. Children and their parents should be educated to the symptoms associated with recurrences or new lesions of active retinochoroiditis. The perception of floatters must alert children as an early sign of intraocular inflammation associated with vitritis.

However, before the age of 7 years, children are frequently unable to report symptoms associated with active chorioretinis.

For the purpose of our current long term prospective study of the ophthalmic outcome of congenital toxoplasmosis, we perform repeated eye examinations every 3 months in the first year, twice a year in the second year and every year until the age of 7. In the general practice of ophthalmology, the first manifestations of active ocular toxoplasmosis are usually observed between 15 and 30 years of age and occasionally in older patients. For example, in a Dutch study of 149 patients with active toxoplasmic retinochoroiditis, the mean age of patients was 27 years [2]. Numerous adult cases of ocular toxoplasmosis, secondary to acquired infection, are documented [3-5]. Among late cases of active retinochoroiditis, the percentage secondary to a congenital infection is unknown, but the assessment of the definitive ophthalmic outcome of congenital toxoplasmosis requires a long term follow-up.

Ophthalmic outcome

Data from experimental models

Experimental models of ocular toxoplasmosis have yielded different results according to the virulence of the strains of Toxoplasma gondii and the modes of infection. In the murine model of congenital infection investigated by Dutton et al. [6], cataracts and/or severe active uveitis was generally observed. In this study, as in humans, the severity of disease was not correlated to serological titres against Toxoplasma gondii. In an acquired murine model of T. gondii infection using the avirulent ME 49 strain, cysts could be observed in the retina, including in the absence of surrounding tissue damage or secondary inflammation (Figs 7-9) [7]. These findings confirm that cysts may remain latent and inapparent in the eye. Data from this experimental model highlight the need for a long term ophthalmic follow-up in children with congenital toxoplasmosis, even when the initial fundus examination is normal.

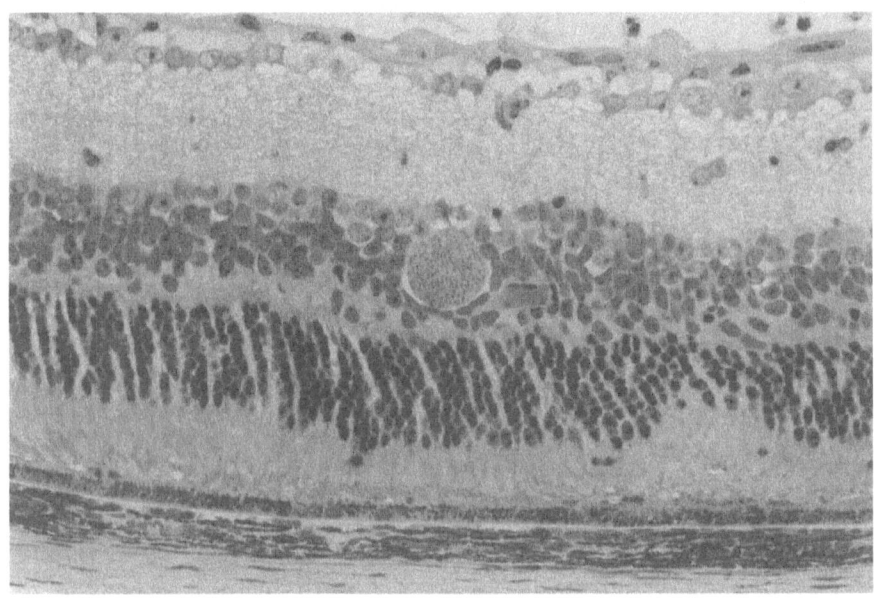

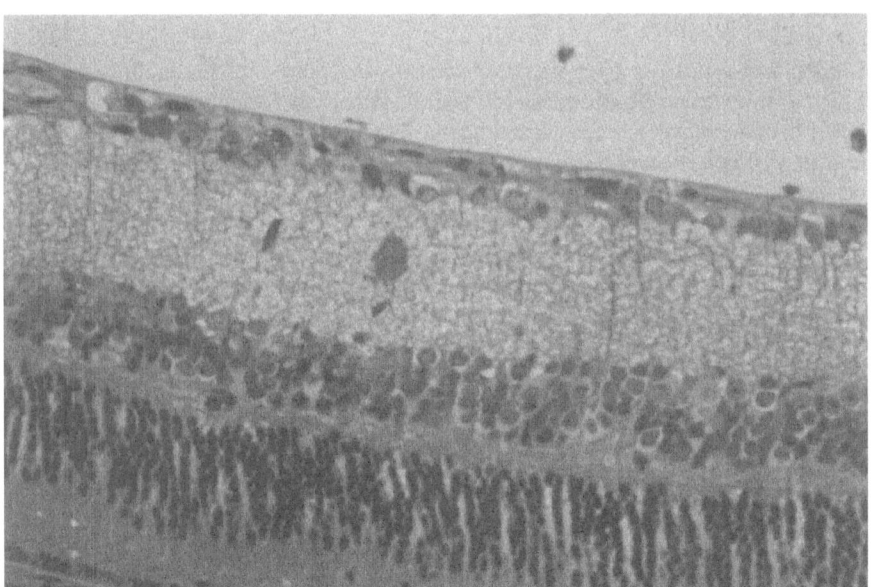

Figs. 7, 8. Intraretinal quiescent toxoplasmic cysts in a murine model of experimental toxoplasmosis (From [7])

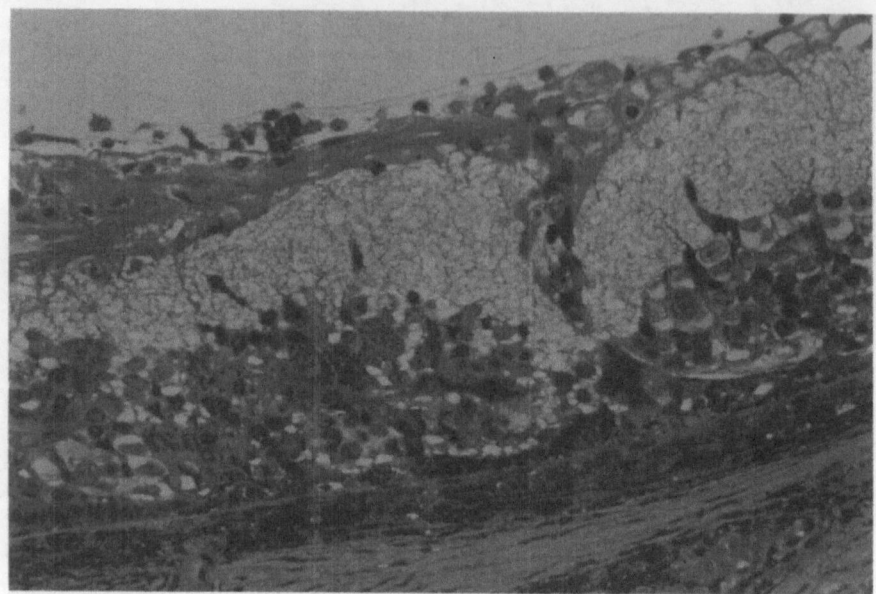

Fig. 9. Intraretinal toxoplasmic cyst and active chorioretinitis in a murine model of experimental toxoplasmosis (From [7])

Ocular toxoplasmosis in the fetus

Ultrasound studies are unable to detect *in utero* signs of ocular infection. In France, the screening program for the diagnosis of congenital toxoplasmosis leads to cases of pregnancy termination. In our study of the histopathological features of the eyes of fetuses infected by *Toxoplasma gondii*, the severity of ocular lesions was correlated with the intensity of pathologic changes in the central nervous system [8]. Retinal necrosis and marked chorioretinal inflammation, despite the absence of bradyzoite, were characteristic findings at these early stages of the infection. The reasons leading to extensive retinal destruction as a sequelae of congenital disease, but uncommonly as a result of adult acquired infection have not yet been elucidated [9]. The mechanisms favoring macular localizations of toxoplasmic scars in congenitally infected children are unknown, but the predilection for this small area of the retina may be related to its particular vascularization.

Ophthalmic outcome in neonates

France and Austria are the only countries in which a systematic screening to detect congenital toxoplasmic infection is implemented. In France the cost of the program for the prevention of toxoplasmosis is estimated approximately as 84 million Euros per year [10]. Serological testing for *Toxoplasma* is required by law in France since 1978 for all women to obtain a wedding licence. Yet, there is a discrepancy between the resources devoted in France to the prevention of ocular toxoplasmosis and the paucity of data available regarding the effects of this program in terms of ophthalmic outcome. Although it is generally admitted by French ophthalmologists that ocular toxoplasmosis is now less frequent and less severe than two decades ago, no large scale epidemiological survey was put in place to validate these claims. The number of cases of ocular toxoplasmosis per year in France, past or present, is unknown.

Table 1 presents ophthalmic outcomes in French, Dutch and US studies of congenital toxoplasmosis. Since recurrences of active retinochoroiditis or new lesions may appear at a later age, eye findings in neonates do not reflect the definitive ophthalmic outcome of congenital toxoplasmosis. Only one study, by Koppe *et al.* has a 20-year follow-up [11, 12]. In this report, 12 congenitally infected children continued to be examined every year until they were aged 20 years. At birth, 4 babies had a retinochoroiditis and 1 had parasites in his placenta and cerebrospinal fluid. Only these 5 children were treated, while 7 symptomless children were not treated. Twenty years later, only 2 subjects had no sign of retinochoroiditis.

In another Dutch study, the long-term ocular involvement in severe congenital toxoplasmosis was studied in 17 patients [13]. In addition to retinochoroiditis observed in 100% of patients, abnormalities of the anterior segment were noted in 50% of cases. In these severely handicapped patients, visual acuity was less than 20/200 in 85% of cases.

Couvreur et al. [14] have studied the ophthalmic outcome in 172 congenitally infected children, treated during the first year of life by alternating courses of pyrimethamine-sulfadiazine combination and spiramycin [14]. At birth, 53 (31%) had symptomatic infections, including 38 (22%) with uni- or bilateral retinochoroiditis. The follow-up of these children ranged from 2 to 11 years. At the end of the study, new lesions were observed in 14 cases. The total number of subjects with at least one lesion of retinochoroiditis increased to 41 (24%) cases. In most instances (10 of 14 cases) new lesions were observed before 19 months of age. Given the difficulties associated with ophthalmic examinations of neonates, particularly regarding the peripheral retina, the authors question the fact that these lesions might have been present since birth, but initially undetected.

Mets et al. [1]studied the ophthalmic outcome of 94 congenitally infected children. Treatment by pyrimethamine and sulfadiazine had been given during the first year of life to 76 patients, while 18 "historica" subjects entered the study after age 1 year. All the historical subjects had chorioretinal lesions. The median follow-up of treated children varied between 15 and 52 months according to treatment regimen. At birth, peripheral chorioretinal scars were observed in 56 (74%) of children that were subsequently treated. Among these children, chorioretinal scars were most common in the periphery (58% of cases), and macular scars were observed in 54% of cases. Macular scars were bilateral in 16 cases and 29 % of subjects had bilateral visual impairment, with visual acuity for the best eye of less than 20/40. During the follow-up, recurrences or new lesions were observed in 7 treated children, including one case with a previously normal examination. Serum titres of anti-*Toxoplasma* antibodies were not correlated to recurrences or new eye lesions.

Table 1. Ophthalmic outcome of congenital toxoplasmosis

Authors	Reference	Year	Number of children with proven infections	Treatment	Chorioretinal lesions at birth	Follow-up	Chorioretinal lesions at the end of follow-up
Mets et al.	[1]	1996	76	P. + S. 1 yr postnatal (different regimen)	56/76 (74%)	median 15, 13 & 52 mo. (according to subgroup)	57/76 (75%)
			18	untreated	NA	78 mo.	18/18 (100%)
Koppe et al.	[11, 12]	1989	12	P. + S.: 5 subjects 1 yr postnatal untreated: 7 subjects	4/12 (33%)	20 yrs	9/11 (82%)
Couvreur et al.	[14]	1985	172	P. + S. - spiramycin 1 yr postnatal	38/172 (22%)	64 patients: 2 yrs 59 patients: 3-4 yrs 34 patients: 5-7 yrs 15 patients: 8-11 yrs	41/172 (24%)
Daffos et al.	[16]	1988	15	P. + S. maternal (antenatal) 1 yr post-natal	2/15 (13%)	30 mo.	2/15 (13%)
Brézin et al.	[17]	1998	18	P. + S. maternal (antenatal) 1 yr postnatal	*	median age: 4.5 yrs	7/18 (39%)

P. = pyrimethamine, S. = sulfonamides; * retrospective study; Chorioretinal lesions: uni- or bilateral, scarred or active, posterior pole or periphery.

Recent French studies report on the ophthalmic outcome of congenitally infected children, diagnosed *in utero* [15]. Antitoxoplasmic treatment in these patients has been administered antenatally and one year after birth.

Daffos et al. [16] reported 39 cases of maternal *Toxoplasma* infection diagnosed antenatally. Pregnancies were terminated in 24 cases and continued in 15 cases. Of the 15 fetuses with congenital toxoplasmosis who were carried to term, peripheral retinochoroiditis in 2 cases were the only findings. No other eye manifestations occured during the 30 months follow-up.

We conducted a retrospective study of 18 children for which *Toxoplasma* infection was diagnosed and treated antenatally [17]. Early time intervals for maternal infections were selected (range of intervals: [7-11weeks] to [21-25 weeks]). All mothers had been treated by alternating cures of spiramycin and sulfadiazine-pyrimethamine combination (sulfadoxine-pyrimethamine [Fansidar®] in the earliest cases). Children were treated during one year by sulfadiazine-pyrimethamine combination for 1 year. In this study, the median age of patients was 4.5 years (range 1-11). All children were examined by two ophthalmologists (Brézin and Mets). Out of 18 children, 11 (61%) had no eye manifestations of congenital toxoplasmosis. Scars of the posterior pole were observed in 5 (28%) children. Only one child had a bilateral visual impairment.

Because in countries without a systematic screening for congenital toxoplasmosis asymptomatic cases are undetected, care should be exercised when comparing French results to studies of postnatally diagnosed and treated children. However, the available data argue favorably for the beneficial effects of antenatal and postnatal treatment in congenital toxoplasmosis.

Role of the ophthalmologist for the treatment of congenital toxoplasmosis

Where antenatal diagnoses of toxoplasmosis are performed, ophthalmologists are systematically called on to examine neonates. However, in countries without a screening program for the detection of congenital toxoplasmosis, ophthalmologists may have the leading role for the detection of the infection, if extra-ocular signs are absent or latent. In these countries, the delay before the eye manifestations of the infection are brought to attention is a function of the severity of lesions. Bilateral visual impairment is usually detected in the first months of life, but unilateral macular lesions may not be symptomatic until several years, revealed in particular by strabismus. The ophthalmologist's role for the management of neonates with congenital toxoplasmosis varies according to the mode of diagnosis of the infection and the severity of manifestations. When the diagnosis of congenital toxoplasmosis has not been previously made, the ophthalmologist should refer the patient to pediatricians used to the follow-up of treatments by pyrimethamine and sulfadiazine in neonates. Once the full course of postnatal treatment is completed, ophthalmologists may again prescribe courses of antitoxoplasmic treatment in case of recurrences.

In all cases with signs of retinochoroiditis, the ophthalmologist must assess if lesions are scarred or active. Active lesions of retinochoroiditis, particularly when threatening the fovea, are usually treated, in addition to anti *Toxoplasma* treatment, by short-term oral corticosteroids (0.5 to 1mg/kg/day) until scarring is observed. Severe vitritis which may complicate active retinochoroiditis responds also to corticotherapy.

Whereas the penetration of spiramycin into the eye after oral penetration is insufficient to have an effect on *Toxoplasma*, the penetration of pyrimethamine in the choroid and the retina after oral administration has been shown to be satisfactory in animal models [18, 19]. Gormley et al. [20] have studied *Toxoplasma* infection in the hamster to evaluate the effects of drug therapy on the course of acute disease. Systemically administered atovaquone was compared to conventional therapies (pyrimethamine combined with sulfadiazine, clindamycin, spiramycin). None of the drugs administered altered the course of the acute disease. Retinal cysts were too rarely observed for the effects of these drugs to be evaluated in the eye. Atovaquone alone significantly reduced the number of cerebral *Toxoplasma* cysts.

No clinical trials have been performed in human neonates to validate the effects of treatments on ocular toxoplasmic lesions. In adults with active ocular toxoplasmosis, Rothova et al. [2] compared the effects of 3 triple-drug combinations: (1) pyrimethamine, sulfadiazine and corticosteroids; (2) clindamycin, sulfadiazine and corticosteroids: (3) trimethoprim, sulfamethoxazole and corticosteroids. The only statistically significant effect of treatment was the reduction in size of the retinal inflammatory lesion for 49% of the pyrimethamine-treated patients, compared to 20% of the untreated patients. This treatment benefit may be critical for visual outcome when active lesions are located near the macula. No significant effect of treatment on the duration of inflammatory activity or the recurrence rate was observed. In a survey of practices in the management of ocular toxoplasmosis among members of the American Uveitis Society, the location of lesion near the macula was the most cited factor suggesting that ocular toxoplasmosis should be treated [21]. Only four ophthalmologists surveyed in this study had treated neonatal patients with active ocular disease: all treated every patient, regardless of findings.

So far, atovaquone has only been tested in a limited number of adult patients with active *Toxoplasma* retinochoroiditis and remains untested in neonates [22]. However, the *in vitro* and *in vivo* activity of atovaquone against *Toxoplasma gondii* make this drug a promising alternative to conventional antitoxoplasmic therapies [23].

Conclusion

The mechanism of early ocular damage after *Toxoplasma* infection remains only partly known. Less severe ophthalmic outcome of congenital toxoplasmosis has been reported in France, after antenatal diagnosis and treatment, than in other countries. A meta-analysis must take into account cases asymptomatic at birth, undetected and unreported when no systematic screening is performed. However, available data strongly suggest that antiparasitic treatments, initiated early after the onset of infection, limit the ophthalmic consequences of congenital toxoplasmosis.

References

1. Mets MB, Holfels E, Boyer KM, Swisher CN, Roizen N, Stein L, Stein M, Hopkins J, Withers S, Mack D, Luciano R, Patel D, Remington JS, Meier P, McLeod R (1996) Eye manifestations of congenital toxoplasmosis. Am J Ophthalmol 122:309-324
2. Rothova A, Meenken C, Buitenhuis HJ, Brinkman CJ, Baarsma GS, Boen-Tan TN, de Jong PT, Klaassen-Broekema N, Schweitzer CM, Timmerman Z et al (1993) Therapy for ocular toxoplasmosis. Am J Ophthalmol 115:517-523
3. Ronday MJ, Luyendijk L, Baarsma GS, Bollemeijer JG, Van der Lelij A, Rothova A (1995) Presumed acquired ocular toxoplasmosis. Arch Ophthalmol 113:1524-1529
4. Couvreur J, Thulliez P (1996) Toxoplasmose acquise à localisation oculaire ou neurologique. 49 cas. Presse Med 25:438-442
5. Glasner PD, Silveira C, Kruszon-Moran D, Martins MC, Burnier Junior M, Silveira S, Camargo ME, Nussenblatt RB, Kaslow RA, Belfort Junior R (1992) An unusually high prevalence of ocular toxoplasmosis in southern Brazil. Am J Ophthalmol 114:136-144
6. Dutton GN, Hay J, Hair DM, Ralston J (1986) Clinicopathological features of a congenital murine model of ocular toxoplasmosis Graefe's. Arch Clin Exp Ophthalmol 224:256-264
7. Gazzinelli RT, Brezin AP, Li Q, Nussenblatt RB, Chan CC (1994) *Toxoplasma gondii*: acquired ocular toxoplasmosis in the murine model, protective role of TNF-alpha and IFN-gamma. Exp Parasitol 78:217-229
8. Brézin AP, Kasner L, Thulliez P, Li Q, Daffos F, Nussenblatt RB, Chan CC (1994) Ocular toxoplasmosis in the fetus: Immunohistochemistry analysis and DNA amplification. Retina 14:19-26
9. Roberts F, McLeod R (1999) Pathogenesis of toxoplasmic retinochoroiditis. Parasitology Today 15:51-57
10. Courgenay A (1997) Évaluation du coût de la prévention et de la prise en charge de la toxoplamose congénitale en France. Thèse pour le Diplôme d'État de Docteur en Médecine. Université Paris Val-de-Marne, Faculté de Médecine Créteil
11. Koppe JG, Loewer-Sieger DH, de Roever-Bonnet H (1986) Results of 20-year follow-up of congenital toxoplasmosis. Lancet 1(8475):254-256
12. Koppe JG, Rothova (1989) A Congenital toxoplasmosis. A long-term follow-up of 20 years. Int Ophthalmol 13:387-390
13. Meenken C, Assies J, van Nieuwenhuizen O, Holwerda-van der Maat WG, van Schooneveld MJ, Delleman WJ, Kinds G, Rothova A (1995) A Long term ocular and neurological involvement in severe congenital toxoplasmosis. Br J Ophthalmol 79:581-584
14. Couvreur J, Desmonts G, Aron-Rosa D (1985) Le pronostic oculaire de la toxoplasmose congénitale: rôle du traitement. Sem Hôp Paris 61:1734-1737
15. Hohlfeld P, Daffos F, Thulliez P, Aufrant J, Couvreur J, Mac Aleese D, Descombey D, Forestier F (1989) Fetal toxoplasmosis: Outcome of pregnancy and infant follow-up after *in utero* treatment. J Pediatr 115:765-769
16. Daffos F, Forestier F, Capella-Pavlovsky M, Thulliez P, Aufrant C, Valenti D, Cox WL (1988) Prenatal management of 746 pregnancies at risk for congenital toxoplasmosis. N Engl J Med 318:271-275
17. Brézin AP, Thulliez P, Couvreur J, Nobré R, McLeod R, Mets M (1998) Ophthalmic outcome after pre- and post-natal treatment of congenital toxoplasmosis. Invest Ophthalmol Vis Sci 39-4:2986 [ARVO Abstract]
18. Kaufman HE (1961) The penetration of daraprim (pyrimethionine) into the monkey eye. Am J Ophthalmol 52:402-404
19. Brihaye M, De Meuter F, Tassignon MJ, Braeckman C, Mercier A, Van Hoof F (1980) Étude de la pénétration intra-oculaire de médicaments à effet thérapeutique sur la toxoplasmose. Etude préliminaire. Bull Soc Belge Ophtal 191:39-43
20. Gormley PD, Pavesio CE, Minnasian D, Lightman S (1998) Effects of drug therapy on *Toxoplasma* cysts in an animal model of acute and chronic disease. Invest Ophthalmol Vis Sci 39:1171-1175
21. Engstrom RE Jr, Holland GN, Nussenblatt RB, Jabs DA (1991) Current practices in the management of ocular toxoplasmosis. Am J Ophthalmol 111:601-610
22. Pearson PA, Piracha AR, Sen HA, Jaffe GJ (1999) Atovaquone for the treatment of *Toxoplasma* retinochoroiditis in immunocompetent patients. Ophthalmology 106:148-153
23. Araujo FG, Huskinson J, Remington JS (1991) Remarkable in vitro and *in vivo* activities of the hydroxynaphthoquinone 566C80 against tachyzoites and tissue cysts of *Toxoplasma gondii*. Antimicrob Agents Chemother 35:293-299

3.3. Biological post-natal diagnosis of congenital toxoplasmosis

E. Candolfi, H. Pelloux

Introduction

Specific postnatal diagnosis of CT is crucial in two cases: (i) when clinical signs occur within the first 6 months of life, and no information on the mother's antenatal serostatus is available, and (ii) seroconversion is diagnosed during pregnancy, with or without antenatal diagnosis of CT. The first situation is mainly observed in countries where maternal screening is inexistent [1]. In countries where maternal screening is obligatory (France and Austria) or is done on a regular basis by obstetricians (Belgium, Switzerland, Italy), the slightest suspicion of maternal toxoplasmosis calls for parasitological and immunological testing at birth and during the first year of life [2, 3]. Parasitological and immunological diagnosis of congenital toxoplasmosis is simpler post-natally than *in utero*, owing to the better accessibility of appropriate samples (cord blood, placenta, serum, etc.). However, CT is mainly subclinical, especially in countries with effective screening programs, where treatment of the fetus reduces the risk of major complications [2, 4-6].

Early postnatal diagnosis is of paramount importance to identify infants qualifying for aggressive treatment see chapter 2.4] based on pyrimethamine and sulfadiazine (PS) and to reduce the incidence of ocular sequelae later in life [5-7].

In the last 10 years the extensive use of sophisticated biological methods to detect the parasite or neosynthesized infant antibodies has increased the efficiency of CT diagnosis during the first year of life.This chapter will focus on biological methods (detection of the parasite and immunological assays) used for postnatal diagnosis of congenital toxoplasmosis, and on the interpretation of their results.

Parasite detection

Samples

The parasite can be detected in various samples both at birth and later, such as placenta, cord blood, newborn blood, amniotic fluid and CSF, and also in various tissues at autopsy (brain, skeletal tissues, heart muscle, etc.). Detection of the parasite establishes the diagnosis of congenital toxoplasmosis, with the exception of the placenta (no proof of transmission). The samples most often tested at birth are the placenta and newborn blood.

Placenta

The placenta is easy to collect, and is large enough to provide ample samples. The best volume of placenta to study is not clear. Two hundred grams of tissue is usually taken [8], but samples sent to the laboratory are often smaller, which can cause a loss of sensitivity in the search for *T. gondii*. The methods used are all based on detection of the parasite (mouse inoculation, cell culture and PCR). Few published data have dealt with the diagnostic value of placental *T. gondii* detection for CT [2, 8-10]. Most suggest that sensitivity is not optimal, but the study groups are often of limited size. Furthermore, the results on *T. gondii* detection at birth in umbilical cord blood and placenta are often given together, making it difficult to assess the contribution of placental studies. The use of PCR has improved the results compared to those obtained with inoculation (mouse and/or *in vitro* cell culture) [8]. The question of the absolute " specificity " of *T. gondii* detection in placenta (does it always mean the child is infected?) has long been controversial, but it appears the placenta can be infected without transmission to the fetus [2]. However, detection of *T. gondii* in the placenta provides strong evidence of congenital toxoplasmosis. Thus, examination of the placenta, which is easy to collect and provides a very early sign of infection in the child, is especially useful for countries where antenatal diagnosis is not performed; in addition, positive placental studies will overrule a negative antenatal diagnosis.

Umbilical cord blood

The detection of *T. gondii* in cord blood at birth is done in parallel with placental studies in some laboratories, but no specific results are given in the literature. Published results are those for the detection of *T. gondii* in both placenta and cord blood. The method used in these studies is mainly mouse inoculation.

Newborn blood

Parasite detection in newborn blood is rarely attempted, even though it provides proof of congenital toxoplasmosis. A recent report underlined the usefulness of PCR in this setting [11]. Routine testing of newborn blood is clearly limited by sampling difficulties, and few data are available on the frequency of parasitemia in infected newborns.

Amniotic fluid

Amniotic fluid is not used to detect *T. gondii* at the time of birth, but can be useful (like samples from the foetus) if a pregnancy is terminated .

Cerebrospinal fluid (CSF)

The diagnostic value of *T. gondii* detection in newborns ' and infants ' CSF has been studied by several authors [2, 12, 13]. This approach is not used routinely by all teams, as its sensitivity is not very high. In contrast, the positive predictive values is 100%: *T. gondii* detection in CSF is proof of infection.

Necropsy samples

Necropsy samples (amniotic fluid, ascitis, liver, spleen, brain) are used to establish CT postmortem, after miscarriage or termination. The presence of *T. gondii* in at least one of these samples is proof of fetal infection.

Isolation procedures

These techniques are described and discussed in chapter 2.3 section of this book. Here, we focus only on the characteristics of methods used for perinatal diagnosis.

No major technical advances have been made in the last 40 years. The reference method was and still is mouse inoculation. However, molecular biology methods have significantly increased the sensitivity.

Mouse inoculation

Mouse inoculation can still be considered the "reference method". It remains more sensitive than *in vitro* culture, even if the results take longer to be obtained. At birth, mouse inoculation is used to test the placenta and umbilical cord blood [13]. One advantage of mouse inoculation is that it allows the parasite to be isolated for strain characterisation.

Cell culture

In vitro cell culture has many advantages over mouse inoculation: the results obtained earlier (4 to 6 days instead of weeks) and no animal facilities are required, but its sensitivity remains lower than that of mouse inoculation. Furthermore, with the advent of PCR it is unlikely that *in vitro* cell culture will be still used in the field of congenital toxoplasmosis.

Polymerase Chain Reaction

The methods are the same as those described in the previous chapter on antenatal diagnosis. The main point is that the use of PCR greatly speeds postnatal diagnosis and enables treatment to be started almost immediately. However, the exquisite sensitivity of PCR can make it difficult to interpret results obtained on the placenta [8].

Histopathology

The methods employed are the same as those applied to other biopsy samples and described in other chapters.

Immunological diagnosis

General considerations

At birth, the sensitivity of parasite detection is pretty poor, ranking between 25% [12] and 60.9% [8]. The use of immunological methods is therefore of paramount importance for definitive postnatal diagnosis of congenital toxoplasmosis. Moreover, in European countries with prenatal screening programs, *Toxoplasma*-infected mothers are routinely treated, meaning that most infants infected *in utero* are asymptomatic at birth [2, 3] and that the diagnosis is mainly based on the detection of specific neosynthesized antibodies. Tests based on cell-mediated immunity in the newborn or infant, such as antigen-specific lymphocyte proliferation, can be done in only a very few laboratories worldwide and are therefore outside the scope of this chapter, even if interesting data have been published on the usefulness of such methods after 3 months of age [14].

Infants' serum contains maternal antibodies transmitted through the placenta during gestation. Only IgG crosses the placental barrier, but IgM and IgA may "leak" through the placenta during labor and contaminate the newborn serum sample. This implies that it is crucial to monitor the disappearance of passively acquired Ig of maternal origin. New methods able to detect neosynthesized IgG/IgM in the infant are now well established and, together with standard methods for Ig detection, can be used to diagnose more than 90% of cases of congenital toxoplasmosis during the first 3 months of life.

Samples

Types of sample

Cord blood, maternal blood and newborn blood can be used for antibody detection. Cord blood can be sampled in the form of paper spots, then dried and assayed later [15]. This approach also reduces the frequency of venopuncture during the monthly follow-up in the first year of life [16]. The purity of cord blood is sometimes imperfect, owing to microtransfusion of maternal blood through the placenta during labour. Until now this problem had hindered the use of cord blood for immunological diagnosis. However, methods for comparing the mother-infant antibodies profile have renewed interest in cord blood testing. The use of CSF is limited to the detection of toxoplasmic IgM, which is strongly suggestive of congenital toxoplasmosis [17].

Sampling frequency

The first sample should be cord blood, for both parasitological and immuno-logical diagnosis. Theoretically the second sample should be done 15 days later and the third at one month. Thereafter, monthly testing is sufficient and allows the decay of passively transferred maternal IgG antibodies to be moni-tored for serologic rebound due to neosynthesis by the infant.

Decay kinetics of transmitted maternal antibodies

Mean antibody survival times are 23 days for IgG, 5 days for IgM and 6 days for IgA. Therefore, the detection of antitoxoplasmic IgM and IgA in the infant's blood from 15 days to 3 months after birth is proof of CT. The date of final clearance of maternal IgG antibodies depends on the initial level at birth. Maternal IgG usually disappears after 5 to 10 months of life. Given the IgG half-life, titers (IU/ml) should fall by approximately one-half every month.

Methods

Non comparative antibody detection methods

These methods are the same as those used to detect maternal antibodies, except that some methods are poorly sensitive for IgM. Moreover, some methods require modifications, especially regarding serum dilution, such ISAGA [18]. Infants produce small amounts of antitoxoplasmic IgM and natural IgM, meaning that the cut-off for ELISA tests can be lowered and/or that the infant's serum should be diluted less [19, 20].

Methods for detecting IgG The method must be quantitative, i.e. the dye test or IgG ELISA. The dye test is certainly a reference method but is of limited use in standard laboratories. ELISA is the method of choice for precise and repro-ducible quantification in international units. For a perfect monitoring of anti-toxoplasmic IgG decay, it is necessary to run together the sample serum with the previous sample and, obviously, to use the same assay. In addition, the assays must be done in the same laboratory for a given patient, in order to avoid interlaboratory variations.

Methods for detecting IgM Detection of toxoplasmic IgM is of crucial importan-ce. The method used should be the most sensitive one available. Recent data indicate that ISAGA IgM is the most appropriate test for the detection of anti-toxoplasmic IgM antibodies in infants less than one year old [21, 22]. Fricker-Hidalgo [23] reported 43.3% sensitivity of ELISA IgM, compared to 73% with ISAGA IgM. Similarly, Pinon [24] reported 77% sensitivity with ISAGA IgM.

These data were confirmed in 1998 by a study from the Serology Group of the European Network on Congenital Toxoplasmosis, where the sensitivity of ISAGA was 81.1%, compared to only 64.8% with ELISA (unpublished data). Assays such as IFAT should be discarded, owing to their poor sensitivity in infants less than one year old [17, 18]. In-house and commercial ELISAs are set up to screen adult sera, in which the background, due to natural IgM, is high [25], and must be modified and carefully validated before being used on infants' sera [19, 20, 26].

Methods for detecting IgA The contribution of IgA to early diagnosis of CT has been underlined by many authors [24, 27-30]. The methods used range from ISAGA to immunocapture ELISA. However, recent reports on the comparative sensitivity of ELISA IgA and ISAGA IgA are discordant. According to Patel [28], ISAGA IgA is more sensitive than ELISA IgA, while Foudrinier [29] reported similar sensitivity (about 65%) between ISAGA IgA and an ELISA using a monoclonal antibody directed to SAG1. The 1998 study from the Serology Group of the ENCT confirms this latter result (unpublished data). Moreover, in Foudriniers study, IgA was detected more readily than IgM (65% and 55%, respectively). In contrast, Pinon [24] obtained lower sensitivity with ISAGA IgA than with ISAGA IgM (62% and 69%, respectively); by adding the results for the two isotypes, Pinon found that the sensitivity increased to 73.7% between day 1 and day 30 of life. These data strongly support the use of an antitoxoplasmic IgA detection test (ISAGA or ELISA based on SAG1) as part of the panel of methods for serological diagnosis of CT during the first year of life.

Comparative mother-infant immunological profiles

Owing to the fact that the placenta allows the passage of maternal IgG (and sometimes IgM or IgA), methods based on comparative mother-infant immunological profiles are of paramount importance during the first three months of life. That passage of antibodies through the placenta considerably hinders and delays the immunological diagnosis of congenital toxoplasmosis, leading to non treatment of some infected infants and treatment of some non infected infants. Fortunately, methods for determining the origin of specific antibodies and for distinguishing the infant's neosynthesised IgG from transmitted maternal IgG are now available.

Comparison of the level of specific IgG production ("antibody load") This approach was established by Desmonts [17] and provided a better estimate of transmitted maternal IgG decay by comparing toxoplasmic IgG levels (in IU/ml) to total non specific IgG levels and computing the "specific antibody load". Although the method is purely quantitative, it should be used if methods for comparing mother-infant antibody profiles are not available.

Immunoblotting (IB) Immunoblotting combines electrophoresis of toxoplasmic antigens in denaturing conditions, electrotransfer to a nitrocellulose membrane, and a specific antibody assay (similar to an ELISA) detecting specific epitopes. The result is a band pattern, resulting from precipitation of the substrate on the membrane and revealing the presence of the antigen-antibody complex [31]. Detection of bands in the infant's serum which are absent from the mother's serum points to antibody neosynthesis. Franck and colleagues [32] were the first to demonstrate the usefulness of IB on a large scale. Use of the semi-automatic computer-driven PHAST SYSTEM from Pharmacia has increased the reproducibility of IB [33], and commercial IB kits are now available. Chumpitazi achieved an overall sensitivity of 92.6% and a specificity of 89.1% [33]. In the 1998 multicenter study conducted by the Serology Group of the ENCT, the sensitivity and specificity of IgG+IgM IB were respectively 77.7% and 96%. However, false-positive results can be obtained, and are due to natural IgM, especially in samples from infants over three months and limit the use of IB to sera from infant less than 3 month old.

ELIFA This method makes use of a microporous cellulose acetate membrane in a co-immunoelectrodiffusion procedure to simultaneously study antibody specificity by immunoprecipitation and antibody isotypes by immunofiltration through the membrane of an enzyme-labelled antibody. The filtration step is automated in an ELIFA cell controlled by an automat [24, 34, 35]. The profiles yield four parameters: the number of precipitating arcs, the isotype (IgG or IgM), the comparative specificity by continuity (coalescence) of the arcs present in two serum samples revealing the same antigen involved in the precipitate, and the relative amounts of antibodies with same specificity in each sample. Neosynthesized antibodies are revealed by the presence of specific antibodies present in the neonatal serum and absent from the maternal blood, or by a higher concentration of neonatal antibodies with specificity identical to that of the maternal antibodies. Pinon's team [24] has obtained excellent results using that method, reaching a sensitivity of 90%. The recent study from the European Network on Congenital Toxoplasmosis indicates a similar excellent sensitivity of ELIFA IgG (88.8%) and a specificity of 100%.

Comparison of IB and ELIFA Only Chumpitazi et al. [33] have so far published a valid comparison of the two assays. The overall sensitivity and specificity of the two methods is better than that of other assays for detecting neosynthesized IgG, IgM or IgA. Their semiautomated IB method has better resolution than ELIFA. However, in the 1998 study from the Serology Group of the ENCT, a similar comparison between a manual IB and an ELIFA demonstrated that ELIFA IgG had better sensitivity (88.8%) than IB IgG (65.4%) or even IB IgG+IgM (77.7%) (unpublished data). On the other hand, in that recent ENCT study, IB IgM gave better results than the other methods used for the detection of IgM antibodies (ISAGA and ELISA).

Specificity is a key factor. ELIFA IgG gave the best results of all the methods, except for cord blood in which the natural hemoconcentration prevents the interpretation of precipitating antibody arcs. IB gave false-positive results, especially for IgM, in the study by Chumpitzazi [33], possibly because some natural IgM recognizes toxoplasmic structures. IB IgM should therefore be avoided after three months of life replaced, if necessary, by immuno-capture assays.

Effect of treatment on immunological profiles

Despite recent studies, the data are insufficient to determine the effect of treatment on immunological profiles. Previous investigations suggested that the infant's IgG production was decreased by treatment, especially when infection occurred during labor [36]. Moreover, prenatal diagnosis by PCR on amniotic fluid during the second trimester allows treatment to be started during pregnancy with the combination of pyrimethamine and sulfadoxine; and we and others have observed that small amounts of neosynthesized anti-bodies are produced by these precociously in utero treated infants. Final post-natal serological diagnosis is also delayed by treatment in utero, and this may induce false hopes in the mother and pediatrician: in some cases persistence of toxoplasmic IgG after one year of life and/or a serological rebound is obser-ved as soon as the treatment is alleviated or discontinued, confirming the pre-natal diagnosis of CT [5, 37].

Interpretation of the results

Detection of the parasite in the placenta by PCR, mouse inoculation or patho-logical examination does not unequivocably demonstrate transmission to the fetus. Only detection of the parasite in cord blood, CSF, newborn blood or other tissues within the first 6 months of life can prove CT.

If the antenatal diagnosis was already positive (i.e. detection of *Toxoplasma* by PCR), confirmation at birth of congenital toxoplasmosis by parasite detec-tion in placenta or cord blood or by immunology is not always obtained. Indeed, treatment with the pyrimethamine and sulfadoxine combination may have eradicated the placental infection, decreased parasitemia, and attenua-ted the immunological response. Given the possibility of false-positive results of antenatal diagnosis by PCR, postnatal follow-up is still crucial.

If antenatal or postnatal detection of parasite are negative, apart from cli-nical signs, the following parameters unequivocally confirm CT during immunological follow-up:
- a detection of neosynthesized IgG by comparative mother-infant or infant-infant immunological profiles within the first 6 months of life;
- a rise in antitoxoplasmic IgG titres within first 12 months of life;
- a lack of fall in specific IgG titres;
- antitoxoplasmic IgM and/or IgA detection within the first 6 months of life.

Most often, during postnatal follow-up, the maternal antibodies disappears after 5 to 10 months of life. This first negative antibody test does not prove the absence of parasite transmission to the fetus, meaning that the result should be absolutely confirmed three months later, without treatment during the interval.

Conclusions

Postnatal diagnosis of CT and follow-up of infants suspected of being infected is crucial, particularly in countries where screening of pregnant women and antenatal diagnosis are not performed. In a recent study Abboud [38] pointed out that 46% of mothers fail to comply adequately with postnatal follow-up, increasing the risk of CT misdiagnosis and the risk of complications. Early postnatal diagnosis allows early pyrimethamine-sulfadoxine treatement, which reduces the clinical complications of CT [5, 6, 39]. As stated above, the choice of parasite and antibody detection methods is crucial. If the optimal set of parasitological and immunological methods is chosen, more than 90% of cases of CT can be diagnosed during the first 3 months of life.

References

1. Guerina N, Hsu H, Meissner C, Maguire J, Lynfield R, Stechenberg B, Abroms I, Pasternack M, Hoff R, Eaton R, Grady G, Group TNERTW (1994) Neonatal serologic screening and early tratment for congenital *Toxoplasma gondii* infection. N Eng J Med 330:1858-1863
2. Daffos F, Forestier F, Capella-Pavlovsky M, Thulliez P, Aufrant C, Valenti D, Cox W (1988) Prenatal management of 746 pregnancies at risk for congenital toxoplasmosis. N Eng J Med 318:271-275
3. Peyron F, Wallon M, Bernardoux C (1996) Long-term follow-up of patients with congenital ocular toxoplasmosis. N Eng J Med 334:993-994
4. Desmonts G, Couvreur J (1986) Toxplasmose congénitale. Etude prospective de l'issue de la grossessechez 542 femmes atteintes de toxoplasmose acquise en cours de gestation. Sem Hôp Paris 62:1418-1422
5. McAuley J, Boyer K, Patel S, Mets M, Qwishers C, Roizen N, Wolters C, Stein L, Stein M, Schey W, Remington J, Meier P, Johnson D, Heydeman P, Holfels E, Withers S, Mack D, Brown C, Patton D, McLeod R (1994) Early and longitudinal evaluations of treated infants and children and untreated historical patients with congenital toxoplasmosis : the Chicago collaborative treatment trial. Clin Infect Dis 18:38-72
6. Roizen N, Swisher C, Stein M, Hopkins J, Boyer K, Holfels E, Mets M, Stein L, Patel D, Meir P, Withers S, Remington J, Mack D, Heydemann P, Patton D, Mc Leod R (1995) Neurologic and devol mental outcome in treated congenital toxoplasmosis. Pediatrics 95:11-20
7. Wilson CB, Remington JS, Stagno S, Reynolds DW (1980) Development of adverse sequelae in children born with subclinical congenital toxoplasma infection. Pediatrics 66:764-774
8. Fricker-Hidalgo H, Pelloux H, Racinet C, Grefenstette I, Bost-Bru C, Goullier-Fleuret A, Ambroise-Thomas P (1998) Detection of *Toxoplasma gondii* in 94 placentae from infected women by polymerase chain reaction, *in vivo*, and *in vitro* cultures. Placenta 19:545-549
9. Desmonts G, Couvreur J, Ferrero G, Marcoux M (1974) L'isolement du parasite dans la toxoplasmose congénitale : Intérêt pratique et théorique. Arch Pediatr 31:157-166
10. Pratlong F, Boulot P, Issert E, Msika M, Dupont F, Bachelard F, Sarda P, Viala J, Jarry D (1994) Fetal diagnosis of toxoplasmosis in 190 women infected during pregnancy. Prenat Diagn 14:191-198
11. Bergström T, Ricksten A, Nenomen N, Lichtenstein M,Olofsson S (1998) *Toxoplasma gondii* infection diagnosed by PCR amplification of peripheral mononuclear blood cells from a child and mother. Scand J Infect Dis 30:202-204
12. Desmonts G, Couvreur J (1974) Congenital toxoplasmosis. A prospective study of 378 pregnancies. N Eng J Med 290:1110-1116
13. Berrebi A, Kobuch W, Bessières M, Bloom M, Rolland M, Sarramon M, Roques C,Fournié A (1994) Termination of pregnancy for maternal toxoplasmosis. Lancet 344:36-39
14. Wilson C, Desmonts G, Couvreur J,Remington J (1980) Lymphocyte transformation in the diagnosis of congenital toxoplasma infection. N Eng J Med 302:785-788
15. Eaton R, Petersen E, Seppanen H, Tuuminen T (1996) Multicenter evaluation of a fluorometric enzyme immunocapture assay to detect toxoplasma-specific immunoglobulin M in dried blood filter paper specimens from newborns. J Clin Microbiol 34:3147-3150
16. Patel B, Holliman R (1994) Antibodies to *Toxoplasma gondii* in eluates from filter paper blood specimens. Br J Biomed Sci 51:104-108

17. Remington J, Mac Leod R, Desmonts G (1994) Toxoplasmosis. In: Remington J. and Klein J. (eds) Infectious diseases of the fetus and newborn infant. WB Saunders, Philadelphia
18. Desmonts G, Naot Y, Remington JS (1981) Immunoglobulin M-immunosorbent agglutination assay for diagnosis of infections diseases: diagnosis of acute congenital and acquired *Toxoplasma* infections. J Clin Microbiol 14:486-491
19. Candolfi E, Kien T (1988) Détection des IgM spécifiques dans le diagnostic de la toxoplasmose congénitale par une méthode d'immunopture ELISA sur billes. Détermination des paramètres d'utilisation. Rev Fr Lab 178:43-46
20. Candolfi E, Bessières MH, Marty P, Cimon B, Gandilhon F, Pelloux H, Thulliez P (1993) Determination of a new cut-off value for the diagnosis of congenital toxoplasmosis by detection of specific IgM in an enzyme immunoassay. Eur J Clin Microbiol Infect Dis 12:396-398
21. Duffy K, Wharton P, Johnson J, New L, Holliman R (1989) Assessment of immunoglobulin-M immunosorbent agglutination assay (ISAGA) for detecting *Toxoplasma* specific assay (ISAGA) for detecting toxoplasma specific IgM. J Clin Pathol 42:1291-1295
22. Holliman R, Johnson J (1989) The post-natal serodiagnosis of congenital toxoplasmosis. Serodiag Immunother Infect Dis 3:323-327
23. Fricker-Hidalgo H, Pelloux H, Racinet C, Bost M, Goullier-Fleuret A, Ambroise-Thomas P (1996) Congenital toxoplasmosis: specific IgM in fetal blood, cord blood and in the newborn. Ann Biol Clin 54:165-168
24. Pinon J, Chemla C, Villena I, Foudrinier F, Aubert D, Puygauthier-Toubas D, Leroux B, Dupouy D, Quereux C, Talmud M, Trenque T, Potron G, Pluot M, Remy G, Bonhomme A (1996) Early neonatal diagnosis of congenital toxoplasmosis: value of comparative enzyme-linked immunofiltration assay immunological profiles and anti-*Toxoplasma gondii* immunoglobulin M (IgM) or IgA immunocapture and implications for postnatal therapeutic strategies. J Clin Microbiol 34:579-583
25. Konishi E (1991) Naturally occuring immunoglobulin M antibodies to *Toxoplasma gondii* in Japanese populations. Parasitology 102:157-162
26. Naot Y, Desmont G, Remington JS (1981) IgM Enzyme Linked Immuno Sorbent Assay test for the diagnosis of congenital *Toxoplasma* infection. J Pédiatr 98:32-36
27. Bessières M, Roques C, Berrebi A, Barre V, Cazaux M, Seguela J (1992) IgA antibody response during acquired and congenital toxoplasmosis. J Clin Pathol 45:605-608
28. Patel B, Young Y, Duffy K, Tanner K, Johnson J, Holliman RE (1993) Immunoglobulin-A detection and the investigation of clinical toxoplasmosis. J Med Microbiol 38:286-292
29. Foudrinier M-C, Aubert D, Bonhomme A, Pinon J (1995) Value of specific immunoglobulin A detection by two immunocapture assays in the diagnosis of toxoplasmosis. Eur J Clin Microbiol Infect Dis 14:585-590
30. Decoster A, Gontier P, Demory J,Duhamel M (1995) Detection of anti-*Toxoplasma* immunoglobulin A antibodies by Platelia-Toxo IgA directed against P30 and by IMx Toxo IgA for diagnosis of acquired and congenital toxoplasmosis. J Clin Microbiol 33:2206-2208
31. Partanen P, Turunen H, Paasivuo R, Leinikii P (1984) Immunoblot analysis of *Toxoplasma gondii* antigens by human immunoglobulin G, M and A antibodies at different stages of infection. J Clin Microbiol 20:133-135
32. Franck J, Mary C, Laugier M, Dumon H, Quilici M (1992) Apport du western blot au diagnostic de la toxoplasmose congénitale. Bull Soc F Parasitol 10:3-7
33. Chumpitazi B, Boussaid A, Pelloux H, Racinet C, Bost M, Goullier-Fleuret A (1995) Diagnosis of congenital toxoplasmosis by immunoblotting and relationship with other methods. J Clin Microbiol 33:1479-1485
34. Pinon JM,Gruson N (1982) Interêt des profils immunologiques comparés ELIFA dans le diagnostic précoce de la toxoplasmose congénitale. Lyon Méd 248:27-30
35. Pinon J, Poirriez J, Dupouy D, Quereux C, Garin J, Leroux B (1987) Diagnostic précoce et surveillance de la toxoplasmose congénitale : méthode des profils immunologiques comparés. Presse Méd 16:471-474
36. Alford C Jr, Stagno S,Reynolds DW (1974) Congenital toxoplasmosis : Clinical, laboratory and therapeutic considerations with special reference to subclinical disease. Bull N Y Acad Med 50:160-181
37. Fortier B, Coignard-Chatain C, Dao A, Rouland V, Valat A, Vinatier D, Lebrun T (1997) Etude des poussées cliniques évolutives et des rebonds serologiques d'enfant atteints de toxoplasmose congénitale et suivis durant les 2 premières années de vie. Arch Pédiatr 4:940-946
38. Abboud P, Villena I, Chemla C, Leroux B, Talmud M, Bednarczyk L, Pinon J, Quéreux C (1997) Dépistage de la toxoplasmose congénitale : devenir des grossesses après le diagnostic anténatal. J Gynecol Obstet Biol Reprod 26:40-46
39. Guerina N (1994) Congenital infection with *Toxoplasma gondii*. Pediatr Ann 23:138-151

3.4. Management of and outcome for the newborn infant with congenital toxoplasmosis

R. McLeod, K. Boyer, and the Toxoplasmosis Study Group and Collaborators

Introduction

As part of a National Collaborative Treatment Trial in the USA, based in Chicago, we have developed the following approach to management of the newborn infant with congenital toxoplasmosis. This approach and outcome when it is applied has been described earlier [1-11]. It also has been guided by, and included when possible, the concomitant experience developed in France in which the infected fetus is treated *in utero* by administration of pyrimethamine and sulfadiazine (with leucovorin) to the mother which then cross the placenta [12-16].

Management of congenital toxoplasmosis in the newborn infant

Diagnosis

The evaluations and diagnostic tests we have found useful when congenital toxoplasmosis is suspected in a newborn infant are listed in Table 1 [9]. These studies establish whether or not infection is present and the extent of involvement. When the diagnosis has been established by amniocentesis and PCR to detect the *T. gondii* B1 gene at the 17th week of gestation (or later) and the fetus has been treated by administering pyrimethamine, sulfadiazine and leucovorin to the mother, analysis of CSF is rarely helpful and certain other markers of infection, such as serum *T. gondii* specific IgM, may no longer be present (Fig. 1, Table 2).

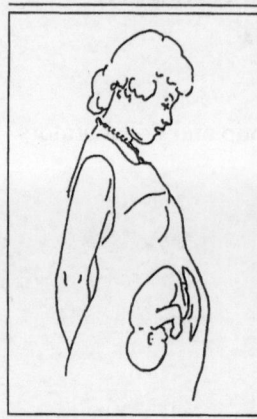

- Diagnosis mother : systematic serologic screening, before conception and intrapartum
- Treatment of mother: if acute serology, spiramycin reduces transmission.
  Untreated [94 (60%) of 154 vs treated 91 (23%) of 388*]
- Treatment of fetus : pyrimethamine, sulfadiazine or termination
  N=54 livebirths; 34 terminaisons**
- Diagnosis fetus : ultradounds, amniocentesis, PCR at ≥ 18 weeks gestation
  Sensitivity 37 (97%) of 38: specificity 301 of 301***
- Outcome: all 54 normal development; initial report was 19% subtle findings:
  7(13%) [intracranial calcifications; 3(6%) chorioretinal scars
  Follow up of 18 yrs (median age 4.5 yrs, range 1-11 yrs): 39% retinal scars, most scars were peripheral****

Fig. 1. Paris approach to prevention, diagnosis and treatment. Adapted from Roberts et al. [9] with minor modifications and permission.
* From Desmonts and Couvreur [12]; ** From Daffos et al. [13]; *** From Hohlfeld et al. [14, 15]; **** From Brezin et al. [16]

Table 1. Evaluation of neonate when serologic tests of mother or the illness of the neonate indicates that diagnosis of congenital toxoplasmosis is suspected or likely

In addition to a careful general examination, when congenital toxoplasmosis is a possible or likely diagnosis, the baby is examined by the following :

Clinical Evaluation and Nonspecific Tests

- By a pediatric ophthalmologist
- By a pediatric neurologist
- CT scan of the brain
- Blood tests
  Complete blood cell count with differential and platelet counts
  Serum total IgM, IgG, IgA, and albumin
- Serum alanine aminotransferase total direct bilirubin
  Cerebrospinal fluid (CSF), cell count, glucose, protein, and total IgG

T. gondii-Specific Tests

- Serum Sabin-Feldman dye test, IgM
  ELISA, IgM ISAGA, IgA ELISA, IgE ELISA/ISAGA (0,5 ml serum, sent to Serology Laboratory, Palo Alto Medical Foundation, 860 Bryant Street, Paolo Alto, CA 94301
- Lumbar puncture: cerebrospinal fluid (CSF) 0,5 ml CSF sent to Serology Laboratory (see above address) for dye test and IgM ELISA
- Sterile placental tissue (100 g in saline, no formalin from near insertion of cord from the fetal side) and newborn blood obtained for inoculation into mice (2 ml clotted whole blood in red topped tube)
- Matenral serum analyzed for antibody detected by dye test, IgM ELISA, IgA ELISA, IgE ELISA/ISAGA, and AC/HS

From Roberts et al. [9] ,with permission

Table 2. Condition of live neonates and positing findings at birth in infants treated according to the Paris algorithm (Fig. 1)

Observations	N°	%
Sublicinal infection	44/54	81
Multiple intracranial calcifications	5/54	9
Single intracranial calcification	2/54	4
Chorioretinitis scar	3/54	6
Abnormal lumbar puncture	1/54	2
Positive findings on inoculation of placenta	23/46	50
Positive cord blood IgM	8/53	15

From Hohlfed et al. [15], with permission

Medical treatment and monitoring this treatment

Our preferred approach, which appears to minimize, but does not always eliminate, serious sequelae, is that developed by Daffos, Thulliez, Holhfeld et al. (Fig. 1 [12-16]). This involves treatment of the fetus *in utero* by administration of pyrimethamine (50 mg once daily), sulfadiazine (3 grams daily, divided as three 1 gram dosages) and folinic acid (leucovorin), (10 mg daily) to the mother. The infant is treated throughout the first year of life with these same medicines as described in Table 3 and Fig. 2. Medicines are formulated as described in Table 4, as there are no pediatric suspensions available. Medications are prepared fresh each week, stored refrigerated, and the dosage is increased as appropriate for weight each week. Prednisone 1mg/kg/day divided bid is administered when there is active intraocular inflammation which threatens vision or if the CSF protein is greater than 1 gram/dl, for as long as these conditions persist. Leucovorin is administered as long as pyrimethamine is administered and for one week after it is discontinued because the half-life of pyrimethamine is approximately 60 hours [11]. Complete blood count with differential is obtained twice weekly (e.g. each Monday and Thursday) while pyrimethamine is administered. Most infants develop a stable neutrophil count of approximately 1,000 neutrophils per mm³. Leucovorin dosage and frequency of its administration is increased if the absolute neutrophil count falls. Ten to 20 mg leucovorin daily has been required to maintain neutrophil counts between 500 and 1,000 per mm³ in some children. Pyrimethamine and sulfadiazine are withheld and leucovorin continued when neutrophil counts are less than 500 per mm³. Dosage of pyrimethamine is maintained at 1mg/kg/day for either two or six months and then this dosage is administered each Monday, Wednesday and Friday for the remainder of the year. At present, this is done in the context of a randomized treatment trial. Pediatricians are cautioned not to use other sulfonamides to treat concomitant bacterial infections such as otitis media, as this may cause profound bone marrow suppression.

Table 3. Treatment of toxoplasmosis

Manifestation of disease	Therapy	Dosage (oral unless specified)	Duration
Congenital toxoplasmosis*	Pyrimethamine*	Loading dose : 2 mg/kg per day for 2 days, then 1 mg/kg/day for 2 or 6 months, then this dose on each Monday, Wednesday, and Friday	1 yr
	and Sulfadiazine* and	100 mg/kg/day in two daily divided doses	1 yr
	Leucovorin (folinic acid)*	10 mg three times weekly†	1 yr
	Corticosteroids (prednisone)§	1 mg/kg/day in two daily divided doses	Until resolution elevated (≥ 1 g/dl) cerebro-spinal fluid protein level or active cho-rioretinitis that threatens vision

From Roberts et al. [9], with permission

* Optimal dosage, fesibility, toxicity currently being evaluated or planned in ongoing U.S. National Collaborative Treatment Trial (773-834-4152)

† Adjusted for megaloblastic anemia, granulocytopenia, or thrombocytopenia; blood counts, including platelets, should be monitored as described in text

§ Corticosteroids should be continued until signs of inflammation (high CSF protein > 1 g/dl) or active chorioretinitis that treatens vision have subsided, dosage then can be tapered and discontinued; use only in conjunction with pyrimethamine, sulfadizine, and leukovorin

Table 4. Oral suspension formulations for pyrimethamine and sulfadiazine in the US

Pyrimethamine: 2 mg/ml suspension
1. Crush FOUR 25 mg pyrimethamine tablets in a mortar to a fine powder
2. Add 10 cc of syrup vehicle
3. Transfer mixture to an amber bottle
4. Rinse mortar with 10 cc of sterile water and transfer
5. Add enough of the serum vehicle to q.s. to 50 ml final volume
6. Shake very well until this is a fine suspension
7. Label and give a 7 day expiration
8. Store refrigerated

Sulfadiazine: 100 mg/ml suspension
1. Crush TEN 500 mg sulfadizine tablets in a mortar to a fine powder
2. Add enough sterile water to make a smooth paste
3. Slowly triturate the syrup vehicle close to the final volume of 50 ml
4. Transfer the suspension to a larger amber bottle
5. Add sufficient syrup vehicle to q.s. to 50 ml final volume
6. Shake well
7. Label and give a 7 day expiration
8. Store refrigerated

Materials
1. Pyrimethamine 25 mg tablets (Daraprim, Glaxo Wellcome Inc.) NDC #0173-0201-55
2. Sulfadiazine 500 mg tablets (Eon Labs Manufacturing, Inc.) NDC #00185-0757-01
3. Syrup vehicle: suggest 2% sugar suspension for pyrimethamine. If the infant is not lactose intolerant 2% sugar suspension can be 2 grams lactose per 100ml distilled water. Suggest for sulfadiazine suspension use simple syrup flavored with or alternatively cherry syrup.

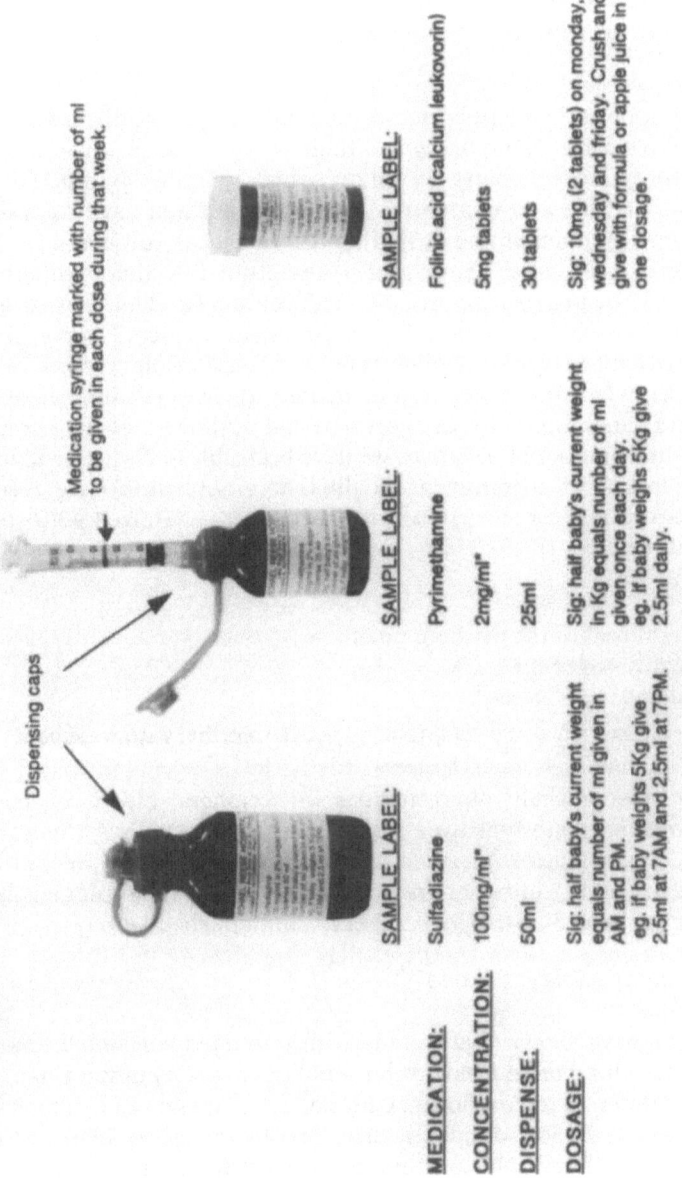

Fig 2. Method used in the U.S. National Collaborative (Chicago) Study for preparing and administering pyrimethamine, sulfadiazine, and leucovorin to infants. From McAuley et al. [1], with permission

Adjunctive therapy

Prompt correction of obstructive hydrocephalus is imperative [3, 4, 7-10]. Adjunctive early intervention strategies to assist cognitive and motor development and vision, physical therapy, occupational therapy and family support are utilized as needed.

Anticonvulsant treatment

Administration of anti-epileptic medications in the context of medicines to treat toxoplasmosis each presents their own unique problem [1]. Phenobarbital induces hepatic enzymes, which degrade pyrimethamine, shortening its half-life and increasing the dosage required to achieve therapeutic levels of pyrimethamine [11]. Dilantin displaces sulfonamides from albumin. Tegretol can cause neutropenia, in a setting in which pyrimethamine is already a bone marrow suppressant. Valproic acid and its derivatives are not considered to be safe to administer to infants under 2 years of age. Experience with the newer anti-epileptic medications for infants is more limited. In general, when anti-epileptic medications for infants were needed, we have utilized Phenobarbital for as short a period of time as we have considered feasible. In a number of instances we have been able to discontinue its use as active toxoplasmic meningoencephalitis or encephalitis have resolved [3, 4]. Hypsarrythmia secondary to toxoplasmosis has resolved with steroid (ACTH) treatment [3].

Outcome of treatment of the newborn infant with congenital toxoplasmosis

Response of systemic signs and symptoms of active infection with treatment

Rash, hepatosplenomegaly, abnormalities in peripheral blood cell counts, thrombocytopenia, abnormal liver function tests and other systemic malfunctions of congenital toxoplasmosis generally resolve within weeks of initiation of treatment [1], although in a few instances hepatosplenomegaly has persisted for prolonged times [McLeod et al., unpublished].

Neurologic and Neuroradiologic Outcome

Earlier studies have shown that infants with untreated congenital toxoplasmosis and generalized or neurologic abnormalities at presentation almost uniformly develop mental retardation, seizures, spasticity, and visual impairment and approximately 20-30% develop hearing loss by the age of 4 years [17]. In earlier decades, children with untreated, subclinical disease at birth subsequently have developed seizures, significant cognitive and motor deficits, and diminution in cognitive function over time [18]. Ophthalmologic lesions occurred in approximately 90% of such children by adolescence [18, 19].

Initially, to determine neurologic, cognitive and motor outcomes for children with congenital toxoplasmosis who were treated for approximately one year with pyrimethamine and sulfadiazine, systematic, prospective and longitudinal neurologic, cognitive and motor evaluations were performed. Thirty-six individuals with congenital toxoplasmosis were evaluated. These infants were born between December 1981 and January 1991. They were treated with pyrimethamine and sulfadiazine for approximately one year beginning in the first months of life. This study presenting our early results was described previously [4] and methods and results were as follows: Medication compliance was documented. These children were evaluated in a standardized manner. This was done in a single center by the same physicians and study group during the children's first months of life, and when the children were approximately 1, 3.5, 5, 7.5, 10, 15 and 20 years of age. Cognitive function of the congenitally infected children was compared with the cognitive function of one of their siblings, who was nearest in age and of the same sex, when such siblings older than 3.5 years were available for study.

We found that signs of active central nervous system infection (e.g., CSF pleiocytosis, hypoglycorrhachia, elevated CSF protein, and in some instances, seizures and motor abnormalities) resolved during therapy. Perinatal seizures were noted for six of the 36 children. We were able to discontinue anticonvulsant therapy without recurrence of seizures for four children within the first months of life. Two additional children developed new seizures at 3 and 5 years of age. There was resolution of tone and motor abnormalities by one year of age in 12 of 20 infants who exhibited abnormalities of tone and motor function at their initial, neonatal evaluation.

In this initial analysis [4], by February 1992, 29 of the 36 children were evaluated at one year of age. Twenty-three (79%) of these children had a mean ± s.d. (range) Mental Developmental Index (MDI) of 102 ± 22 (59-140). For six (21%) of these children, the measure of their cognitive function was < 50. There was no significant difference over time in results of sequential IQ tests, performed at 1 1/2 year intervals ($p > 0.05$). There were seven children with quantifiable MDIs who were compared with their sibling controls. These seven children had scores of 87 ± 11 (68-97) and their siblings had scores of 112 ± 15 (85-132) ($p = 0.008$). For 17 of 18 children without hydrocephalus and 6 of 8 children with obstructive hydrocephalus responsive to shunting (Fig. 3) neurologic and developmental outcomes were normal or near normal. Children with hydrocephalus *ex vacuo* present at birth, and usually those with high CSF proteins (> 1 gram/dl) and/or lack of response to shunting procedures, have done less well.

In this early analysis, for most of these treated children, neurologic and developmental outcomes were significantly better than outcomes reported for untreated children or those treated for only 1 month ($p < 0.001$). There was no significant deterioration in neurologic and cognitive function of the treated children tested sequentially, although level of cognitive function for treated children was less than for their uninfected siblings ($p < 0.008$). The general trends described above have continued as we have treated and followed additional congenitally infected infants, and these favorable treatment out-

comes justify systematic identification and treatment of pregnant women
with acute gestational *Toxoplasma* infection and young infants with congenital toxoplasmosis.

In addition, as described earlier [5], we determined natural history of
intracranial calcifications detected with cranial computed tomography scans
in children with treated congenital toxoplasmosis between January 1982 and
March 1994. Cranial computed tomography (CT) was performed for 56

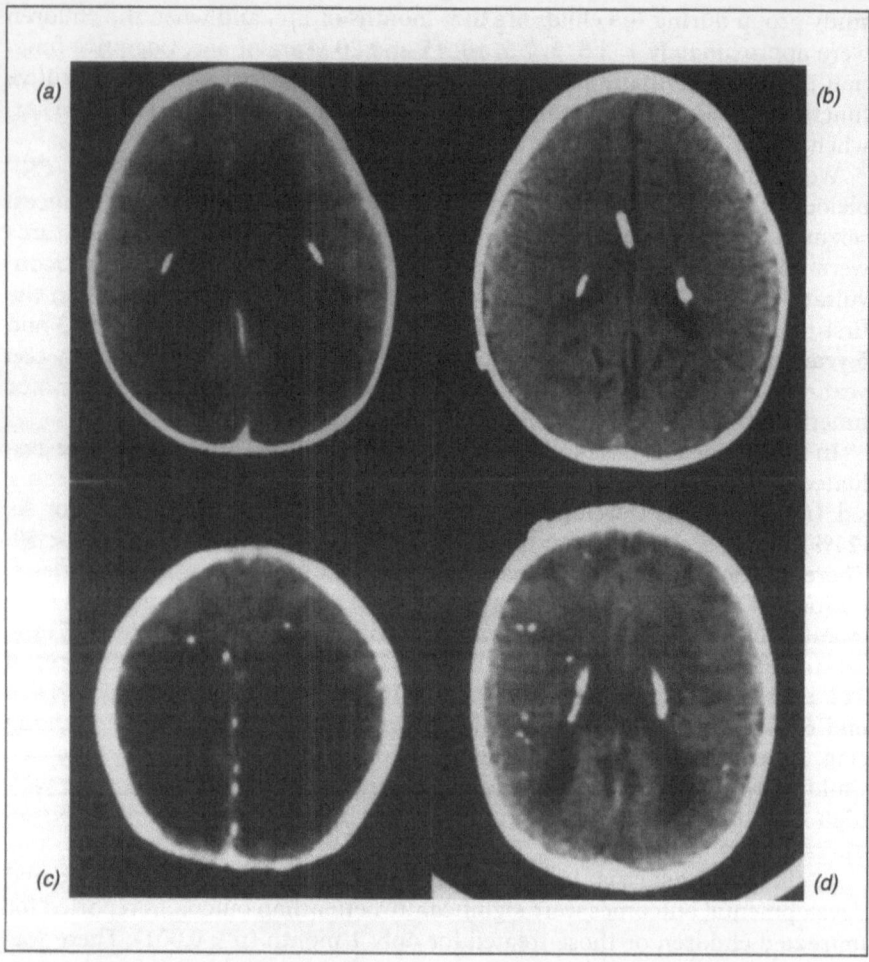

Fig. 3. Cranial CT scans of two infants one represented in (a) and (b), the other in (c) and
d) before (a and c) and after (b and d) placement of ventriculoperitoneal shunts. Both
infants have developed normally. CT scans and the subsequent normal development of these
children indicate that it is not possible to predict ultimate cognitive outcome from the initial appearance of the CT scan. From Boyer and McLeod [8], with permission

infants with treated congenital toxoplasmosis. These studies were performed when the children were newborn and approximately 1 year old. We noted locations and sizes of intracranial calcifications. There were 40 newborns with intracranial calcifications. By 1 year of age, calcifications diminished or resolved in 30 (75%) and remained stable in 10 (25%) of these treated children (e.g., as seen in the representative examples in Fig. 4).

Ten (33%) of 30 children whose calcifications diminished versus 7 (70%) of 10 children with stable calcifications received less intensive antimicrobial treatment than the other treated children. In contrast, a small number of children who were untreated or treated (1 month), had intracranial calcifications that remained stable or increased during their first year of life. Diminution or resolution of intracranial calcifications was unexpected. This remarkable finding in children with treated, congenital toxoplasmosis, is consonant with their improved neurologic functioning. Response to shunt procedures has varied. In some instances, favorable responses are quite remarkable (Fig. 3).

Ophthalmologic outcome

In our study we also determined the natural history of treated and untreated congenital ocular toxoplasmosis, and defined the impact of this infection on vision [6-10]. In recent descriptions of this experience [6], we characterized ninety-four patients who were studied in a consistent, systematic, prospective, and longitudinal manner. Briefly, as summarized in [6], seventy-six congenitally infected children were treated with pyrimethamine and sulfadiazine beginning in the newborn period (or perinatally) for approximately 1 year. Eighteen individuals entered our study after their first year of life and had not been treated during the first year of life ("historical patients"). In all patients, chorioretinal scars were the most common eye finding (Fig. 5, Table 5). They occurred most commonly in the peripheral retina (58% of treated and 82% of historical patients). Macular scars were present in 54% of treated patients and 41% were bilateral. Macular scars were present in 76% of historical patients and 23% were bilateral. In the presence of macular lesions visual acuity ranged from 20/20 to 20/400 [6].

Twenty-nine percent of the patients followed from the newborn period and treated had bilateral visual impairment and visual acuity for their best eye less than 20/40. When eye lesions were quiescent, causes for this visual impairment included macular scars and dragging of the macula secondary to a peripheral lesion, retinal detachment, optic atrophy, cataract, amblyopia, and phthisis (tables 5, 6).

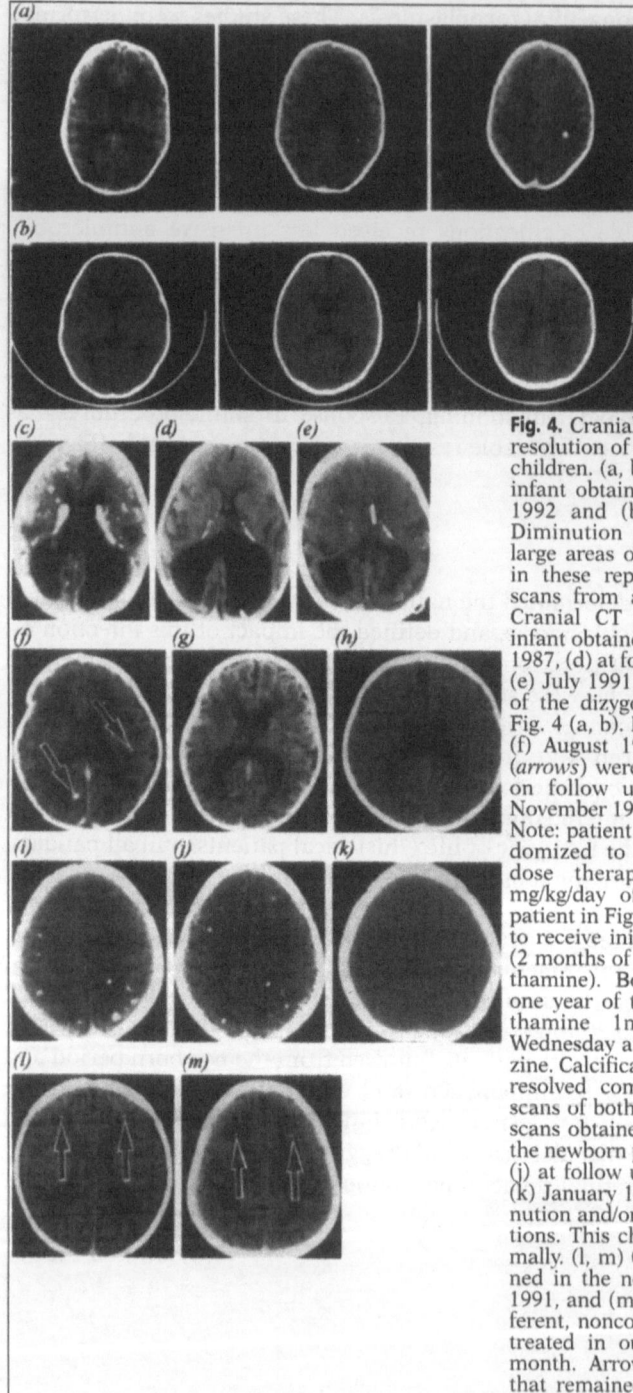

Fig. 4. Cranial CT scans demonstrate resolution of calcifications in treated children. (a, b) CT scans in a treated infant obtained (a) at birth, August 1992 and (b) August 1993. (c-e) Diminution and/or resolution of large areas of calcification are seen in these representative cranial CT scans from another treated infant. Cranial CT scans in this treated infant obtained (c) at birth, February 1987, (d) at follow up, May 1988, and (e) July 1991. (f-h) Cranial CT scans of the dizygotic twin of patient in Fig. 4 (a, b). Newborn scan obtained (f) August 1992. The calcifications (*arrows*) were seen to have resolved on follow up scans obtained (g) November 1992 and (h) August 1993. Note: patient in Fig 4 (a, b) was randomized to receive initial higher dose therapy (6 months of 1 mg/kg/day of pyrimethamine) and patient in Fig 4 (f-h) was randomized to receive initial lower dose therapy (2 months of 1 mg/kg/day of pyrimethamine). Both infants completed one year of treatment with pyrimethamine 1mg/kg each Monday, Wednesday and Friday and sulfadiazine. Calcifications were seen to have resolved completely in cranial CT scans of both twins. (i-k) Cranial CT scans obtained for another infant in the newborn period (i) January 1993, (j) at follow up, February 1993, and (k) January 1994, demonstrate diminution and/or resolution of calcifications. This child has developed normally. (l, m) Cranial CT scans obtained in the newborn period (l) May 1991, and (m) August 1992, in a different, noncompliant child who was treated in our study for only one month. Arrows mark calcifications that remained the same size. From Patel et al. [5], with minor modifications and permission

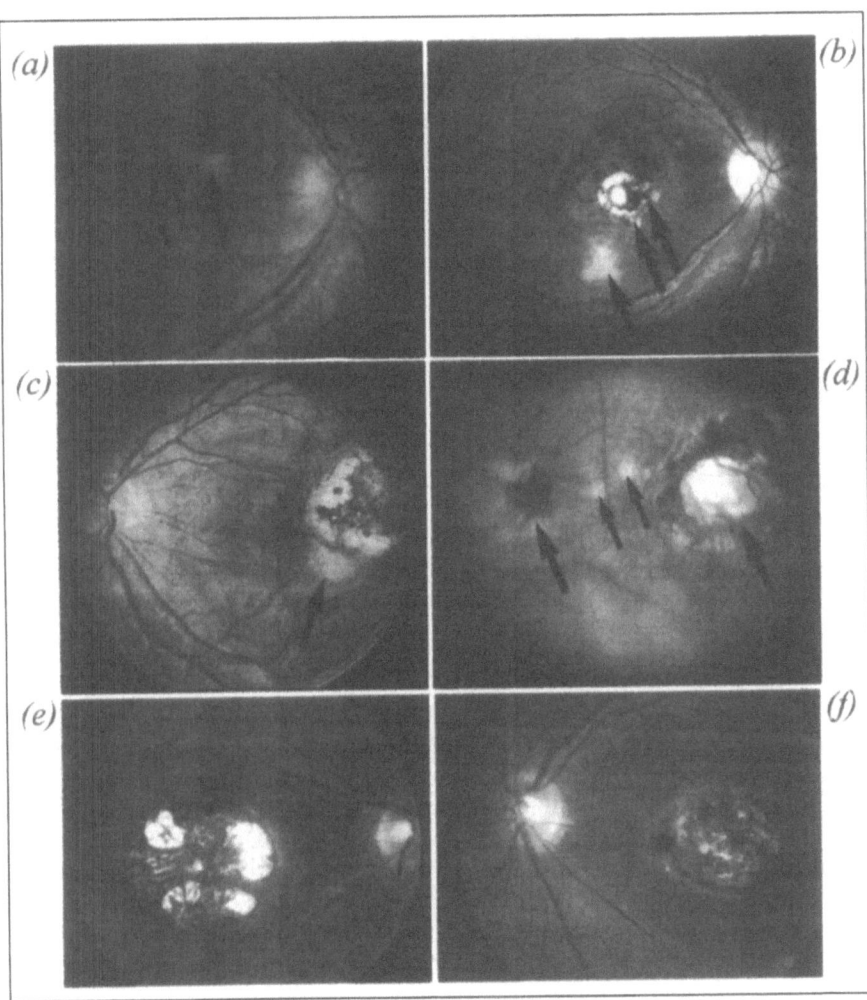

Fig. 5. Toxoplasmic chorioretinitis and scars. (a, b) Two examples of active and quiescent retinal lesions. Active lesions satellite quiescent pigmented scars. (a) Right eye of 4-year-old patient showing an active lesion (*single arrow*) nasal to an old pigmented chorioretinal scar (*double arrow*). It is noteworthy that visual acuity in this eye is 20/30. (b) Right eye of 12-year-old patient showing an active lesion (*arrow*) inferior to an old chorioretinal scar (*double arrows*). (c) Subretinal neovascularization. Left eye of a 6-year-old patient. The central chorioretinal scar has a contiguous chorioretinal neovascular membrane (*arrow*). (d) Newer lesions (*small arrows*) satellite old pigmented scars (*large arrows*). (e, f) Macular scars with similar appearance associated with different visual acuities in the same individual. (e) Right eye, visual acuity is 20/200. (f) Left eye, visual acuity is 20/60. Figs. (a-c, e, f) from Mets et al. [6], with permission

Table 5. Ophthalmologic manifestations of congenital toxoplasmosis

	Treated patients	Historical patients	Total
	Number with finding (%) n = 76	Number with finding (%) n = 18	Number with finding (%) n = 94
Strabismus	26 (34	5 28)	31 (33)
Nystagmus	20 (26)	5 (28)	25 (27)
Microphthalmia	10 (13)	2 (11)	12 (13)
Phtisis	4 (5)	0 (0)	4 (4)
Microcornea	15 (20)	3 (17)	18 (19
Cataract	7 (9)	2 (11)	9 (10)
Vitritis (active)	3 (4)*	2 (11)	5 (5)
Retinitis (active)	6 (8)	4 (22)	10 (11)
Chorioretinal scars	56 (74)	18 (100)	74 (79)
- Macular	39/72 (54)†	13/17 (76)	52/89 (58)
- Juxtapapillary	37/72 (50)	9/17 (53)	46/89 (52)
- Peripheral	43/72 (58)	14/17 (82)	57/89 (64)
Retinal detachment	7 (9)	2 (11)	9 (10)
Optic atrophy	14 (18)	5 (28)	19 (20)

* Two additional patients, not included in this table, were receiving treatment and retino-choroiditis had resolved, but vitreous cells and veils persisted at time of examination.
† Numerator represents number with finding. Denominator represents n, unless otherwise specified. Number in parentheses is percentage. Patients with bilateral retinal detachment in whom the location of scars was not possible were exluded from the denominator.
From Mets et al. [6], with permission

Recurrences occurred in both treated (13%, 7/54) and previously untreated historical patients (44%, 8/18) (table 6). The total, median, and range of years of follow-up during which recurrences were observed were as follows: 189 years (total), 5 years (median), and 3 to 10 years (range) for treated children, and 160 years (total), 11 years (median) and 3-24 years (range) for historical untreated patients [6]. New lesions occurred contiguous to older scars [5] and also in previously normal retina. Within 10 to 14 days of initiation of pyrimethamine and sulfadiazine therapy, active lesions became more sharply demarcated, sometimes pigmented, and thus appeared to become quiescent.

We conclude [6] that many children with congenital toxoplasmosis already have substantial retinal damage when they are born, with consequent loss of vision. Nonetheless, in the presence of large macular scars, vision may be remarkably good. With treatment, active lesions become quiescent.

In a study [16] in which a subsequent ophthalmologic evaluation was similar to that performed in the US,18 children with congenital toxoplasmosis who were treated in utero were examined by a US (M. Mets) and a French (A. Brezin) ophthalmologist. This was done to assess the effect of maternal and post-natal anti-*Toxoplasma* treatment when a prenatal diagnosis of toxoplasmosis was made, and to facilitate a direct comparison of the US postnatal and prenatal/postnatal approach used in France and in the US when possible. Only cases in which maternal infection was documented to have developed during the first half of the pregnancy were included. Disease was

Table 6. New or recrudescent retinal lesions in treated and historical patients which occurred after 1 year of age

Group	Patient number	Age (years) noted*	Previous eye lesion	Active	Location	Visual acuity before; after	Serology during relapse
Treated	7	6[A], 10[A]	no, yes	yes	perimacular, peripheral†	20/20; 20/206	not acute, n/a
	9	5[A]	no	no	posterior pole	nl; 20/50	n/a
	12	3[A], 10[A]	no, yes	yes	peripheral, peripapillary†	20/20; 20/30	not acute
	13	7[b]	yes	yes**	perimacular†	6/400; 20/200	not acute
	15	3[A]	yes	no	peripheral†	20/30; 20/30	n/a
	19	5[C], 8[C]	yes	yes**	peripheral†	20/20; 20/20	not acute
	21	4[A]	yes	no	perimacular†	abnl; 1/30	not acute
Historical	20	3[A]	yes	yes**	peripheral	1/30; 20/400	not acute
	25	10[A]	yes	no	peripheral	20/400; 18/200	not acute
	27	7[A]	yes	no	perimacular	3/30; 5/30	n/a
	42	10[A]	yes	yes**	perimacular†	20/30; 20/30	not acute
	46	24[A]	yes	yes**	perimacular†	20/60; 20/60	not acute
	62	11[C], 13[C], 15[B]	yes	yes**	perimacular, peripheral	20/20; 20/15	n/a
	82	16[A]	yes	yes**	peripapillary	20/400; 20/400	not acute
	89	12[B]	yes	yes**	perimacular	20/100; n/a	not acute

n/a, not available; nl, normal; abnl, abnormal. Patient numbers are those used in publications from the U.S. National Collaborative Study Group
* [A]Recurrence documented at visit in Chicago; [B]recurrence documented by history, photographs reviewed in Chicago, and [C]recurrence documented by history only
† Satellites earlier lesion; § Quantitative visual acuity measured using Snellen chart or Allen cards; ** Symptoms present during active disease.

From Mets et al. [6], with permission

first suspected due to the mother's seroconversion, with monitoring performed routinely in France. Toxoplasmic infection of the fetus was confirmed by analysis of fetal blood or amniotic fluid [13, 16]. Pregnant women received a regimen of alternating pyrimethamine-sulfadiazine and spiramycin until their infants were born. Treatment of children for toxoplasmosis was initiated at birth and continued during the first 12 months of life in most cases. Median age of the children was 4.5 years (range 1-11) when they were evaluated by A. Brezin and M. Mets (who also has evaluated most of the US children). No lesions were found in either eye in 11/18 (61%) of the children. Unilateral and bilateral chorioretinal scars were observed in 3/18 (17%) and in 4/18 (22%) of the cases, respectively. Only one case with bilateral macular lesions, with severe visual impairment, was seen. The localization of the scars was only in the periphery for 5 eyes, in the posterior pole but non foveal for 3 eyes, and foveal or juxta-foveal for 3 eyes. *In utero* diagnosis of congenital toxoplasmosis allowed for early therapeutic intervention, and our results suggested that prenatal treatment decreased the frequency and severity of chorioretinal lesions compared to those of comparable children treated only postnatally in the US (Table 5, [6]), although the incidence of retinal lesions was greater than that described earlier for retinal examinations near birth in such children [12, 16].

The advantage of prenatal treatment (Fig. 1) also was emphasised to us by our evaluation of histopathological features in the eyes of fetuses and infants with congenital toxoplasmosis [Roberts et al., manuscript submitted]. In this study eyes from fetuses, premature infants and a 2 year old child with congenital toxoplasmosis were examined using light microscopy and with immunohistochemistry to identify inflammatory cells and *T. gondii*. In these tissues, retinitis, retinal necrosis, retinal pigment epithelial disruption and choroidal inflammation and congestion and optic neuritis were noted. One fetal eye had retinal rosettes at the edge of a scar. There were T cells and parasites in retinal lesions and choroid. There are important implications of this work for treatment. Specifically, as ocular toxoplasmosis causes irreversible damage to the retina in utero and the fetus and infant mount inflammatory responses which may contribute to ocular damage, serological screening programs and *in utero* therapy [12-16] are needed to help to prevent ocular damage from this congenital infection.

Audiologic outcome

Educationally significant hearing loss has been reported to occur in 10% to 30% of children with congenital toxoplasmosis. As part of a pilot study to assess feasibility and safety of prolonged therapy for congenital toxoplasmosis, auditory function of 30 congenitally infected infants and children was evaluated [2]. Serial testing was performed beginning within 2 months of birth. Evaluation at an earlier age than previously possible was feasible due to availability of auditory brainstem response (ABR) testing. Six (20%) of 30 infants had mild to moderate conductive type hearing loss associated with otitis media. No infant or child had sensorineural hearing loss. The better outcome we observed (Table 7) compared to previous reports of a 15% to 26% incidence of sensorineural hearing loss and 10% to 15% incidence of educationally significant, bilateral hearing impairment. Outcome may be related to early initiation and/or prolonged institution of antimicrobial therapy [2]. Continued follow-up to date in larger numbers of children has not revealed progressive hearing impairment in any child and thus appears to verify the preliminary findings reported earlier [2].

Table 7. Definitions of hearing impairment and outcome in reported studies of hearing in cases of congenital toxoplasmosis

	Définitions						
	Present study						
Degree of hearing impairment	ABR (dB/HL)	Audiogram (dB/HL)	Wilson et al.	Eichenwald	Present Study	Wilson et al	Eichenwald
Normal	≤ 20	0-20	< 25 dB*	not available	104	14	not available
Mild	> 20-40	25-40	25-50 dB	not available	0	3	not available
Moderate	> 40-60	> 40	51-80 dB	not available	0	2	not available
Severe	> 60	> 70-90	not found	not available	0	0	not available
Profound		> 90	not found	"deaf"	0	0	15
Total					104	19	105

Adapted from McGee et al [2] with minor modifications and permission.
* Defined as "hearing reception threshold" in Remington et al [7]

Comparisons with the untreated disease or disease treated only one month and between shorter and longer treatment with 1 mg/kg pyrimethamine daily

Comparisons of outcomes of earlier untreated children or children treated only one month with children in our study (with 2 or 6 months of 1 mg/kg dosages of pyrimethamine followed by this dosage on Monday, Wednesday and Friday, and sulfadiazine), are in Tables 8a-b and 9a-d.

Medication toxicity and alternative medicines

We observed no irreversible medicine toxicity in infants, which precluded the use of pyrimethamine and sulfadiazine, which are the most active of the available antimicrobial agents [11, 21]. Potentially therapeutic levels of pyrimethamine [11] were achieved by the medication regimens described herein. As we noted that CSF pyrimethamine levels were 10 to 25% of serum levels [11], it seems reasonable that serum concentrations of pyrimethamine should be in excess of 250 ng/ml (trough), in order to achieve therapeutic levels of pyrimethamine in CSF, retina and cerebral tissues, based on *in vitro* testing of the standard laboratory (RH), Type I, *T. gondii* strain (Fig. 6, [11, 21]). To our knowledge, multiple strains of *T. gondii* have not been tested in this manner *in vitro* or in animal models *in vivo*. Serum concentrations in excess of 250ng/ml were not consistently present longer than 48-72 hours after a dose of 1 mg/kg of pyrimethamine given to infants, at steady state (Fig. 6).

Table 8a. Development of adverse sequelae in children born with subclinical congenital *Toxoplasma* infection

	Group 1[a] (n = 13)	Group 2[b] (n = 11)
Ophthalmologic finding		
– No sequelae	2	0
– Retinochoroiditis		
• Bilateral		
Bilateral blindness	0	5
Unilateral blindness	3	3
Moderate unilateral visual loss	0	1
Minimal or no visual loss	5	1
• Unilateral		
Minimal or no visual loss	3	0
Mean age at onset (yr)	3.67	0.42
Range	0.08-9.33	0.25-1.00
Recurrences of active chorioretinitis	3	2
Neurological finding[c]		
– No sequelae	8	3
– Major sequelae		
• Hydrocephalus	0	1
• Microcephaly	1	1
• Seizures	1	3
• Severe psychomotor retardation	1	2
– Minor sequelae		
• Mild cerebellar dysfunction	2	4
• Transiently delayed psychomotor development	2	2
Other abnormality		
– Sensorineural hearing loss		
• Moderate unilateral	1 of 10	1 of 9
• Mild unilateral	1 of 10	0 of 9
• Mild bilateral	1 of 10	1 of 9
– Precocious puberty	2	2
– Premature thelarche	0	1
– Miscellaneous	3	1.

From Wilson et al [18], with permission
[a] No abnormalities found on extensive newborn evaluation based on awareness of a diagnosis of congenital toxoplasmosis; [b] No abnormalities found on a routine newborn physical examination; [c] Eighty-six percent of eight children who were tested had sequentially lower intelligence quotient scores

Table 8b. Signs and symptoms ocurring before diagnosis or during the course of untreated acute congenital toxoplasmosis in 152 infants and 101 of these same patients after 4 years or more of follow-up[a]

Signs and symptoms	Frequency of Occurence in Patients with	
	Neurologic disease[b]	Generalized disease[c]
Infants	N = 108	N = 44
Retinochoroiditis	102 (94)a	29 (66)
Abnormal spinal fluid	59 (55)	37 (84)
Anemia	55 (51)	34 (77)
Jaundice	31 (29)	35 (80)
Splenomegaly	23 (21)	40 (90)
Convulsions	54 (50)	8 (18)
Fever	27 (25)	34 (77)
Intracranial calcification	54 (50)	2 (4)
Hepatomegaly	18 (17)	34 (77)
Lymphadenopathy	18 (17)	30 (68)
Vomiting	17 (16)	21 (48)
Hydrocephalus	30 (28)	0 (0)
Diarrhea	7 (6)	11 (25)
Pneumonitis	0 (0)	18 (41)
Microcephalus	14 (13)	0 (0)
Eosinophilia	6 (4)	8 (18)
Rash	1 (1)	11 (25)
Abnormal bleeding	3 (3)	8 (18)
Hypothermia	2 (2)	9 (20)
Cataracts	5 (5)	0 (0)
Glaucoma	2 (2)	0 (0)
Optic atrophy	2 (2)	0 (7)
Microphthalmia	2 (2)	0 (7)
Children 4 years old (or more)	N = 70	N = 31
Mental retardation	62 (89)	25 (81)
Convulsions	58 (83)	24 (77)
Spasticity and palsies	53 (76)	18 (58)
Severely impaired vision	48 (69)	13 (42)
Hydrocephalus or microcephalus	31 (44)	2 (6)
Deafness	12 (17)	3 (10)
Normal	6 (9)	5 (16)

From Eichenwald [17], with permission. [a] Data indicate numbers of patients, with percentages in parentheses; [b] Patients with central nervous system diseases in the first year of life; [c] Patients with non-neurologic diseases during the first 2 months of life

Table 8c. Comparison of ophthalmologic, developmental and audiologic outcomes with postnatal treatment[a]

Author(s), year of publication [ref.]	Treatment	N° studied	Mean age in years when data tabulated (range)	Ophthalmologic			Neurologic		Audiologic
				Lesions[b]	Vision[c]	New[d]	Cognitive	Motor of seizures	
Eichenwald, 1959 [17]	0 or 1 mo P, S[e]	104	4 (minimum)	NA[f]	0,42, 67[g]	NA	50, 81, 89[g]	0, 58, 76[g]	0, 10, 17[g]
Wilson et al., 1980 [18]	0 or 1 mo, P, S	23	8.5 (1-17)	93	47	22	55 (20 severe)	20	22,30[a]
Koppe et al., 1986 [19]	0 or 1 mo P, S	12	20 (NA)	80	NA	NA	0	0	NA
Labadie and Hazeman, 1984 [20]	0	17	1 (NA)	28	NA	NA	NA	NA	NA
Couvreur et al., 1984 [21]	1 yr P, S, Sp[i]	172	NA (2-11)	NA	NA	8	NA	NA	NA
Hohlfeld, 1989 [15]	Prenatal, 1 yr P, S, Sp	43	NA (0.5-4)	12	NA	NA	0	0	NA
Villena, 1998 [23]	F[j], SP	47	NA [born 1980-89]	–	–	15/45 (33)[k]	–	–	–
	1 yr F	19	NA [born 1990-96]	–	–	2/18 (11)	–	–	–
	2 yrs F	12	NA [born 1990-97]	–	–	1/11 (9)	–	–	–
Peyron, 1996 [24]	F[l]	121	12 (5-22)	–	–	37/121 (31)	–	–	–
Chicago study (historical patients)	0	7	5.6 (2-10)	100	86	29	25	25	14
Chicago study (treated patients)	Most for 1 yr P, S	37[m]	3.4 (0.3-10)	81	81	8	0,24[h]	0,24	0

[a] Adapted from McAuley et al. [1], with permission; [b] Lesions = any chorioretinal lesions; [c] Vision = vision impaired; [d] New = new lesions; [e] P = pyrimethamine, S = sulfonamides; [f] NA = not available; [g] Subclinical, generalized, neurologic; [h] Subclinical, generalized/neurologic; [i] Sp = spiramycin; [j] F = Fansidar® (in utero, and postnatally pyrimethamine 1.25 mg/kg each 14 days); [k] Number with finding/number in group (%); [l] F = Fansidar® (in utero, and postnatally pyrimethamine 6 mg/5 kg each 10 days). Small numbers also treated in utero; [m] These data are for the first 37 children studied prior to May 1991

Table 9b. Ages of patients in US National Collaborative Study*

	All patients		Patients ≥ 5 years old	
	Mean ± s.d.	Range	Mean ± s.d.	Range
Historical patients	13.9 ± 8.9	5.4-33.4	15.3 ± 8.9	5.4-33.4
Treatment A: feasibility	11.7 ± 1.1	10.0-14.3	11.7 ± 1.1	10.0-14.3
randomized	5.7 ± 1.9	1.9-8.8	7.7 ± 0.9	6.2-8.8
Treatment C: feasibility	0.5 ± 4.8	0.5-15	12.7 ± 3.2	10.5-15.0
randomized	5.4 ± 2.0	09-10.0	7.5 ± 1.3	6.2-10.0

* Historical patients were untreated patients diagnosed after one year of age. Treated children received 2 months (Treatment A) or 6 months (Treatment C) of daily pyrimethamine and sulfadiazine, followed by pyrimethamine on Monday, Wednesday and Friday and continued daily sulfadiazine for the remainder of the year of therapy

There is a large experience in Europe with administration of pyrimethamine/sulfadoxine (Fansidar®) to pregnant women and children to treat toxoplasmosis and serum pyrimethamine and sulfadoxine levels have been determined [22-27]. Serum levels of pyrimethamine were approximately 350 ng/ml peak and 25 ng/ml trough following administration of 1.25mg/kg pyrimethamine to infants each 14 days [22]. Certain outcomes associated with administration of this regimen of Fansidar® each 10-14 days either alone for the first one or two years of life or with spiramycin (presumably in alternate treatment with Fansidar® as was standard at the time, although this is not stated in the manuscript) have been described [23]. These authors and others suggest that such treatments may have reduced, but not eliminated, sequelae such as retinal lesions and visual loss, when treated children are compared with those in the literature [23, 24]. These authors suggest that treatments with more Fansidar® might have resulted in fewer ocular sequelae, but apparently there was no prospective randomization, clear correlation with antimicrobial agent levels, and no statistical analyses of these data were reported [23].

Fansidar® is a more convenient regimen to administer than daily pyrimethamine and sulfadiazine and when Fansidar® was administered each 14 days there was no reported hematological toxicity from the pyrimethamine [23]. This contrasts with relatively frequent, reversible neutropenia necessitating careful hematologic monitoring of children treated with the US regimen. There was no reported serious toxicity in this experience [23, 24] with Fansidar® although the numbers of patients described would not have been sufficient to detect the idiosyncratic, serious and life threatening, although infrequent, toxicity of pyrimethamine/sulfadoxine (Fansidar®) that has been reported with its use in other settings [28]. The long half-life of sulfadoxine leads to its presence in sera and tissues for prolonged times. This has led others considering its use for treatment of toxoplasmosis or other conditions to express concern about the potential increased danger in using Fansidar®, with possible prolongation of potentially life threatening sulfonamide toxicity. Further, a direct comparison of the relative efficacy of pyrimethamine with sulfadoxine versus sulfadiazine *in vitro* demonstrated that sulfadoxine was somewhat less effective than sulfadiazine (Fig. 7, [29]). The clinical significance of these differences, if any, remain to be determined.

Table 9c. Endpoints for US National Collaborative Study for children ≥ 5 years old

	Mild						Severe					
	% in Literature 5 yrs, 10 yrs	Historical Patients*	Feasibility	Treatment A Randomized	Feasibility	Treatment C Randomized	% in Literature 5 yrs, 10 yrs	Historical Patients	Feasibility	Treatment A Randomized	Feasibility	TreatmentC Randomized
Vision < 20/20	25, 50	11/14 (79)	0/4 (0)	0/3 (0)	0/0 (0)	0/0 (0)	70, 70	10/10 (100)	7/9 (78)	8/9 (89)	1/2 (50)	6/9 (67)
New retinal lesions	25, 85	5/9 (56)	0/4 (0)	1/3 (33)	0/0 (0)	0/0 (0)	50, 90	4/9 (44)	3/9 (33)	1/8 (13)	2/2 (100)	0/9 (0)
Motor abnormality	10, 10	0/14 (0)	0/4 (0)	0/3 (0)	0/0 (0)	0/0 (0)	60, 60	1/10 (10)	3/9 (33)	2/9 (22)	0/2 (0)	1/9 (11)
IQ < 70	0-50, 0-50	0/13 (0)	0/4 (0)	0/3 (0)	0/0 (0)	0/0 (0)	90, > 90	1/10 (10)	4/9 (44)	4/9 (44)	0/2 (0)	1/9 (11)
ΔIQ ≥ 15	50, 50	0/5 (0)	0/4 (0)	1/3 (33)	0/0 (0)	0/0 (0)	95, 95	0/8 (0)	0/9 (0)	2/9 (22)	0/2 (0)	1/9 (11)
Hearing loss	30, 30	0/14 (0)	0/4 (0)	0/3 (0)	0/0 (0)	0/0 (0)	30, 30	0/10 (0)	0/9 (0)	0/9 (0)	0/2 (0)	0/9 (0)

* Number with abnormality/number in group (% affected). See Table 9b for description of groups. No differences between treatment regimens achieved statistical significance ($p > 0.05$ using Fischer Exact test)

Table 9d. Toxicity is measured as episodes of reversible neutropenia requiring temporary with holding of medications

	N° of episodes medication withheld (mean ± s.d. [range])	Number who stopped medication/ N° in group who have completed one year of therapy (%)	N° of children who stopped medications temporarily/N° in group (%) Feasibility	N° of children who stopped medications temporarily/N° in group (%) Randomized	Discontinued medications due to neutropenia ≥ 4 times
Treatment A	1.8 ± 1.1 [1-4]	11/32 (34)	6/14 (43)	11/34 (32)	4
Treatment C	3.8 ± 3.1 [1-11]	17/48 (35)	1/4 (25)	10/28 (36)	5

See Table 9b for description of groups

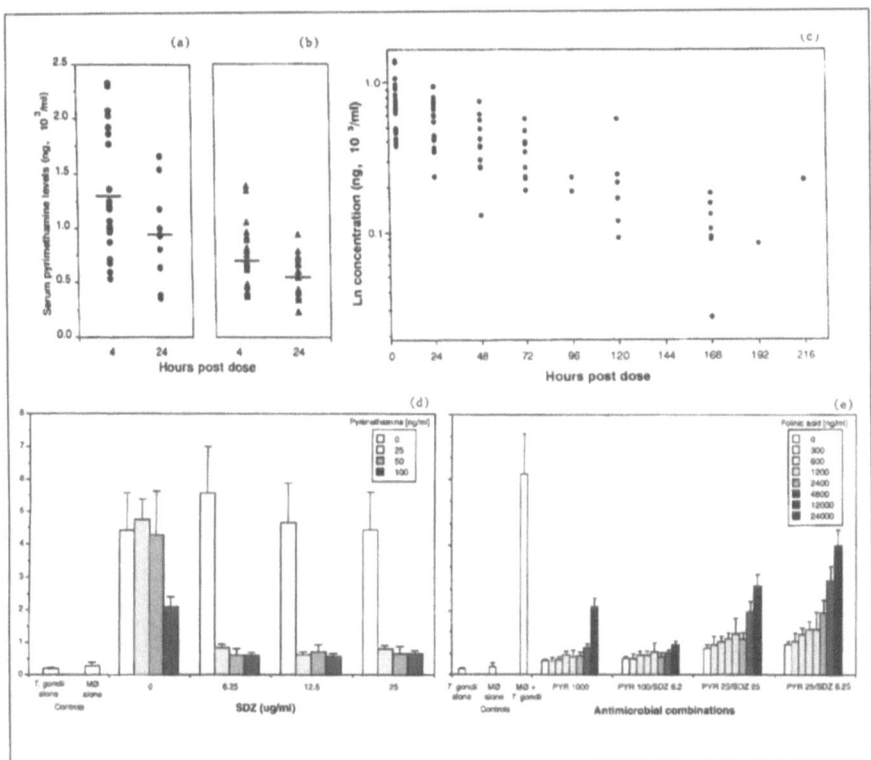

Fig. 6. Pyrimethamine pharmacokinetics. (a) Pyrimethamine serum levels (4 and 24 hours post dose) of children given 1 mg of pyrimethamine per kg daily. (b) Pyrimethamine serum levels (4 and 24 hours post dose) of children given 1 mg of pyrimethamine per kg on Monday, Wednesday and Friday of each week. Values for children taking Phenobarbital are not included. (c) Pyrimethamine serum levels of the entire study population of infants taking 1 mg of pyrimethamine per kg on Monday, Wednesday, and Friday of each week. Values for children taking Phenobarbital are not included. (d) Effects of pyrimethamine (alone and with sulfadiazine [SDZ] on [3H] uracil incorporation by intracellular *T. gondii*. (e) Effects of various concentrations of folinic acid on the antimicrobial activity of pyrimethamine and sulfadiazine on intracellular *T. gondii*; MØ mouses peritoneal macrophages. From McLeod et al. [11], with permission

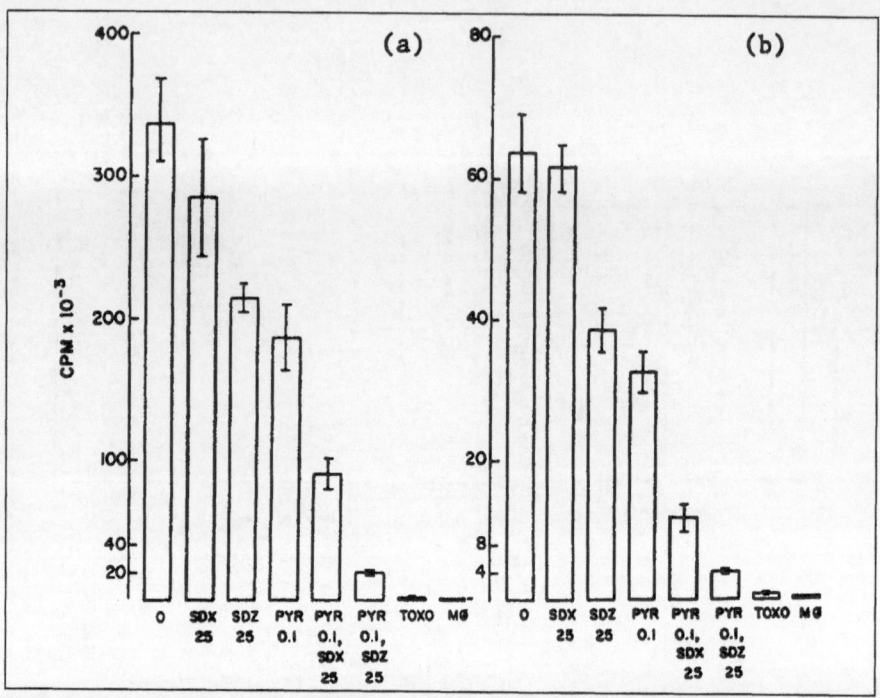

Fig. 7. Comparison of sulfadiazine and sulfadoxine effects on growth of the RH strain of *T. gondii in vitro*. These studies were performed in a study of usefulness of (a) a macromethod and (b) a micromethod in evaluating the effects of antimicrobial agents on *T. gondii*. SDX, sulfadoxine; SDZ, sulfadiazine; PYR, pyrimethamine; TOXO, *T. gondii* alone; MØ, macrophages alone. Concentrations of antimicrobial agents are shown in micrograms per milliliter, data are means ± standard deviation for four replicate wells. From Mack and McLeod [21], with permission

Because we have no direct experience with use of Fansidar® or medicines other than pyrimethamine/sulfadiazine and leucovorin for the treatment of congenital toxoplasmosis in the newborn, and for the reasons above, at the present time we cannot recommend using medicines besides pyrimethamine, sulfadiazine, and leucovorin as "first line" treatment for congenital toxoplasmosis in the newborn. Other medicines or medical regimens such as clindamycin and pyrimethamine together have been used as "second line" medicines in other settings.

Resources

Available resources are listed in Table 10. These include Diagnostic Reference Laboratories, Treatment Trials, Educational Materials, Early Intervention Programs, and Parent/Family Support.

Table 10. Some pertinent resources and phone numbers

Reference laboratory for serology, isolation and PCR (US)	650-853-4828
Reference laboratory for serology, isolation and PCR (France)	33-1-40-44-39-41
FDA for IND number to obtain spiramycin for treatment of a pregnant woman (US)	301-827-2335
Spiramycin (Rhone Poulenc) for treatment of a pregnant woman (US)	610-454-8469
Congenital Toxoplasmosis Study Group (US)	773-834-4152
Education pamphlet/The March of Dimes (US)	312-435-4007
Information concerning AIDS and congenital toxoplasmosis (US)	305-243-6522
Information for European families (UK)	44-0171-713-0663
Educational information on the Internet	http://www.iit.edu/~toxo/pamphlet

The Future

The single most needed improvement in management of congenital toxoplasmosis is medicine(s) able to eradicate latent bradyzoites. A better understanding of the metabolism of bradyzoites and also of the constituents of the cyst wall may provide the needed information to begin to rationally develop antimicrobial agent targeted against components of bradyzoites and thus the medicines needed to eradicate bradyzoites.

Acknowledgements

This work was supported by National Institutes of Health Grant R01-TMP-AI 27530, The United Airlines Foundation, Angel Flight, The Huffy and the Buchanan Family, United to Save Children, Gerico, and Hyatt Hotel Corporation Foundation, the Research and Education Foundation of the Michael Reese Medical Staff, the Michael Reese Institute Council, and The Research to Prevent Blindness Foundation (University of Chicago). Rima McLeod, MD is the Jules and Doris Stein Research to Prevent Blindness Professor at the University of Chicago. We also gratefully acknowledge the cooperation of the patients in the US National Collaborative Treatment Trial and their families and the primary physicians of these patients.

References

1. McAuley J, Boyer K, Patel D et al (1994) Early and longitudinal evaluations of treated infants and children and untreated historical patients with congenital toxoplasmosis: the Chicago Collaborative Treatment Trial. Clin Infect Dis 18:38-72
2. McGee T, Wolters C, Stein L et al (1992) Absence of sensorineural hearing loss in treated infants and children with congenital toxoplasmosis. Otolaryngol Head Neck Surg 106(1):75-80
3. Swisher CN, Boyer K, McLeod R et al (1994) Congenital Toxoplasmosis. Sem. Ped. Neurol 1(1):4-25
4. Roizen N, Swisher C, Stein M et al (1995) Neurologic and Developmental Outcome in treated congenital toxoplasmosis. Pediatrics 95:11-20
5. Patel DV, Holfels EM, Vogel NP et al (1996) Resolution of intracerebral calcifications in children with treated congenital toxoplasmosis. Radiology 199:433-440

6. Mets M, Holfels E, Boyer KM et al (1996) Eye manifestations of congenital toxoplasmosis. Am J Ophthalmol 122:309-324
7. Remington JS, McLeod R, Desmonts G (1995) In: Remington JS, Klein J (eds).
   Infectious Diseases of the fetus and newborn infant. 4th Ed, WB Saunders, Philadelphia,
   pp 140-267
8. Boyer KM, McLeod RL (1996) *Toxoplasma gondii* (Toxoplasmosis). In: Long SS, Prober
   CG, Pickering LK (eds). Principles and Practice of Infectious Diseases. Churchill
   Livingstone, New York, pp. 645-672
9. Roberts F, McLeod R, Boyer K (1998) Toxoplasmosis. In: Katz S, Gershon A, Hotez P
   (eds) Krugman's Infectious Diseases of Children - 10th Ed. Mosby, St. Louis, MO, pp. 538-
   570
10. McLeod R (1994) Treatment of Congenital Toxoplasmosis. Plenary Symposium:
    Advances in Therapy of Protozoal Infections. ICAAC, Orlando, Florida
11. McLeod R, Mack D, Foss R et al (1992) Levels of pyrimethamine in sera and cerebros-
    pinal and ventricular fluids from infants treated for congenital toxoplasmosis.
    Antimicrob Ag Chemother 36(5):1040-1048
12. Desmonts G, Couvreur J (1974) Congenital Toxoplasmosis: A prospective study of 378
    pregnancies. NJEM 290(20):1110-1116
13. Daffos F, Forestier F, Capella-Pavlovsky M, Thulliez P, Aufrant C, Valenti D, Cox W (1988)
    Prenatal management of 746 pregnancies at risk for congenital toxoplasmosis. NEJM
    318(5):271-275
14. Hohlfeld P, Daffos, F, Costa J-M, Thulliez P, Forestier F, Vidaud M (1994) Prenatal dia-
    gnosis of congenital toxoplasmosis with a polymerase-chain reaction test on amniotic
    fluid NEJM 331(11):695-699
15. Hohlfeld P, Daffos F, Thulliez P, Aufrant C, Couvreur J, MacAleese J, Descombey D
    ,Forestier F (1989) Fetal Toxoplasmosis: Outcome of pregnancy and infant follow-up
    after in utero treatment. J Pediatrics 115(5):765-769
16. Brezin AP, Thulliez P, Couvreur J, Nobre R, McLeod R, Mets M (1998) Ophthalmic out-
    come after pre- and post-natal treatment of congenital toxoplasmosis. ARVO
17. Eichenwald HF (1959) A study of congenital toxoplasmosis with particular emphasis on
    clinical manifestations, sequelae and therapy. In: Siim JC (ed) Human Toxoplasmosis.
    Munksgaard, Copenhagen, p. 41
18. Wilson CB, Remington JS, Stagno S, Reynolds DW (1980) Development of adverse
    sequelae in children born with subclinical congenital toxoplasma infection. Pediatrics
    66(5):767-774
19. Koppe JG, Loewer-Sieger DH, de Roever-Bonnet H (1986) Results of 20-year follow-up
    of congenital toxoplasmosis. Lancet 1:254-256
20. Labadie MD, Hazemann JJ (1984) Apport des bilans de santé de l'enfant pour le dépis-
    tage et l'etude épidémiologique de la toxoplasmose congénitale. Annales de Pediatrie
    31(10):823-828
21. Couvreur J, Desmonts G, Aron-Rosa D (1984) Le prognostic oculaire de la toxoplasmo-
    se congénitale: rôle du traitment. Annales de Pediatrie 31(10):855-858
22. Dorangeon PH, Fay R, Marx-Chemla C, Leroux B, Harika G, Dupouy D, Quereux C,
    Choisy H, Pinon JM, Wahl P (1990) Passage transplacentaire de l'association pyrimé-
    thamine-sulfadoxine lors du traitement anténatal de la toxoplasmose congénital. La
    Presse Medicale 19(44):2036
23. Villena I, Aubert D, Leroux B, Dupouy D, Talmud M, Chemla C, Trenque T, Schmit G,
    Quereux C, Guenounou M, Pluot M, Bonhomme A, Pinon JM (Reims Toxoplasmosis
    Group) (1998) Scan J Infect Dis 30:295-300
24. Peyron F, Wallon M, Bernardoux C (1996) Long-term follow-up of patients with conge-
    nital ocular toxoplasmosis. NEJM 334(15):993-994
25. Dorangeon PH, Marx-Chemle C, Quereux C, Fay R, Leroux B, Dupouy D, Choisy H,
    Pinon JM, Wahl P (1992) Les risques de l'association pyriméthamine-sulfadoxine dans le
    traitement anténatal de la toxoplasmose. J Gynecol Obstet Biol Reprod 21:549-556
26. Matsui D (1994) Prevention, diagnosis and treatment of fetal toxoplasmosis. Fetal Drug
    Ther 21:675-689
27. Barbosa J and Ferreira L (1978) Sulfadoxine-pyrimethamine (Fansidar) in pregnant
    women with *Toxoplasma* antibody titers. Curr Chemother 1:134-135

28. Zitelli BJ, Alexander J, Taylor S, Miller KD, Howrie DL, Kuritsky JN, Perez TH, Van Thiel DH (1987) Fatal hepatic necrosis due to pyrimethamine-sulfadoxine (Fansidar®). Annals Int Med 106:393-395

29. Mack DG, McLeod R (1984) New micromethod to study the effect of antimicrobial agents on *Toxoplasma gondii*: comparison of sulfadoxine and sulfadiazine individually and in combination with pyrimthamine and study of clindamycin, metronidazole and cyclosporin A. Antimicrob Ag Chem 26(1):26-30

3.5. Recurrent ocular disease in congenital toxoplasmosis: clinical manifestations

A. ROTHOVA

Introduction

Ocular involvement in toxoplasmosis (of both, congenital and postnatal origins) manifests itself in the majority of patients during the late chronic stage of the infection and does not complicate the acute stage of the disease [1]. Of the congenitally infected children only a small proportion (less than 15%) have apparent ocular involvement in the (acute) perinatal period; however, long-term follow-up demonstrated that about 80% to 100% of these infected children developed late neurological and/or ocular sequelae [2-4]. This indicates that congenitally infected children, including those with subclinical infections without any signs and symptoms of the disease at birth, regularly develop late ocular involvement, even after an interval of many years (most typically during the teenage years and young adulthood) [5].

Recurrent ocular disease in congenital and acquired infection

Chronic toxoplasmosis (of both congenital and postnatal origins) is characterized by the presence of inactive bradyzoites in tissue cysts in contrast to active and proliferating tachyzoites, which are typical of the acute stage. The equilibrium between the proliferating and dormant stages of the parasites is regulated by the cellular immunity; when this is suppressed, reactivation of the disease may follow [6]. During the chronic phase of ocular toxoplasmosis (OT), short and usually self-limiting periods of parasite reactivation in the eye regularly occur and cause the typical presentation of recurrent toxoplasmic chorioretinitis. The exact cause and pathogenesis of recurrences of OT are not known. Stage conversion of the parasite is a crucial process in OT, which is still not fully understood; switch mechanisms from latent to proliferative forms are obscure and numerous hypothetical triggers were suggested such as the immune response and hormonal status of the host, HLA type, autoimmune or hypersensitivity reactions against exposed toxoplasmic antigens as well as parasite-related factors as a mechanical rupture of the cyst due to parasite multiplication, release of toxins or lytic enzymes by the parasite, or reinfections with other parasite strains [7-14]. Recurrent toxoplasmic retinitis is thought to occur when the cyst located in the retina ruptures and liberated parasites multiply in the surrounding cells and cause an inflammatory reaction in the retina and choroid. Although the ocular disease has two distinct routes of infection (congenital and postnatal), clinical and laboratory features in patients with late recurrent disease are not specific; so, the discrimination between the recurrent congenital and recurrent postnatal infections is not possible [15]. Therefore, the relative frequency of congenital and postnatal routes of infection in recurrent OT has not yet been identified.

The exact percentage of congenitally infected patients with recurrent relapses or with new manifestations of ocular disease in previously unaffected eyes is not known, but probably includes the majority of children with congenital disease [2, 4, 5, 16]. Of the congenitally infected children who received either short-term treatment or were untreated after birth, about 80% had ocular disease diagnosed in the course of a long-term follow-up [2, 4]. In a study with a 20-year follow-up, the highest frequency of visual loss due to recurrences was noted between 12 and 18 years of age [4, 5]. The recurrence rate of OT in congenitally infected children who received long-term treatment (usually one year) seemed to be lower than in those who remained untreated [16, 18, 19], but the follow-up of patients treated in the long-term was shorter than for those not treated, so the question of whether long-term treatment really reduces future recurrences of OT cannot be answered yet (Table 1).

In addition, in the earlier studies the new manifestations of ocular disease in previously normal eyes were not included among recurrences so that the exact percentages of those with late ocular disease activity is not known. Of consecutive adult patients with OT, 50% developed recurrences within 3 years and furthermore, the recurrence rate was not dependent on the treatment given [17]. The high-risk factors for recurrent disease are not known and identification of the patients who will develop the recurrent form of OT is at present not feasible. The prediction of location of future attacks is not possible, but satellite dark dots documented by indocyanine green angiography (though not visible on fluorescein angiography or clinical examinations) were associated with the future location of recurrences in 2 patients [20]. The prevention of reactivation of ocular disease by long-term administration of antiparasitic drugs, needed for those with ocular disease and immunosuppression, was never systematically examined in immunocompetent patients.

In the majority of immunosuppressed patients OT is due to primary infections; however, the reactivation of preexistent OT by immunosuppression was also reported [21, 22]. The reactivation of quiet toxoplasmic scar with systemic prednisone medication was occasionally described [23, 24].

Table 1. Visual loss in ocular toxoplasmosis in relation to treatment and follow-up

Study [Ref.]	Number of infected patients	Selection of cases	Number with ocular toxoplasmosis	Average follow-up (years range)
[19]	94	n p	76*	5 (3-10)
[16]	121	p	37	12 (5-22)
[5]	22	p	8 9	13 18
[2]	24	n p**	22	8.5 (1-17)

Table 1. Continued

Study [Ref.]	Legal blindness		Visual acuity 20/40	
	treated cases (%)	not treated cases (%)	treated cases (%)	not treated cases (%)
[19]	5/58 (9)	6/18 (33)*	39/58 (67)	14/18 (78)*
[16]	10/37 (27)	–	not specified	–
[5]	–	1/8 (13)	–	not specified
	–	4/9 (44)	–	not specified
[2]	–	12/22 (55%)	–	11/22 (50)

np, not prospective; p, prospective; ptns, patients; ns , not specified; * ocular disease was a criterium for selection in the not treated cases; ** all patients had subclinical toxoplasmosis at birth

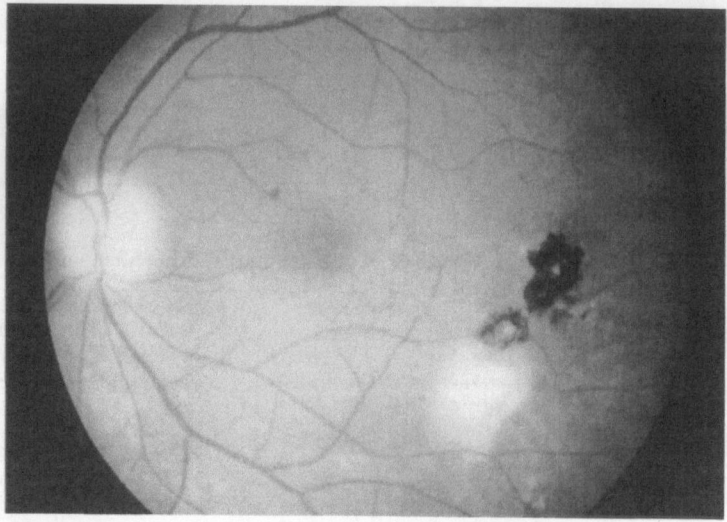

Fig. 1. Recurrent toxoplasmic chorioretinitis. Active lesion with fuzzy margins adjacent to old inactive hyperpigmented scars. Macular area is not affected

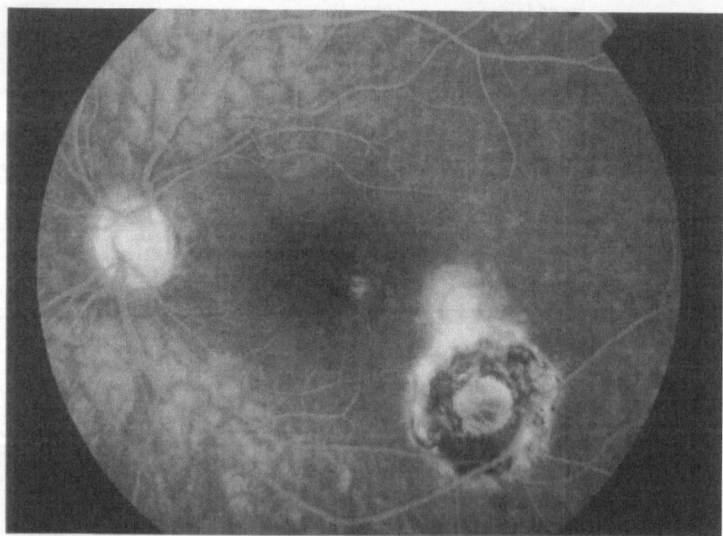

Fig. 2. Fluorescein angiogram of a small area of active retinitis adjacent to larger inactive scar, illustrating the typical satellite formation of new inflammatory lesion. Note the secondary changes of retinal pigment epithelium in the macula, which are the result of long-standing macular edema

Clinical manifestations

The typical manifestation of recurrent OT consists of focal necrotizing retinitis in combination with old atrophic chorioretinal scars (Figs. 1 and 2) [6]. The most characteristic location of the active lesion is on the margin of an old inactive atrophic scar, but this typical satellite formation is not always present and solitary chorioretinal lesions may also occur (Fig. 3). This suggests that tissue cysts may also be present in the areas of the retina, which appeared normal on fundoscopy. The active lesions are characterized by an overlying vitreous inflammatory reaction, the appearance of which was classically described as "headlights in the fog". The active lesions are usually oval or circular, the affected retina is yellowish white due to the necrosis and associated edema (Fig. 4). Active lesions might be accompanied by vasculitis and sometimes haemorrhages, located usually in the retinal areas adjacent to the inflammatory lesion (Fig. 5) [25]. Fluorescein angiography demonstrates an early blockage with subsequent leakage of the dye from the active lesion (Fig. 6) [26]. Indocyanine green angiography documents retinal involvement larger than that visible on fluorescein angiograms and on fundoscopy [27].

Granulomatous anterior uveitis, frequently with elevated eye pressure, may also be present, and may sometimes even mask the posterior segment lesion. This anterior segment reaction is thought to represent an "overspill" from the posterior segment or to be a secondary immunological reaction [6], but toxoplasmic iritis has sporadically been documented [28]. Less typical features include extensive retinal necrosis, papillitis, neurouveitis and scleritis (Fig. 7) [29, 30]. The juxtapapillary lesion (Fig. 6) may cause an arcuate

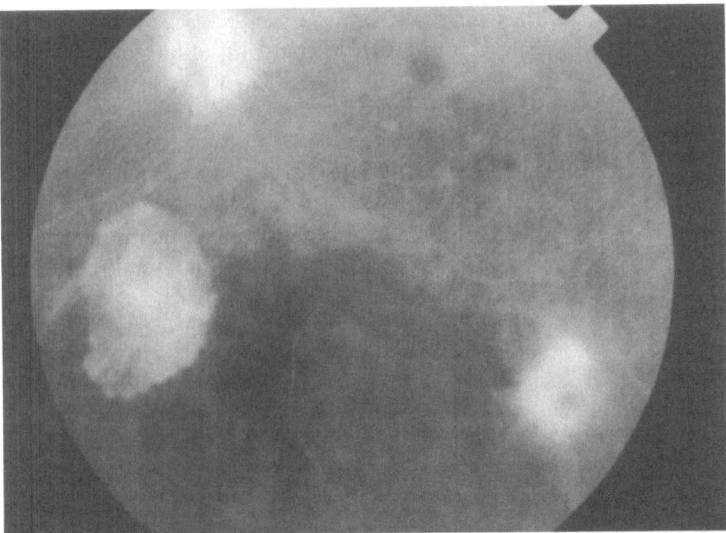

Fig. 3. Late phase fluorescein angiogram of 2 solitary toxoplasmic lesions (the larger inactive scar is located below the optic disc and smaller active lesion is situated below the macular area). Note the secondary macular edema and papillitis

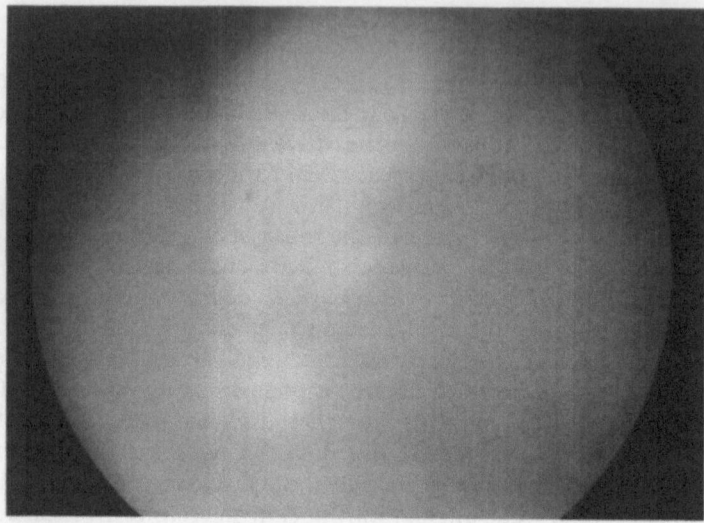

Fig. 4. Large active toxoplasmic lesion located above the optic disc. The loss of details on the photograph is due to associated inflammatory reaction in the vitreous

visual field defect, which may be very troublesome if it involves an area important for reading and other near-distance activities. Sometimes (partial) papillitis (Figs. 6 and 7) develops and may be complicated by secondary optic disc atrophy. Clinical presentation of OT as multiple punctate lesions located deep in the retina has also been described [31]. The resolution of these multiple lesions may leave a typical toxoplasmosis scar.

OT is (in patients with a normal immune system) a self-limiting disease, and when not treated, the inflammatory lesion first enlarges for a period of one to two weeks and then gradually subsides. The active lesion usually heals in 6-10 weeks [17]. The typical scar shows atrophy of the retina and has hyperpigmented borders (Fig. 8). Atypical scars may be encountered in cases treated early (Fig. 5). The patients demonstrate a visual field defect corresponding to the location of the scar.

Bilateral disease was reported in about 35% of the congenital cases [19]; in our series of 150 patients with OT, 58 (39%) had bilateral involvement. In immunocompetent persons the ocular disease is almost never simultaneously active in both eyes. The finding of the typical scar in the contralateral eye may be contributory in the diagnostic process [1].

Symptoms

The most common symptoms in patients with OT are black floating spots in the affected eye. Blurred vision is common due to intraocular inflammato-y reaction. If the macula or optic nerve are involved, vision may be severely reduced. Ocular pain and redness may also be manifest in those with accompanying anterior segment inflammation.

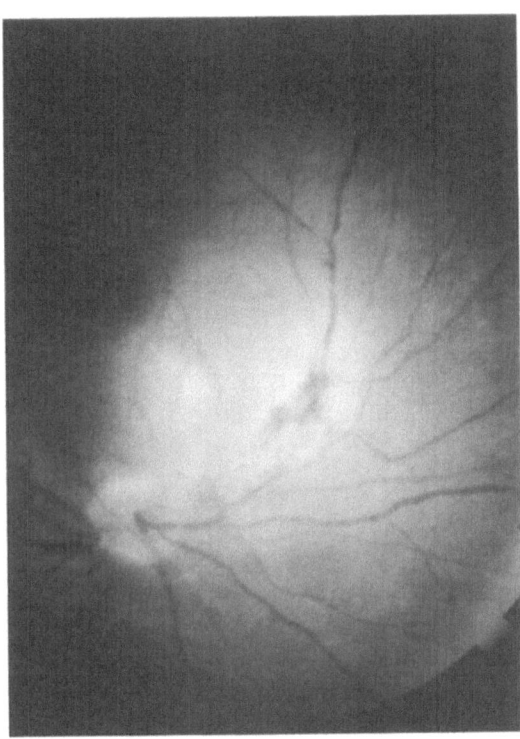

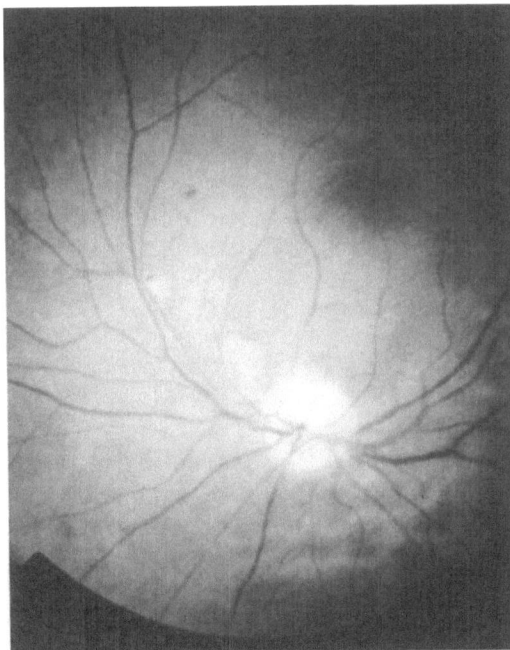

Fig. 5. Toxoplasmic chorioretinitis: active and inactive stage of the disease. **Upper** Active bullous toxoplasmic lesion with associated haemorrhages and secondary vasculitis (note the irregular filling of the retinal vein, which crosses to the inflammatory lesion); **Lower.** The same retinal lesion 4 months after presentation. Patient was treated early with antiparasitic agents and systemic corticosteroids. Note the small scar and restoration of the previously affected vessels

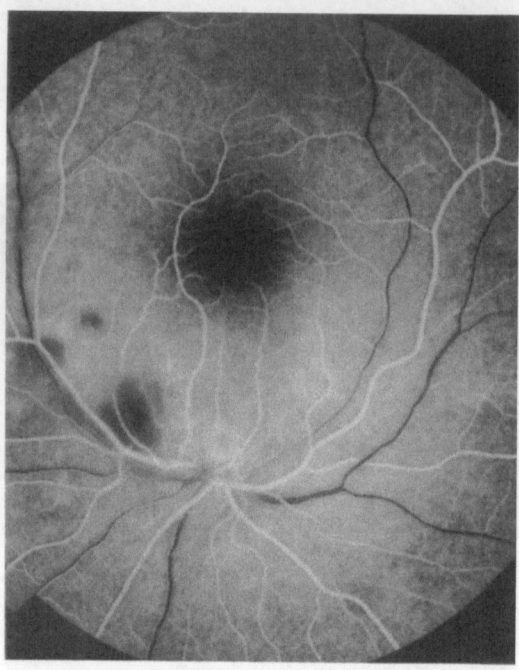

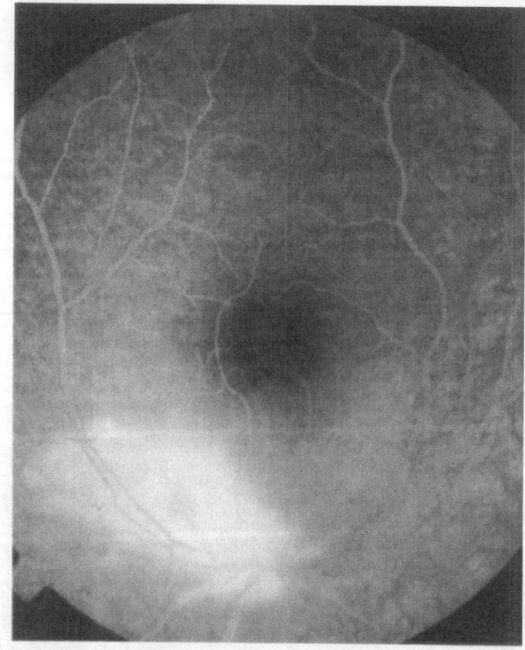

Fig. 6. Fluorescein angiogram of toxoplasmic chorioretinitis. **Upper.** Early phase of fluorescein angiogram of active toxoplasmic lesion located above the optic disc documents the hypofluorescent areas; **Lower** Late phase of fluorescein angiogram of the same eye showing the intense staining in the area of retinitis and leakage of dye from the optic disc and surrounding major retinal vessels

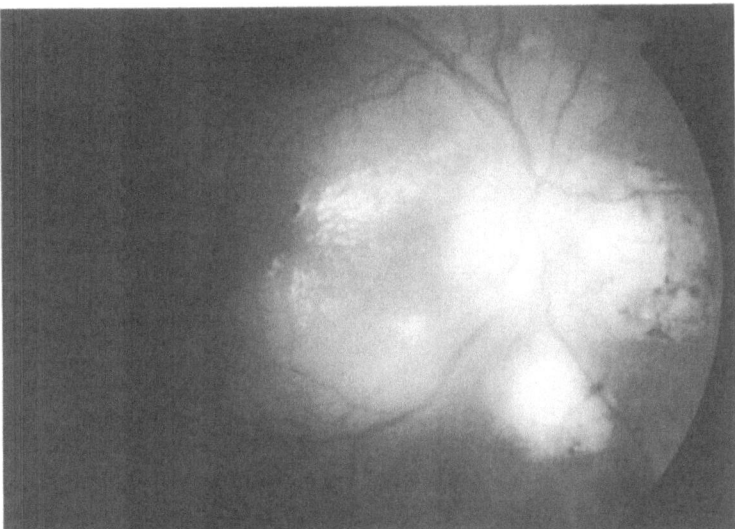

Fig. 7. Toxoplasmic chorioretinitis with swollen optic disc and macular scar. Note also two old chorioretinal scars encroaching on the optic disc. Angiography revealed papillitis with active retinal lesion just below the optic disc and no abnormalities in the macula. Six months later the atrophic scar developed and the exudates disappeared from the macular area

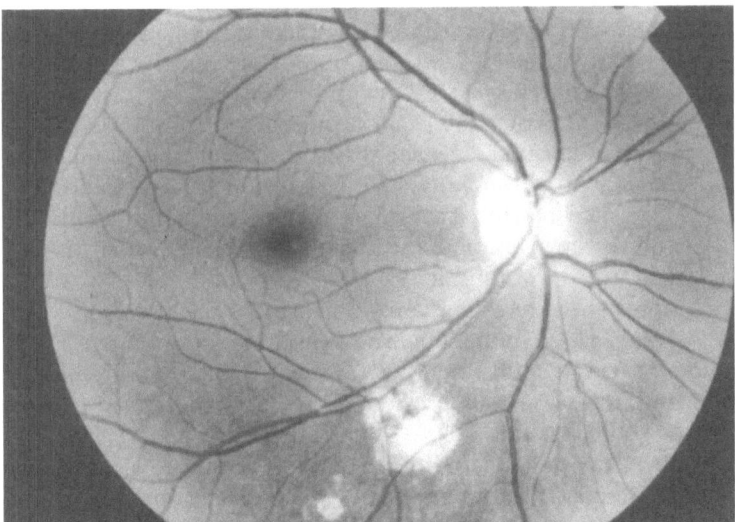

Fig. 8. Atrophic toxoplasmic chorioretinal scar with hyperpigmented borders. Retinal vessels cross the scar

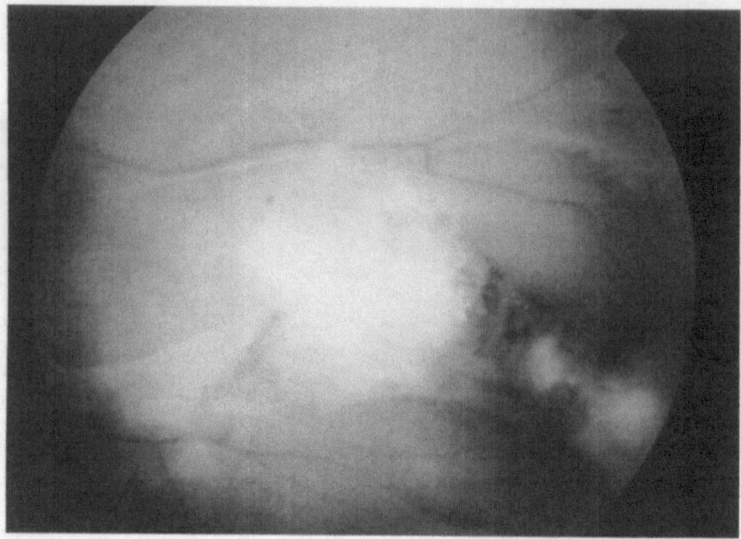

Fig. 9. Toxoplasmic scar with retinal traction. Note the associated retinal folds lifting the retina

Visual prognosis and complications

The most important complication of ocular toxoplasmosis is a permanent loss of visual acuity; this occurred in 27% of treated children with congenital toxoplasmosis with 12-year follow-up and in 44% of untreated children with congenital disease with 18-year follow-up (Table 1) [5, 19]. In our series of 157 patients with OT (congenital and acquired infections), visual acuity of less than 0.1 (legal blindness) was identified in at least one eye in 39 patients (25%) and visual acuity of less than 0.3 (visual impairment) in additional 18 patients (12%). The cause of visual impairment was predominantly the location of the inflammatory lesion in the macula (41/57, 72%). Surprisingly, retinal detachment was the second major cause of visual loss in OT (6/57, 11%). Retinal traction, caused by the organization of vitreous opacities or by retinal scarification may lead to retinal pucker and eventual detachment (Fig. 9). The development of retinal detachment was associated with the presence of myopia, severe inflammation and previous vitrectomy and laser treatment of inflammatory retinal lesions [32].

During the active stage of the disease, visual acuity is usually decreased due to the inflammatory debris in the eye. When the retinal lesion is located in the macula, a definitive loss of central visual acuity may follow. When the lesion is situated peripherally, the visual prognosis is excellent. In patients with severe intraocular inflammation or in those with lesions located near the macula, an associated macular edema may affect the central acuity (Fig. 3). Other complications involve predominantly retinal vessels and include subretinal and choroidal neovascularizations, chorioretinal anastomoses and branch artery or vein occlusions (Fig. 10). Focal periarterial or perivenous exudates may also occur, usually adjacent to the lesion, but vasculitis in the remote retinal areas was also described (Fig. 11) [25]. Associated structural ocular anomalies such as microphthalmus, nystagmus, strabismus, and iris or optic atrophy are typical of severe congenital disease [33, 34].

The curious associations between congenital ocular toxoplasmosis and Fuchs' heterochromic uveitis and retinal pigmentations resembling retinitis pigmentosa were reported [35-37].

Management of recurrent OT

The diagnosis of recurrent OT is usually based on clinical grounds solely and is therefore presumptive. The reason why the majority of ophthalmologists make clinical diagnosis only, lies in the fact that ocular disease, which typically occurs during the chronic phase of toxoplasmosis, has no characteristic serological findings. Therefore, the more invasive diagnostic method of analyzing of intraocular fluids is needed for the definitive proof of OT. The demonstration of local synthesis of toxoplasma antibodies in the eye by intraocular fluid analysis is an extremely valuable diagnostic tool (Goldmann-Witmer coefficient) [38]. The value of polymerase chain reaction for the diagnosis of OT in intraocular fluids is not yet well defined. Until now positive results were found in about one third of patients with otherwise proven ocular OT [39-41]. The traditional treatment for recurrent OT consists of various combinations of antiparasitic drugs given usually for 4 to 8 weeks, depending on the clinical features; the most common agents used are pyrimethamine, clindamycin and sulphonamide, sometimes in combination with corticosteroids to alleviate the inflammatory reaction [17, 42, 43]. The role of this treatment for an individual attack of recurrent OT in an immunocompetent patient is probably limited; furthermore, this type of treatment has probably no value in preventing recurrences [17]. To date, the prevention of recurrent OT attacks is not feasible, although newly developed drugs decreased the number of cysts in experimental and animal studies [44, 45]. The administration of corticosteroids during the primary systemic (and ocular) infection was associated with a higher recurrence rate [23]. For further reading see chapter 3.6.

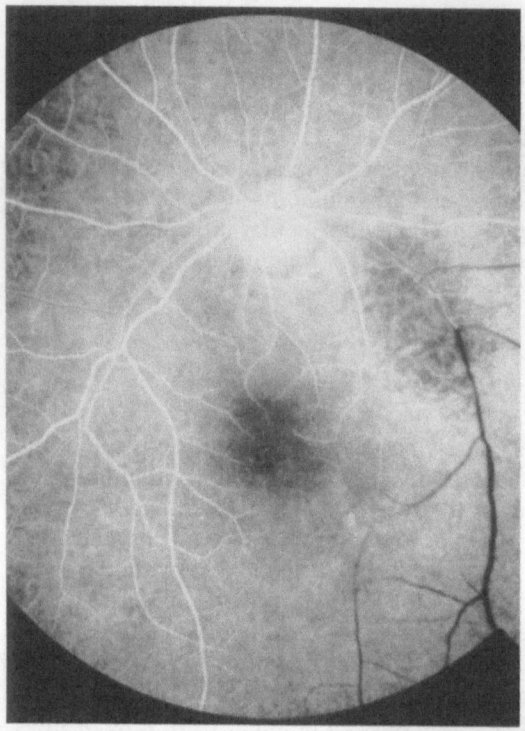

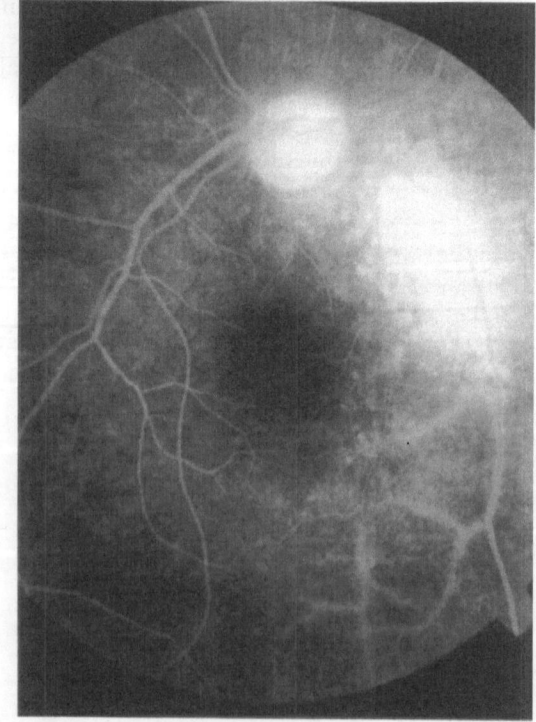

Fig. 10. Branch retinal venous occlusion caused by acute toxoplasmic chorioretinitis. **Upper.** Early phase of fluorescein angiogram revealed venous obstruction located at the site of the toxoplasmic lesion; **Lower** Late phase angiogram documents the leakage from the retinal inflammatory lesion and from the retinal vessels peripheral to the occlusion site

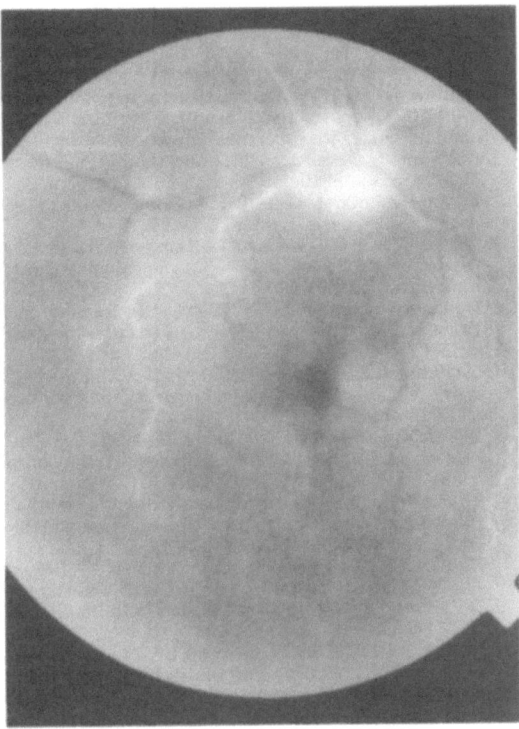

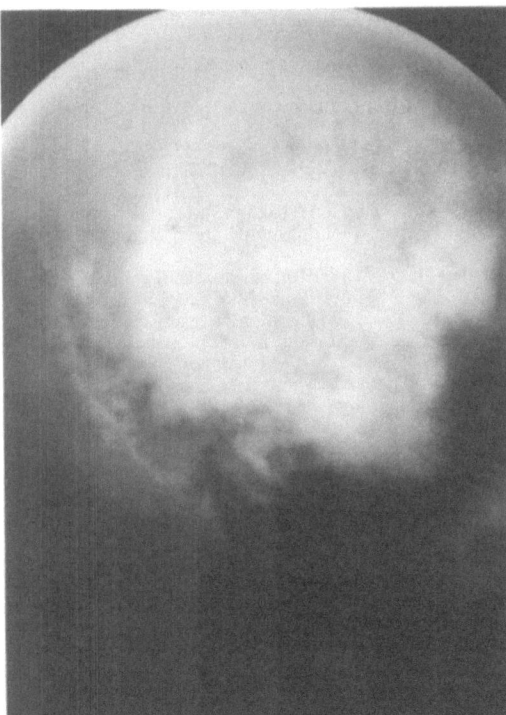

Fig. 11. Large toxoplasmic lesion with severe secondary inflammatory reaction. **Upper.** Diffuse periarterial exudation extending from the optic disc into the retinal periphery; **Lower.** Associated toxoplasmic lesion was located in the temporal periphery. Note the beginning of hyperpigmentation on the border of the lesion

References

1. Rothova A (1992) Ocular involvement in toxoplasmosis. Br J Ophthalmol 77:371-377
2. Wilson CB, Remington JS, Stagno S, Reynold DW (1980) Development of adverse sequelae in children born with subclinical *Toxoplasma* infection. Pediatrics 66:767-774
3. Desmonts G, Remington JS, Couvreur J (1987) Congenital toxoplasmosis. In: Stern L, Vert P (eds) Neonatal medicine. Masson Publ Comp, pp 662-678
4. Koppe JG, Loewer-Sieger DH, de Roever-Bonnet (1986) Results of 20 year follow-up of congenital toxoplasmosis. Lancet 1:254-256
5. Loewer-Sieger DH, Rothova A, Koppe JG, Kijlstra A (1984) Congenital toxoplasmosis: a prospective study based on 1821 pregnant women. In: Saari KM (ed) Uveitis update. Elsevier, Amsterdam, pp 203-207
6. Holland G, O'Connor GR, Belfort R Jr, Remington JS (1996) Toxoplasmosis. In: Pepose JS, Holland GN, Wilhelmus KR (eds). Infectious ocular diseases. Mosby-Year Book Inc, pp 1183-1223
7. Nussenblatt RB, Mittal KK, Fuhrman S, Sharma SD, Palestine AG (1989) Lymphocyte proliferative responses of patients with ocular toxoplasmosis to parasite and retinal antigens. Am J Ophthalmol 107:632-641
8. Wyler DJ, Blackman HJ, Lunde MN (1980) Cellular hypersensitivity to toxoplasmal and retinal antigens in patients with toxoplasmal retinochoroiditis. Am J Trop Med Hyg 29:1181-1186.
9. Whittle RM, Wallace GR, Whiston RA, Dumonde DC, Stanford MR (1988) Human retinal antibodies in toxoplasma retinochoroiditis. Br J Ophthalmol 82:1017-1021
10. Pavesio CE, Lightman S (1996) Toxoplasma gondii and ocular toxoplasmosis: pathogenesis. Br J Ophthalmol 80:1099-1107
11. Rao NA, Font RL (1997) Toxoplasmic retinochoroiditis: electron microscopic and immunofluorescence studies of formalin-fixed tissue. Arch Ophthalmol 95:273-277
12. O'Connor GR (1983) Factors related to initiation and recurrence of uveitis. Am J Ophthalmol 96:577-599
13. Meenken C, Rothova A, de Waal LP, van der Horst AR, Mesman BJ, Kijlstra A (1995) HLA typing in congenital toxoplasmosis. Br J Ophthalmol 79:494-497
14. Smith JE, McNeil G, Zhang YW, Dutton S, Biswas-Hughes G, Appleford P (1996) Serological recognition of Toxoplasma gondii cyst antigens. In: Gross U (ed). *Toxoplasma gondii*. Springer-Verlag Berlin Heidelberg, pp 67-73
15. Rothova A, van Knapen F, Baarsma GS, Kruit PJ, Loewer-Sieger DH, Kijlstra A (1986) Serology in ocular toxoplasmosis. Br J Ophthalmol 70:615-22
16. Peyron F, Wallon M, Bernardoux C (1996) Long-term follow-up of patients with congenital ocular toxoplasmosis N Eng J Med 334:993-994
17. Rothova A, Meenken C, Buitenhuis HJ et al (1993) Therapy for ocular toxoplasmosis. Am J Ophthalmol 115:517-523
18. Couvreur J, Nottin N, Desmonts G (1980) La toxoplasmose congénitale traitée. Annales de Pédiatrie 27:647-652
19. Mets MB, Holfels E, Boyer KM, Swisher CN, Roizen N, Stein L, Stein M, Hopkins J, Withers S, Mack D, Luciano R, Patel D, Remington JS, Meier P, McLeod R (1997) Eye manifestations of congenital toxoplasmosis. Am J Ophthalmol 123:1-16
20. Bernasconi O, Auer C, Herbort CP (1997) Recurrent toxoplasmic retinochoroiditis. Significance of perilesional satellite dark dots seen by indocyanine green angiography. Ocul Immunol Inflamm 5:207-211
21. Holland GN, Engstrom RE, Glasgow BJ et al (1998) Ocular toxoplasmosis in patients with the acquired immunodeficiency syndrome. Am J Ophthalmol 106:653-667
22. Peacock JE Jr, Greven CM, Cruz JM, Hurd DD (1995) Reactivation of toxoplasmic retinochoroiditis in patients undergoing bone marrow transplantation: is there a role for chemoprophylaxis? Bone Marrow Transplant 15:983-987
23. Bosch-Driessen EH, Rothova A (1998) Sense and nonsense of corticosteroid administration in the treatment of ocular toxoplasmosis. Br J Ophthalmol 82:858-860
24. Morhun PJ, Weisz JM, Elias SJ, Holland GN (1996) Recurrent ocular toxoplasmosis in patients treated with systemic corticosteroids. Retina 16:383-387
25. Theodossiadis P, Kokolakis S, Ladas I, Kollia AC, Chatzoulis D, Theodossiadis G (1995) Retinal vascular involvement in acute toxoplasmic retinochoroiditis. Int Ophthalmol 19:19-24
26. Iijima H, Tsukahara Y, Imasawa M (1995) Angiographic findings in eyes with active ocular toxoplasmosis. Jpn J Ophthalmol 39:402-410
27. Auer C, Bernasconi O, Herbort CP (1997) Toxoplasmic retinochoroiditis: new insights provided by indocyanine green angiography. Am J Ophthalmol 123:131-133
28. Rehder JR, Burnier M, Pavesio CE et al (1988) Acute unilateral toxoplasmic iridocyclitis in an AIDS patient. Am J Ophthalmol 106:740-741
29. Fish RH, Hoskins JC, Kline LB (1993) Toxoplasmosis neuroretinitis. Ophthalmology 100:1177-1182

30. Tandon R, Menon V, Das GK, Verma L (1995) Toxoplasmic papillitis with central retinal artery occlusion. Can J Ophthalmol 30:374-376
31. Friedman CT, Knox DL (1969) Variations in recurrent active toxoplasmic retinochoroiditis. Arch Ophthalmol 81:481-493
32. Bosch-Driessen EH, Stilma JS, Karimi S, Rothova A (1999) Retinal detachment in ocular toxoplasmosis. (Submitted manuscript)
33. De Jong PTVM (1997) Ocular toxoplasmosis; common and rare symptoms and signs. Int Ophthalmol 13:391-397
34. Meenken C, Assies J, van Nieuwenhuizen O, Holwerda-van der Maat WG, van Schooneveld MJ, Delleman WJ, Kinds G, Rothova A (1995) Long term ocular and neurological involvement in severe congenital toxoplasmosis. Br J Ophthalmol 79:581-584
35. Schwab IR (1991) The epidemiologic association of Fuchs' heterochromic iridocyclitis and ocular toxoplasmosis. Am J Ophthalmol 111:356-362
36. La Heij E, Rothova A (1991) Fuchs's heterochromic cyclitis in congenital ocular toxoplasmosis. Br J Ophthalmol75:372-373
37. Silveira C, Belfort R Jr, Nussenblatt R et al (1989) Unilateral pigmentary retinopathy associated with ocular toxoplasmosis. Am J Ophthalmol107:682-683
38. De Boer JH, Verhagen C, Bruinenberg M, Rothova A, De Jong PTVM, Baarsma GS, Lelij van der A, Ooyman FM, Bollemeijer JG, Derhaag PJFM, Kijlstra A (1996) Serologic and Polymerase Chain Reaction Analysis of Intraocular Fluids in the Diagnosis of Infectious Uveitis. Am J Ophthalmol 121:650-658
39. Khalifa el KS, Roth A, Roth B, Arasteh KN, Janitschke K (1994) Value of PCR for evaluating occurrence of parasitemia in immunocompromised patients with cerebral and extracerebral toxoplasmosis. J Clin Microbiol 32:2813-2819
40. Garweg J, Boehnke M, Koerner F (1996) Restricted applicability of the polymerase chain reaction for the diagnosis of ocular toxoplasmosis. Ger J Ophthalmol 5:104-108
41. Aouizerate F, Cazenave J, Poirier L, Verin P, Cheyrou A, Begueret J, Lagoutte F (1993) Detection of *Toxoplasma gondii* in aqueous humour by the polymerase chain reaction. Br J Ophthalmol 77:107-109
42. Lam S, Tessler HH (1993) Quadruple therapy for ocular toxoplasmosis. Can J Ophthalmol 28:58-61
43. Engstrom RE, Holland GN, Nussenblatt RB, Jabs DA (1991) Current practices in the management of ocular toxoplasmosis. Am J Ophthalmol 111:601-610
44. Huskinson-Mark J, Araujo FG, Remington JS (1991) Evaluation of the effect of drugs on the cyst form of toxoplasma gondii. J Infect Dis 164:170-177
45. Gormley PD, Pavesio CE, Minnasian D, Lightman S (1998) Effects of drug therapy on *Toxoplasma* cysts in an animal model of acute and chronic disease. Invest Ophthalmol Vis Sci 39:1171-1175

3.6. Laboratory diagnosis of ocular toxoplasmosis: serological and PCR based analysis of ocular fluids

A. Kijlstra

Inflammation of the uvea is a sight threatening disease affecting people in the prime of their life. Infectious as well as non infectious mechanisms play a role in the pathogenesis of uveitis. Toxoplasmosis, which is caused by the protozoan parasite *Toxoplasma gondii*, is the most common cause of posterior uveitis in many countries [1, 2]. Epidemiological studies have indicated that the incidence of toxoplasmic retinochoroiditis may range from 0.6% in an area in the USA to up to 20% in southern Brazil [3, 4].

In most affected individuals, ocular toxoplasmosis is considered a late manifestation of a congenital infection. New data are becoming available indicating that ocular toxoplasmosis, as a result of postnatally acquired infection, may be more prevalent than initially thought.

The rate of ocular lesions following recent epidemics of postnatally acquired toxoplasmosis range between 4% and 19% [5, 6]. On the other hand, congenital infection with *Toxoplasma* may lead to a rate of 80% of ocular lesions [7]. Although definite proof is still lacking there is circumstantial evidence that treatment strategies between the postnatally acquired and congenital form of ocular toxoplasmosis should be different [8].

In congenitally acquired disease the parasite resides in the retina during the development of the embryo and can remain there for years in its encysted stage without causing problems to the visual system and without marked stimulation of the systemic anti-parasitic immune response, and possibly leading to a low level of circulating anti-*Toxoplasma* antibodies.

The diagnosis of ocular toxoplasmosis is based on the characteristic clinical picture of a focal necrotizing retinitis. Most cases seen by an ophthalmologist represent recurrent disease and show a typical clinical picture of a characteristic scar with a border or satellite activity. Cases presenting with a primary lesion may however be more difficult to diagnose.

Atypical presentation occurs in elderly patients, or can sometimes be caused by mistreatment with high doses of immunosuppressive drugs, making it very difficult to distinguish from other causes of uveitis. In other cases an intense inflammatory response in the vitreous may obscure the retina making fundoscopy impossible.

In cases presenting as a diagnostic dilemma, the clinical diagnosis can be confirmed by detecting toxoplasma antibodies in the blood. In congenital disease, titres may be low and sometimes barely detectable. In an earlier study we showed that all patients with ocular toxoplasmosis had circulating antibodies against the parasite as detected by an ELISA [9].

Case reports have been documented however showing the absence of antibodies in the blood of patients. This may be due to the fact that patients with the congenital form of ocular toxoplasmosis have low levels of antibodies which may not be detected by certain techniques.

The presence of IgG *Toxoplasma* antibodies in serum is however not of great importance in view of the fact that many healthy individuals also have these antibodies resulting in a low specific diagnostic value. Nevertheless, recent data challenge the pessimistic view on the value of serological techniques to confirm a diagnosis of ocular toxoplasmosis. High serum IgG titers against the parasite may point to recent acquired disease manifesting itself as primary ocular toxoplasmosis (Ongkosuwito et al, manuscript in preparation). Others have also observed that serological analysis of blood samples often contains markers of a previous episode of acquired toxoplasmosis [10]. It should be kept in mind however that patients with ocular sarcoidosis, which is an entity that should be included in the differential diagnosis, may have an aberrant serum IgG response including very high titers against *Toxoplasma*. For the uveitis, specialist *Toxoplasma* serology should give an answer to the question whether the patient has ever been infected with *Toxoplasma*. If this is negative, one may exclude toxoplasmosis as a causal agent. If the test is positive it is compatible with the diagnosis of ocular toxoplasmosis but the disease may still be due to various other causes. In these cases additional proof may be obtained by analysing an aqueous humour sample for the presence of locally produced *Toxoplasma* antibodies and/or the presence of *Toxoplasma* DNA. Since treatment of the various uveitis entities should often be started as soon as possible, it is not wise to await the natural course of the disease and not pursue further diagnostic procedures.

Although invasive, we and others have proposed anterior chamber paracentesis as a safe procedure to obtain further clues to the diagnosis of the inflammatory event. A recent survey by van der Lelij et al. [11], who analyzed 360 anterior chamber paracenteses did not reveal serious complications. As yet no case reports have been published describing endophthalmitis following a diagnostic anterior chamber procedure in a uveitis patient. On the other hand, endophthalmitis following a paracentesis in case of retinal vein occlusion has been reported.

This observation can be explained as follows. Blood aqueous barrier breakdown in uveitis probably results in the presence of sufficient intraocular antibodies preventing bacterial infection, which is not the case in a quiet eye with a retinal vein occlusion. Normal aqueous humour contains very low IgG levels (approximately 10 µg/ml) which may be insufficient to neutralise bacteria accidentally introduced into the eye during a paracentesis.

Determination of local intraocular antibody production has been shown to be a specific and sensitive method to confirm the diagnosis of ocular toxoplasmosis [12]. To determine local antibody production it is necessary to obtain a paired blood and ocular fluid sample, taken on the same day. The amount of ocular fluid obtained during anterior chamber paracentesis ranges between 100 and 200 µl, which in combination with a few millilitres of serum is sufficient to perform a large number of tests.

Various techniques can be used to detect *Toxoplasma* antibodies in these paired blood/ocular fluid samples. In our laboratory we chose the commercially available indirect immunofluorescence method, whereby only small amounts of sample are needed. Routinely antibodies are tested against Herpes simplex virus, Varicella zoster virus and *Toxoplasma gondii*. Various dilutions of serum and intraocular fluid are incubated for « hour on a slide with virus-infected-cells to determine the titre of anti-viral antibodies. Slides coated with formalin fixed *Toxoplasma* parasites were employed to detect *Toxoplasma* antibodies. After a short washing procedure a second incubation with Fluorescein labelled anti-human IgG takes place and slides are scored. The highest dilution still giving a positive result under the Fluorescence microscope is defined as the titre of antibodies present in the serum, aqueous or vitreous.

Antibodies detected in the ocular fluid can originate from the peripheral blood, due to blood ocular barrier breakdown or may be produced within the eye itself. To discriminate between the two it is necessary to relate the specific antibodies to the total amount of Immunoglobulin G present in the blood and ocular fluid. By means of the Radial Immuno Diffusion method according to Mancini, both local and serum IgG levels can be simply quantitated.

Intraocular synthesis of antibodies is considered to have taken place if the relative amount of specific antibodies compared to the total IgG level found in the ocular fluid exceeds that measured in a paired serum sample.

The quotient of the relative amount of antibodies is called the Goldmann-Witmer Coefficient (C). Theoretically a C higher than 1 would indicate a local production of antibodies within the eye. In view of the variability in the results of the various measurements, a C higher than 3 is considered significant. Each laboratory should define its own cut-off level of this coefficient. In our laboratory we compared the C coefficients obtained in patients retrospectively diagnosed as ocular toxoplasmosis with cases caused by either Herpes simplex or Varicella zoster virus. This resulted in a specificity of 100% and a sensitivity of 75% when taking a cut-off level of 3.0. When a patient is clinically suspected of ocular toxoplasmosis whereby analysis of ocular fluid cannot support such a diagnosis, testing for Herpes viruses has often revealed a positive test result leading to a change in the initial clinical diagnosis and involving a change in the therapeutic approach. Therefore it is extremely important to also involve testing for the Herpes viruses [13].

If sufficient material is available, DNA is isolated and PCR tests for Herpes simplex, Varicella zoster, Cytomegalovirus and *Toxoplasma gondii* are performed. We prefer to isolate DNA using silica absorption and elution techniques to eliminate PCR inhibitors present in ocular fluids. Others have advocated boiling samples to eliminate PCR inhibitors but this procedure may be disastrous for the *Toxoplasma* antibody activity residing in the ocular fluid. The PCR test for *Toxoplasma gondii* is only positive in approximately 25% of immunocompetent patients, whereby almost all of the DNA positive patients also had evidence of local intraocular toxoplasma antibody production. In immunocompromised patients presenting with an atypical ocular toxoplasmosis we have more often observed patients with *Toxoplasma* DNA in their eyes in the absence of a detectable antibody production. The above experience has led us to prefer serology over DNA analysis when the amount of available ocular fluid was limited.

Recently, we have also included intraocular *Toxoplasma* IgA antibody production in our routine testing of patients suspected for ocular toxoplasmosis [14]. This test is only performed after all other procedures (local IgG testing for *Toxoplasma* and Herpes viruses, PCR testing for *Toxoplasma* DNA and Herpes virus DNA) have proven negative. A recent study performed by our laboratory has indicated that 15% of ocular toxoplasmosis cases referred to our diagnostic centre could be diagnosed by virtue of an isolated local IgA response against the parasite.

Analysis of the *Toxoplasma* antibody repertoire by immunoblotting has shown that the intraocular antibody response of patients with recurrent ocular toxoplasmosis differs from the systemic response [15]. Ocular toxoplasmosis patients have a characteristic set of antibodies in their ocular fluid as detected by this technique. Since the immunoblotting technique is laborious and needs a large volume of ocular fluid, it will only replace the traditional methods of comparing antibody titers, when the sensitivity of the immunoblotting procedure is markedly improved, thereby using less sample volume.

In conclusion, it can be stated that aspiration of an ocular fluid sample is a safe and helpful procedure, since the present combined serological and PCR testing can confirm the diagnosis of ocular toxoplasmosis in almost 90 percent of cases.

Acknowledgements

I would like to thank Dr. Jenny Ongkosuwito for critically reading the manuscript.

References

1. Holland GN, O'Connor GR, Belfort R Jr, Remington JS (1996) Toxoplasmosis. In: Pepose JS, Holland GN, Wilhelmus KR (eds) Ocular Infection and Immunity-1996. Mosby Year Book Inc St Louis, Missouri
2. Pavesio CE, Lightman S (1996) *Toxoplasma gondii* and ocular toxoplasmosis: pathogenesis. Br J Ophthalmol 80:1099-1107
3. Smith RE, Ganley JP (1972) Ophthalmic survey of a community. 1. Abnormalities of the ocular fundus. Am J Ophthalmol 7:1126
4. Glasner PD, Silveira C, Kruszon-Moran D et al (1992) An unusually high prevalence of ocular toxoplasmosis in Southern Brazil. Am J Ophthalmol 114:136
5. Teutsch SM, Juranek DD, Sulzer A et al (1979) Epidemic toxoplasmosis associated with infected cats. N Engl J Med 300:695-699
6. Bowie WR, King AS, Werker DH et al (1997) Outbreak of toxoplasmosis associated with municipal drinking water. Lancet 350:173
7. Loewer-Sieger DH, Rothova A, Koppe JG, Kijlstra A (1984) Congenital toxoplasmosis, a prospective study based on 1821 pregnant women. In: Saari KM, (ed.) Uveitis Update. Amsterdam, Elsevier Science Publishers, Amsterdam

8. Bosch-Driessen EH, Rothova A (1998) Sense and nonsense of corticosteroid administration in the treatment of ocular toxoplasmosis. Br J Ophthalmol 82:858-860
9. Rothova A, Van Knapen F, Baarsma GS, Kruit PJ, Loewer- Sieger DH, Kijlstra A (1986) Serology in ocular toxoplasmosis. Br J Ophthalmol 70:615-622
10. Montoya JG, Remington JS (1996) Toxoplasmic chorioretinitis in the setting of acute acquired toxoplasmosis. Clin Inf Dis 23:277-282
11. van der Lelij A, Rothova A (1997) Diagnostic anterior chamber paracentesis in uveitis: a safe procedure? Br J Ophthalmol 81:976-979
12. Kijlstra A, Luyendijk L, Baarsma GS et al (1996) Aqueous humor analysis as a diagnostic tool in *Toxoplasma* uveitis. Int Ophthalmol 13:383-386
13. De Boer JH, Verhagen C, Bruinenberg M et al (1996) Serologic and polymerase chain reaction analysis of intraocular fluids in the diagnosis of infectious uveitis. Am J Ophthalmol 121:650-658
14. Ronday MJH, Ongkosuwito JV, Rothova A, Kijlstra A (1999) Intraocular anti-*Toxoplasma gondii* IgA antibody production in patients with ocular toxoplasmosis. Am J Ophthalmol 127:294-300
15. Klaren VNA, Van Doornik CEM, Ongkosuwito JV, Feron EJ, Kijlstra A (1998) Differences between intraocular and serum antibody responses in patients with ocular toxoplasmosis. Am J Ophthalmol 126:698-706

4.1. Epidemiology of infection in pregnant women

R. GILBERT

Introduction

How best to prevent symptoms and disability due to congenital toxoplasmosis is a question which has caused controversy among clinicians for the last 3 decades. At the core of the debate is uncertainty about the effectiveness of prenatal treatment on the risk of congenital toxoplasmosis and of prenatal and postnatal treatment on the risk of long term clinical sequelae. The uncertainty exists because no controlled trials have been conducted and no comparative, observational studies have adequately taken account of the effect of gestation at maternal infection on the risk of congenital infection or clinical sequelae. Differing interpretations of the available evidence have resulted in a variety of preventive strategies. In Britain and Norway, there is an explicit policy not to screen [1, 2], while in France, monthly prenatal testing of susceptible women is mandatory [3]. In Austria [4] and Italy [5], susceptible women are re-tested every 3 months while Denmark [6], Poznan (Poland) and Massachusetts [7] have chosen to operate neonatal, rather than prenatal screening programmes.

The aim of this chapter is to highlight the most reliable and up to date information on the risks of infection in the mother and her child and of clinical sequelae. This information is relevant to policy makers, clinicians and women making decisions about whether to undergo testing. Finally, I will highlight gaps in knowledge which need to be addressed in order to develop effective preventive strategies.

Risk of infection in pregnant women

Prevalence of past infection

Congenital toxoplasmosis occurs in babies born to women who acquire infection for the first time during pregnancy. Congenital infection following preconceptional infection [8-10] or reactivation of latent infection in immunocompetent women [11-13] is exceptional and limited to a few case reports. The risk of infection during pregnancy therefore depends on the prevalence of past infection and the incidence of infection in susceptible pregnant women.

Studies published in the past 10 years on the prevalence of past infection in pregnant women are shown in Table 1. The highest rates occur in central and southern European and Francophone countries and decrease further north in Europe. The USA has comparable rates to north-west Europe but prevalence is higher in the southern states [14]. Differences across the world have been reviewed elsewhere [15]. In brief, central and south America and sub-Saharan Africa have similar rates to southern Europe. Lower rates are found in the Far East. Part of the variation between studies is explained by the different tests used or different age distributions. However, regional differences are marked and consistent and likely to reflect true differences in the risk of past infection. Several studies show that the principal factors determining variation within country are secular trends, altitude, latitude, and country of birth or ethnic group [14, 16-23]. Within Europe, there is no consistent evidence of rural-urban variation in infection [18, 24, 25].

There is strong evidence from studies based in the same geographical area, that prevalence of past infection, reflected by *Toxoplasma* IgG, has fallen over the past 3 decades (see Table 2). Modelling of changes in prevalence according to age and time in South Yorkshire, UK [26] suggests that seroprevalence in the 20-40 age group is largely attributable to the high incidence of infection during childhood. In other words, the decline in the prevalence of infection in pregnant women is due to a cohort effect. The prevalence in women aged 40 in 1999 is mainly attributable to a higher incidence of infection between 1959 and 1979 than experienced by women aged 20 in 1999 between 1979 and 1999. As the decline in childhood ceased about 20 years ago, seroprevalence in pregnant women may be about to level off.

In the past, regional differences in the prevalence of susceptibility were cited as justification for differing policies regarding screening. For example, when prenatal screening was made mandatory by law in France, only 13% of women were susceptible and required re-testing throughout pregnancy compared with 80% in the UK [14]. Nearly 50% are now susceptible in France, more than doubling the costs of re-testing.

Incidence of infection in susceptible women

The fact that more pregnant women are susceptible does not necessarily mean that more infections occur, as the incidence of infection in susceptible pregnant women may have also declined. However, information on the incidence of infection in pregnancy should be interpreted with caution. Unless based on a geographically defined population, incidence rates are easily exaggerated by referral of infected women to specialist centres. In addition, few studies are explicit about the delay between negative and positive IgG tests or take account of these in the rates reported [27]. Thirdly, the tests and titres used to define maternal infection, high titre, rising titre, or seroconversion, can substantially alter the chance of being classified as infected or not [28, 29]. A further complication is that tests detecting recent infection have become more sensitive which may explain why, in some studies, seroconversion rates in susceptible women appear to have increased [30].

Table 1. Prevalence of *Toxoplasma* IgG antibodies in pregnant women

Study	Country and year of survey	Pregnant women (No.)	% IgG positive
Ancelle et al. [16]	France (all), 1995	13,459	54%
Berger et al. [42]	Switzerland, Basel 1986-1994	30,000	29%
Jaquier et al. [20]	Switzerland, (most), 1990-1991	9,059	46%
Buffolano et al. [43]	Italy, Naples 1993	3,518	40%
Valcavi et al. [44]	Italy, Parma 1987-1991	19,432	49%
Roos et al. [45]	Germany, Wurzburg, 1989-1990	2,104	42%
Aspock and Pollak [46]	Austria, Vienna, 1981-1991	167,041	43%
Conyn van Spaedonck [47]	Netherlands, 1987	28,049	45%
Ljungstrom et al. [17]	Sweden, 1987-1988: north south	3,654	12% 26%
Foulon et al. [48]	Belgium, 1979-1990	11,286	56%
Allain et al. [25]	UK, Eastern, 1992	13,000	8%
Zadik et al. [49]	UK, Sheffield, 1989-1992	1,621	10%
Lappalainen et al. [50]	Finland, south 1988-1989	16,733	20%
Jenum et al. [18]	Norway, 1992 north south	35,940	7% 13%
Lebech et al. [51]	Denmark, 1992	5,402	27%
Decavalas et al. [52]	Greece, 1987	217	52%
Remington et al. [14]	USA, 7 different regions 1986-1993	10 to 30%	
Walpole [53]	Australia, Western 1986-1989	10,207	35%
Galvan-Ramirez et al. [54]	Mexico, NA	350	35%
Guimares et al. [19]	Brazil, Sao Paulo, 1989	1,286	59-78%
Altintas et al. [55]	Turkey, Agean region, 1991-1995	2,287	55%
Sun et al. [56]	China, Chengdu, NA	1,211	39%
Ashrafunnessa et al. [57]	Bangladesh, NA	286	38%

NA : not available

Given these concerns, incidence rates in susceptible pregnant women given in Table 3 are restricted to those derived from recent population-based studies which include only seroconverting women or those with low IgG avidity in the numerator. All incidence rates are adjusted for a 9 month pregnancy and range from 3 to 8/1000 susceptible pregnancies.

Table 2. Change in prevalence of *Toxoplasma* IgG in pregnant women over time

Country [Ref.]	Years	IgG positive
Switzerland, Geneva [58]	1973-75	87%
	1976-78	73%
	1979-81	60%
	1982-84	51%
	1985-87	47%
France, Paris [16, 32]	1965	86%
	1966	75%
	1969	80%
	1974	76%
	1974-81	81%
	1977-82	55%
	1981-82	57%
	1995	62%
France, Liege [30]	1966-75	70%
	1976-81	62%
	1982-87	47%
UK, South Yorkshire [26]	1969-73	22%
	1976-79	18%
	1981-85	14%
	1988-90	8%
Sweden, Stockholm [59]	1969	34%
	1979	30%
	1987	18%

Table 3. Incidence of *T. gondii* infection in susceptible pregnant women.

Study	Number of non-immune pregnant women (% of all pregnant women)	Number of T. gondii infected women	Incidence /1000 T. gondii antibody negative pregnant women
Conyn van Spaendonck Netherlands 1987[3] [47,60]	15,427 (55%)	55	5.4
Lappalainen et al. [61][2,3] Finland 1988-1989	13,336 (80%)	28	3.4
Lebech et al. [62][4] Denmark 1992-1996	64,708 (72%)	141	2.9
Ancell et al. [16][1,3] France 1995	5943 (46%)	32	8.1

1   Only "certain" diagnoses of primary infection included. "Probable" infections not included as, in a substantial proportion, infection may have occurred before pregnancy;
2   Only women with seroconversion or low IgG avidity included;
3   Mean observation period approximately 26 weeks;
4   Mean observation period 30 weeks
    Note: all incidence rates are adjusted for a 9 month pregnancy

Risk of clinical sequelae due to congenital infection

Women who acquire infection during pregnancy are faced with decisions about whether to undergo antibiotic treatment, amniocentesis and possibly, termination of pregnancy. These decisions should be based on reliable estimates of the risks of mother to child transmission of infection and symptoms or disability due to congenital toxoplasmosis which take account of gestation at maternal infection.

Risk of mother to child transmission of infection

The risk of congenital toxoplasmosis increases with gestation at maternal infection. Although this relationship has been a consistent finding, rates reported from case series in French centres vary from 3% to 11% for the first trimester, 16% to 30% for the second trimester, and 29% to 52% for the third trimester [31-34]. Such variation is partly due to analysis of women according to trimester of pregnancy, within which the risk may vary substantially. Secondly, some studies include a mix of women identified by seroconversion or rising IgG titres [31-33]. Thirdly, methods for defining gestation at infection are not given and may vary between studies. Fourthly, many studies are subject to selection bias due to inadequate confirmation of congenital infection particularly in terminations or fetal losses, and differential follow up of infected and uninfected children. Fifthly, studies include treated and untreated women. Lastly, a particular problem in referral centres is the inclusion of women referred due to suspected infection or damage in the fetus. Such referral bias leads to overestimation of the transmission and sequelae risks, respectively.

The population-based cohort studies shown in Table 4 minimise these biases but are based on small numbers. However, a recent collaborative study between Lyon and London by Dunn et al. [35] provides more precise and reliable estimates of the risk of congenital toxoplasmosis and can be used for counselling women. The study includes only women who unambiguously acquired infection during pregnancy and minimises selection bias by exclusion of mother-child pairs in whom referral was prompted by suspicion of congenital infection and minimising loss to follow up (8% at 1 year). Nearly all (94%) women were treated. Diagnosis of congenital infection was based on persistence of toxoplasma specific IgG beyond 12 months of age or positive PCR or culture for fetal losses. Congenital infection was excluded if IgG became negative after discontinuation of treatment. The risks of congenital toxoplasmosis and clinical signs are given for gestation at seroconversions estimated by means of a probabilistic statistical model which considers the dates of the last negative and first positive tests and whether the baby was infected or developed clinical signs. As the date of maternal infection is not detectable, estimates are based on the date of seroconversion – the first day when IgM would be detected assuming the mother was tested every day.

Overall, the risk of congenital toxoplasmosis is 29% but this masks a steep increase with gestation (see Fig. 1). The risk is low in early pregnancy and only 6% (3-9%) at 13 weeks gestation. Thereafter the risk rises sharply reaching 40% (34-46%) at 26 weeks, 72% (61-80%) at 36 weeks and 81% just before delivery.

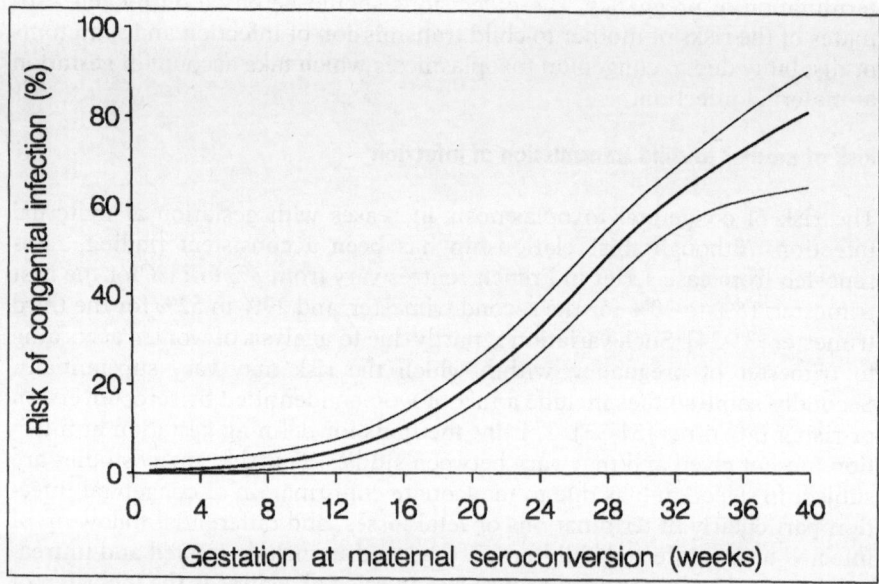

Fig. 1. Risk of congenital infection by gestational age at maternal seroconversion. Thin lines represent 90% confidence interval [35]

Risk of clinical sequelae in congenitally infected children

In the study by Dunn et al [35], 33 of the 153 congenitally infected children (22%) had at least one of the following clinical signs by 3 years of age: intracranial calcification, retinochoroiditis or hydrocephalus. Development of clinical signs was strongly related to gestation at maternal seroconversion, declining from an estimated 61% (37-83) at 13 weeks, to 25% (19-31) at 26 weeks, and 9% (4-16%) at 36 weeks (see Fig. 2).

Risk of clinical signs in children exposed to maternal infection

For pregnant women with a diagnosis of acute *Toxoplasma* infection, knowledge of the risks of clinical sequelae is not relevant as they first need to decide whether to undergo prenatal diagnosis or not. The risk of clinical signs in a fetus born to an infected woman is obtained by multiplying the risk of congenital infection by the risk of signs among congenitally infected children. For example, at 26 weeks gestation the risk of maternal-fetal transmission is 40% and the risk of clinical signs in an infected fetus is 25%. The overall risk is therefore 10% (0.4x0.25). If this calculation is repeated for all gestational ages, an "n" shaped distribution is produced which reaches a maximum of

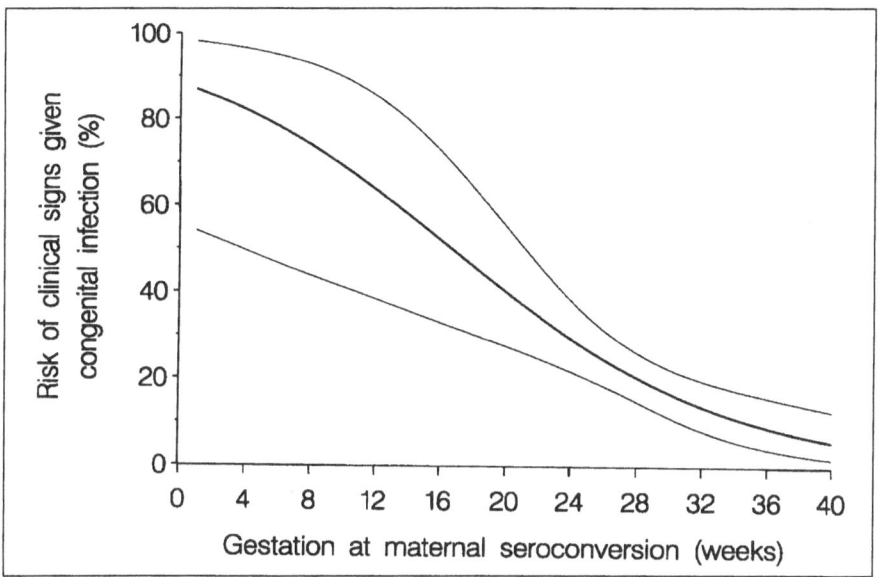

Fig. 2. Risk of developing clinical signs (not necessarily symptomatic) before age 3 years given congenital infection, according to gestation at maternal seroconversion. Thin lines represent 90% confidence interval [35]

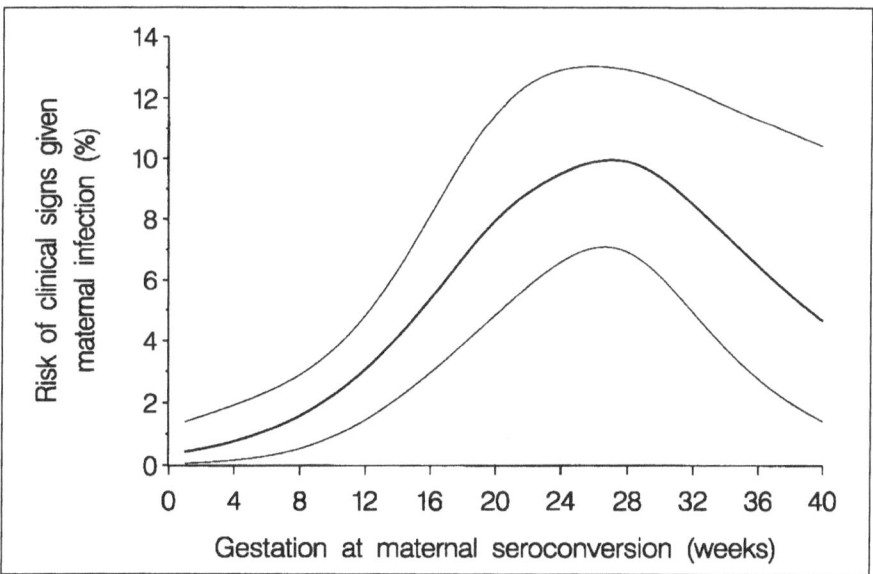

Fig. 3. Risk of developing clinical signs (not necessarily symptomatic) before age 3 years given maternal infection, according to gestation at maternal seroconversion. Thin lines represent 90% confidence interval [35]

10% at 24-30 weeks gestation (see Fig. 3). In the second and third trimesters the risk never falls below 5% and is 6% just before delivery.

Consistency of results

Previous studies show a similar trend in the risk of congenital infection with gestation but produce a flatter curve due to the broad gestational groupings. Desmonts and Couvreur [34] estimated the overall risk of congenital infection to be 30% (145/489) and the risk of subclinical, benign and severe clinical signs according to first, second and third trimesters at maternal infection to be 7% (8/120), 8% (19/241), and 6% (8/128), respectively. The overall risk for clinical signs was 7%, close to the rate observed by Dunn et al. [35]. Population-based cohort studies also report similar overall risks of mother to child transmission and clinical sequelae (see Table 4). However, comparisons between studies should be made with caution. Differences may be due to length of follow-up, intensity of examination, definition of signs, and most importantly, gestation at maternal infection.

Effect of prenatal treatment

Adjustment for gestation at maternal infection is particularly important in the investigation of the effect of screening and treatment schedules and has been reported in 2 studies. In a collaborative, 5 centre study, Foulon et al. [36] found no effect of prenatal treatment on transmission but a marked reduction in the risk of clinical signs with any treatment given. Although the study included referral centres for prenatal diagnosis, they made no attempt to exclude women referred due to suspicion of infection or signs in the fetus. Selection bias may therefore account for the relatively high transmission rate (44%) and rate of clinical signs at 1 year (14%) reported for women infected at a mean gestation of 20 weeks. Selection bias may also account for the apparent effect of treatment on clinical signs: untreated mothers missed by screening who have affected children may have been more likely to be included than those with unaffected children. Desmonts and Couvreur examined the effect of prenatal treatment with pyrimethamine and sulfadiazine on sequelae in children born to treated mothers compared with children born to untreated mothers infected at a similar gestation. They reported no difference in the risk of clinical sequelae [37].

Clinical relevance

Information from the study by Dunn et al. [35] on the risk of giving birth to a child with clinical signs due to toxoplasmosis can be used to help women decide about amniocentesis, treatment and termination. In practice the date at seroconversion is not known, only the date of the last negative test and the first positive test. Upper and lower limits for risk can therefore be given. For example, if seroconversion occurred between 12 and 20 weeks the risk of clinical signs in treated women is 3-8% and, if fetal infection has been diagnosed, 40-64%. In 2 recent French studies, over half the treated women had infection diagnosed during the first trimester [31, 33]. This would usually be based on tests for recent infection, such as IgM, rising IgG titre, and IgG avidity, performed at pregnancy booking. In this situation, Dunn et al. [35] provide only an upper estimate of the risks. For example, a woman with a positive test at 12 weeks gestation would have a risk of giving birth to a child with clinical signs of 3% or less depending on how well the test predicts postconceptional infection. This risk must be balanced against the risk of fetal loss of 0.9% associated with amniocentesis [38].

Finally, clinical signs do not necessarily result in functional impairment. The risk of giving birth to a child with functional impairment due to congenital toxoplasmosis is essential to enable women to make informed decisions about interventions in pregnancy. No studies have reliably measured the risk of functional impairment according to gestation at maternal infection, and information from population-based cohorts is based on small numbers (see Table 4) with poorly defined criteria for impairment.

Public health implications

From the public health perspective, the burden of disability is determined by the birth prevalence of congenital toxoplasmosis and the risk of impairment in congenitally infected children. Rates of birth prevalence of congenital toxoplasmosis derived from population-based cohort studies are given in Table 4 and range from 1-4/10.000 live births. Extrapolation of the incidence rate of "certain" maternal infections derived from Ancelle et al. [16] (Table 3) and the transmission risk observed in seroconverting women by Dunn et al. [35] (29%), gives an estimated birth prevalence of congenital toxoplasmosis in France of 10/10.000 live births. Data shown in Table 4 are limited by small numbers and length of follow up. However, of 103 congenitally infected children followed in the 5 studies shown, so far only 3 are reported to have neurological impairment and 13 unilateral visual impairment.

How much the burden of disease due to congenital toxoplasmosis might be altered by prenatal screening and treatment is not known. However, prenatal screening programmes are associated with a substantial clinical cost. Some women may be treated, investigated or even have their pregnancies terminated [5] unnecessarily due to IgM positive results reflecting infection before pregnancy or false positive results [25]. 1 French study reported that for every 1000 live births 0.2 medical terminations are carried out for toxoplasmosis [40]. Confirmation of infection by reference laboratories reduces these risks. Secondly, prenatal diagnosis of fetal infection involves amniocentesis which is associated with an average 0.9% risk of fetal loss due to the procedure [38]. Projections by Bader et al. [39] suggest that, even if prenatal treatment reduced the risk of congenital toxoplasmosis by 60%, many more fetuses would miscarry due to amniocentesis than infected babies avoided. Thirdly adverse effects of treatment can occur in the mother and cannot be ruled out in the fetus [14]. Lastly, infection in pregnancy raises anxieties which persist beyond birth and are not easily allayed. Absence of congenital toxoplasmosis cannot

Table 4. Birth prevalence of congenital toxoplasmosis and risks of congenital infection and clinical signs in children born to infected women: data from population based cohort studies

Study, country and year of study	Birth prevalence /10.000 liveborn (95% confidence interval)[a]	Risk of mother to child transmission of infection	Risk of child with clinical signs in infected women	Number of children with retinochoroiditis (visual impairment)[b]	Number with intracranial calcification or hydrocephalus (neurological impairment)	Length of follow-up
Koppe [28,63][c]	N/A	12/38 (32%)	9/38 (24%)	9 (4)	(0)	20 years
Conyn van Spaendonck [47] Netherlands 1987	4.3 (2.2 - 7.5)	12/44 (27%)	4/44 (9%)	3 (1)	1 (0)	2 years
Lappalainen [61] Finland 1988-1989	2.4 (0.7 - 6.1)	4/14 (29%)	2/14 (14%)	1 (N/A)	2 (1)	5 years
Guerina[d] [7] USA 1986-199	0.8 (0.6 - 1.1)	N/A	N/A[e]	12 (8)	14 (1)	1-6 years
Lebech et al. [62][d] Denmark 1992-1996	3.0 (1.5 - 5.0)	27/141 (19%)	5/141 (3.5%)	4 (N/A)	2 (1)	18 months

N/A = not available; a) confidence intervals derived from Poisson distribution; b) based on reports of visual impairment or macular lesion: c) no clear definition of maternal infection given; d) all women untreated; e) 19/48 congenitally infected children developed 1 or more signs (intracranial calcification/retinochoroiditis)

be diagnosed for certain until the child is 12 months old [41], and infected children, including those without clinically evident disease, live with the risk sight-impairing eye lesions throughout child and adulthood.

Future research

Reliable information is needed on the effectiveness of prenatal treatment on the risks of mother to child transmission of *Toxoplasma* infection and on the risk of clinical signs. Clinical trials to address these questions would require the enrolment of whole countries and are unlikely to be feasible. Instead, a longitudinal cohort study – EMSCOT (European Multicentre Study on Congenital Toxoplasmosis) – was established in 1997 to address questions of prenatal treatment effectiveness and provide reliable data on the risks of long term clinical sequelae. The study has recruited over 1300 mother-child pairs in 14 centres in 7 European countries. Analyses will exploit the variation in prenatal treatment delay inherent in screening schedules involving monthly, 3 monthly or neonatal testing in the collaborating centres.

Unfortunately, EMSCOT will not be able to address the important question of the effect of postnatal treatment on long term symptoms and signs, particularly in infants without signs at birth. This question can only be adequately addressed by a multicentre trial of postnatal treatment.

References

1. Eskild A, Oxman AP, Magnus A, Bjorndal S, Bakketeig LS (1996) Screening for toxoplasmosis in pregnancy: what is the evidence of reducing a health problem? J Med Screen 3:188-194
2. Multidisciplinary Working Group (1992) Prenatal screening for toxoplasmosis in the UK. Royal College of Obstetricians and Gynaecologists, London
3. Thulliez P (1992) Screening programme for congenital toxoplasmosis in France. Scand J Infect Dis Suppl 84:43-45
4. Aspock H, Pollak A (1992) Prevention of prenatal toxoplasmosis by serological screening of pregnant women in Austria. Scand J Infect Dis Suppl 84:32-37
5. Buffolano W, Sagliocca L, Fratta D, Tozzi A, Cardone A, Binkin N (1994) Prenatal toxoplasmosis screening in Campania region, Italy. Ital J Gynaecol Obstet 6:70-74
6. Lebech M, Petersen E (1992) Neonatal screening for congenital toxoplasmosis in Denmark: presentation of the design of a prospective study. Scand J Infect Dis Suppl 84:75-79
7. Guerina NG, Hsu HW, Meissner HC, Maguire JH, Lynfield R, Stechenberg B, Abroms I, Pasternack MS, Hoff R, Eaton RB et al (1994) Neonatal serologic screening and early treatment for congenital *Toxoplasma gondii* infection. The New England Regional Toxoplasma Working Group see comments. N Engl J Med 330:1858-1863
8. Pons JC, Sigrand C, Grangeot Keros L, Frydman R, Thulliez P (1995) Congenital toxoplasmosis: transmission to the fetus of a pre-pregnancy maternal infection. Presse Med 24:179-182
9. Desmonts G, Couvreur J, Thulliez P (1990) Congenital toxoplasmosis. 5 cases of mother-to-child transmission of pre-pregnancy infection. Presse Med 19:1445-1449
10. Marty P, Le-Fichoux Y, Deville A, Forest H (1991) Congenital toxoplasmosis and preconceptional maternal ganglionic toxoplasmosis (letter). Presse Med 20:387
11. Fortier B, Aissi E, Ajana F, Dieusart P, Denis P, Martin de Lassalle E, Lecomte Houcke M, Vinatier D (1991) Spontaneous abortion and reinfection by *Toxoplasma gondii* (letter). Lancet 338:444
12. Hennequin C, Dureau P, N'Guyen L, Thulliez P, Gagelin B, Dufier JL (1997) Congenital toxoplasmosis acquired from an immune woman. Pediatr Infect Dis J 16:75-77
13. Holliman RE (1994) Clinical sequelae of chronic maternal toxoplasmosis. Reviews in Medical Microbiology 5:(1)47-55
14. Remington JS, McLeod R, Desmonts G (1995) Toxoplasmosis. In: Remington JS, Klein J (eds). Infectious diseases of the fetus and newborn. 4th ed, WB Saunders, Philadelphia, pp 140-267
15. Zuber P, Jacquier P (1995) Epidemiology of toxoplasmosis: the world situation. Schweiz Med Wochenschr (Suppl) 65:19S-22S

16. Ancelle T, Goulet V, Tirard-Fleury V, Baril L, Mazaubrun C du, Thulliez P, Wcislo M, Carme B (1996) La Toxoplasmose chez la femme enceinte en France en 1995. Résultats d'une enquête nationale périnatale. Bulletin Épidemiologique Hebdomadaire 51:227-229

17. Ljungstrom I, Gille E, Nokes J, Linder E, Forsgren M (1995) Seroepidemiology of *Toxoplasma gondii* among pregnant women in different parts of Sweden. Eur J Epidemiol 11:149-156

18. Jenum PA, Kapperud G, Stray Pedersen B, Melby KK, Eskild A, Eng J (1998) Prevalence of *Toxoplasma gondii* specific immunoglobulin G antibodies among pregnant women in Norway. Epidemiol Infect 1:87-92

19. Guimaraes AC, Kawarabayashi M, Borges MM, Tolezano JE, Andrade Junior HF (1993) Regional variation in toxoplasmosis seronegativity in the Sao Paulo metropolitan region. Rev Inst Med Trop Sao Paulo 35:479-483

20. Jacquier P, Hohlfeld P, Vorkauf H, Zuber P (1995) Epidemiology of toxoplasmosis in Switzerland: national study of seroprevalence monitored in pregnant women 1990-1991. Schweiz Med Wochenschr (Suppl) 65:29S-38S

21. Jeannel D, Niel G, Costagliola D, Danis M, Traore MB, Gentilini M (1988) Epidemiology of toxoplasmosis among pregnant women in the Paris area. Int J Epidemiol 17:595-602

22. Gilbert RE, Tookey PA, Cubitt WD, Ades AE, Masters J, Peckham CS (1993) Prevalence of toxoplasma IgG among pregnant women in west London according to country of birth and ethnic group (see comments). BMJ 306:185

23. Zuber PL, Jacquier P, Hohlfeld P, Walker AM (1995) Toxoplasma infection among pregnant women in Switzerland: a cross-sectional evaluation of regional and age-specific lifetime average annual incidence. Am J Epidemiol 141:659-666

24. Ades AE, Parker S, Gilbert R, Tookey PA, Berry T, Hjelm M, Wilcox AH, Cubitt D, Peckham CS (1993) Maternal prevalence of Toxoplasma antibody based on anonymous neonatal serosurvey: a geographical analysis. Epidemiol Infect 110:127-133

25. Allain J, Palmer C, Pearson G (1998) Epidemiological study of latent and recent infection by *Toxoplasma gondii* in pregnant women from a regional population in the UK. J Infect 36:(2)189-196

26. Ades A, Nokes DJ (1993) Modeling age – and time – specific incidence from seroprevalence: toxoplasmosis. Am J Epidemiol 137:1022-1034

27. Ades AE (1992) Methods for estimating the incidence of primary infection in pregnancy: a reappraisal of toxoplasmosis and cytomegalovirus data. Epidemiol Infect 108:367-375

28. Koppe JG, Kloosterman GJ, de Roever-Bonnet H, Eckert-Stroink JA, Loewer-Sieger DH, de Bruijne JL (1974) Toxoplasmosis and pregnancy, with a long-term follow-up of the children. Europ J Obstet Reprod Biol 4:101-110

29. Sever JL, Ellenberg JH, Ley AC, Madden DL, Fuccillo DA, Tzan NR, Edmonds DM (1988) Toxoplasmosis: maternal and pediatric findings in 23,000 pregnancies. Pediatrics 82:181-192

30. Horion M. Thoumsin H, Senterre J, Lambotte R (1990) 20 years of screening for toxoplasmosis in pregnant women. The Liege experience in 20,000 pregnancies. Rev Med Liege 45:492-497

31. Pratlong F, Boulot P, Villena I, Issert E, Tamby I, Cazenave J, Dedet JP (1996) Antenatal diagnosis of congenital toxoplasmosis: evaluation of the biological parameters in a cohort of 286 patients. Br J Obstet Gynaecol 103:552-557

32. Excler JL, Piens MA, Maisonneuve H et al (1985) Toxoplasmosis screening in pregnant women and their newborn. Lyon Med 253:33-38

33. Hohlfeld P, Daffos F, Costa JM, Thulliez P, Forestier F, Vidaud M (1994) Prenatal diagnosis of congenital toxoplasmosis with a polymerase-chain-reaction test on amniotic fluid. N Engl J Med 331:695-699

34. Desmonts G, Couvreur J (1984) Congenital toxoplasmosis. a prospective study of the outcome of pregnancy in 542 women with toxoplasmosis acquired during pregnancy. Ann Pediatr 31:805-809

35. Dunn D, Wallon M, Peyron F, Petersen E, Peckham CS, Gilbert RE (1999) Mother to child transmission of toxoplasmosis: risk estimates for clinical counselling. Lancet 353:1829-1833

36. Foulon W, Villena I, Stray-Pedersen B, Decoster A, Lappalainen M, Pinon JM, Jenum PA, Hedman K, Naessens A (1999) Treatment of toxoplasmosis during pregnancy: a multicentre study of impact on fetal transmission and children's sequelae at age 1 year. Am J Obstet Gynecol 180:410-415

37. Couvreur J, Thulliez P, Daffos F, Aufrant C, Bompard Y, Gesquiere A, Desmonts G (1993) *In utero* treatment of toxoplasmic fetopathy with the combination pyrimethamine-sulfadiazine. Fetal Diagn Ther 8:45-50

38. Tabor A, Madsen M, Obel E, Philip J, Bank J, Norgaard-Pedersen B (1986) Randomised controlled trial of genetic amniocentesis in 4606 low risk women. Lancet i:1287-1293

39. Bader TJ, Macones GA, Asch DA (1997) Prenatal screening for toxoplasmosis. Obstet Gynecol 90:457-464

40. Schneider S, Roussey M, Odent S, Debroise C, Poulain P, Jouan H, Milon J, Betremieux P, Journel H, Le Mee F, Morellec J, le Marec B (1994) Ten year experiences with medically induced abortion. J Gynecol Obstet Biol Reprod 23:157-165

41. Lebech M, Joynson DHM, Seitz HM, Thulliez P, Gilbert RE, Dutton GN, Ovlisen B, Petersen E (1996) Classification system and case definitions of *Toxoplasma gondii* infection in immunocompetent pregnant women and their congenitally infected offspring. Eur J Clin Microbiol Infect Dis 15:799-805

42. Berger R, Merkel S, Rudin C (1995) Toxoplasmosis and pregnancy-findings from umbilical cord blood screening in 30,000 newborn infants. Schweiz Med Wochenschr 125:1168-1173

43. Buffolano W, Del Pezzo M, Avagliano G, Di Costanzo P (1993) Prevalenza degli anticorpi anti-*Toxoplasma* nelle donne campane in eta fertile. Microbiol Medica 8:189-191

44. Valcavi PP, Natali A, Soliani L, Montali S, Dettori G, Checzi C (1995) Prevalence of anti-*Toxoplasma gondii* antibodies in the population of the area of Parma (Italy). Eur J Epidemiol 11:333-337

45. Roos T, Martius J, Gross U, Schrod L (1993) Systematic serologic screening for toxoplasmosis in pregnancy (see comments). Obstet Gynecol 81:243-250

46. Aspock H, Pollak A (1992) Prevention of prenatal toxoplasmosis by serological screening of pregnant women in Austria. Scand J Infect Dis (Suppl) 84:32-37

47. Conyn-van-Spaedonck MAE (1991) Prevention of congenital toxoplasmosis in the Netherlands. (Thesis). National Institute of Public Health and Environmental Protection (Netherlands) ISBN 90-9004179-6

48. Foulon W, Naessens A, Derde MP (1994) Evaluation of the possibilities for preventing congenital toxoplasmosis. Am J Perinatol 11:57-62

49. Zadik PM, Kudesia G, Siddons AD (1995) Low incidence of primary infection with toxoplasma among women in Sheffield: a seroconversion study. Br J Obstet Gynaecol 102:608-610

50. Lappalainen M, Koskela P, Hedman K, Teramo K, Ammala P, Hiilesmaa V, Koskiniemi M (1992) Incidence of primary toxoplasma infections during pregnancy in southern Finland: a prospective cohort study. Scand J Infect Dis 24:97-104

51. Lebech M, Larsen SO, Petersen E (1993) Prevalence, incidence and geographical distribution of *Toxoplasma gondii* antibodies in pregnant women in Denmark. Scand J Infect Dis 25:751-756

52. Decavalas G, Papapetropoulou M, Giannoulaki E, Tzigounis V, Kondakis XG (1990) Prevalence of *Toxoplasma gondii* antibodies in gravidas and recently aborted women and study of risk factors. Eur J Epidemiol 6:223-226

53. Walpole IR, Hodgen N, Bower C (1991) Congenital toxoplasmosis: a large survey in western Australia. Med J Aust 154:720-724

54. Galvan-Ramirez M, Soto Mancilla JL, Velasco Castrejon O, Perez Medina R (1995) Incidence of anti-Toxoplasma antibodies in women with high-risk pregnancy and habitual abortions. Rev Soc Bras Med Trop 28:333-337

55. Altintas N, Kuman H, Akisu C, Aksoy U, Atambay M (1997) Toxoplasmosis in last four years in Agean region, Turkey. J Egypt Soc Parasitol 27:(2)439-443

56. Sun RG, Liu ZL, Wang DC (1995) The prevalence of *Toxoplasma* infection among pregnant women and their newborn infants in Chengdu. Chung Hua Liu Hsing Ping Hsueh Tsa Chih 16:98-100

57. Ashrafunnessa S, Khatun S, Islam M, Huq T (1998) Seroprevalence of *Toxoplasma* antibodies among the antenatal population in Bangladesh. J Obstet Gynaecol Res 24:(2)115-119

58. Bornand JE, Piguet JD (1991) *Toxoplasma* infection. Schweiz Med Wochenschr 121:21-29

59. Nokes DJ, Forsgren M, Gille E, Ljungstrom I (1993) Modelling *Toxoplasma* incidence from longitudinal seroprevalence in Stockholm, Sweden. Parasitology 107:33-40

60. Conyn van Spaendonck MA (1989) Prevention of congenital toxoplasmosis; experience in The Netherlands. Int Ophthalmol 13:403-406

61. Lappalainen M, Koskiniemi M, Hiilesmaa V, Ammala P, Teramo K, Koskela P, Lebech M, Raivio KO, Hedman K (1995) Outcome of children after maternal primary *Toxoplasma* infection during pregnancy with emphasis on avidity of specific IgG. The Study Group Pediatr Infect Dis J 14:354-361

62. Lebech M, Andersen O, Christensen N, Hertel J, Nielsen HE, Peitersen B, Rechnitzer C, Larsen SO, Norgaard-Pedersen B, Petersen E, and the Danish Congenital Toxoplasmosis Study Group (1999) Feasibility of neonatal screening for toxoplasma infection in the absence of prenatal treatment. Lancet 353:1834-1837

63. Koppe JG, Loewer Sieger DH, de Roever Bonnet H (1986) Results of 20-year follow-up of congenital toxoplasmosis. Lancet 1:254-256

4.2. Epidemiology of ocular *Toxoplasma*

M. STANFORD, R. GILBERT

Introduction

Toxoplasma retinochoroiditis is a common cause of posterior uveitis and accounts for 20-90% of patients with posterior uveitis seen in tertiary referral clinics (see Table 1). *Toxoplasma* retinochoroidal lesions are commonly attributed to congenital infection except where there is clear evidence of acquired toxoplasmosis [1-5]. We challenge this view by comparing the epidemiological evidence on the characteristics and risks of ocular disease due to congenital and acquired toxoplasmosis. In summary, although the clinical appearances and serological findings are frequently indistinguishable, the age at onset of signs and symptoms helps to differentiate between congenital and acquired infection. Finally, information on the risks of ocular disease due to congenital and acquired toxoplasmosis provide broad and uncertain estimates but no evidence that the majority of cases are due to congenital infection. On balance, the available evidence suggests that at least two-thirds of *Toxoplasma* ocular disease may be due to acquired infection.

Clinical characteristics

Age at appearance of lesions

Congenital toxoplasmosis

In children with congenital toxoplasmosis, retinochoroidal lesions may be present at birth or develop at any point during child or adulthood. Examinations during infancy are difficult and some "new" lesions detected at older ages may have been present from birth but were missed by the examiner. Five population-based cohort studies [38] of congenitally infected children identified by prenatal or neonatal screening assessed the age at detection of first and subsequent lesions (see Table 2). In 4 studies, 20 of 91 congenitally infected children with retinochoroiditis were followed for 1-6 years [38] and all but 1 [6] had their first lesion detected by 2 years of age. A further, population based cohort study followed 11 congenitally

Table 1. Prevalence of toxoplasmosis in uveitis clinics

Country/City	Population/Hospital based	New patients	% All uveitis	% Posterior uveitis	Reference	Year
Rochester/ Minnesota	Population	52	–	10%	[24]	1962
North Finland	Population	120	3%	40%	[25]	1977
Japan	Clinic	–	4.6%	–	[26]	1979
Iowa/London	Hospital based	172	10%	75%	[27]	1984
Savoy, France	Population (330,000)	51	13%	50%	[28]	1984
Sydney	Clinic	245	3%	20%	[29]	1986
California	Clinic	600	7%	18.3%	[30]	1987
California	Clinic	–	–	46%	[3]	1988
N. Portugal	Clinic	450	9.1%	–	[31]	1990
Rotterdam	Clinic	769	9.6%	40%	[32]	1992
South Brazil	Population	–	–	90%	[18]	1992
Finland	Clinic	1,122	3%	51.6%	[33]	1994
California	Clinic	426	4%	34%	[34]	1996
Sierra Leone	Hospital	93	43%	–	[23]	1996
Singapore	Clinic	260	4%	32%	[35]	1998
Padua, Italy	Clinic	1,522	10%	60%	[36]	1998

Table 2. Risk of retinochoroiditis in children with congenital toxoplasmosis (not adjusted for gestation at maternal infection)

Country of study	Total with congenital toxoplasmosis	Number with retinochoroiditis	Length of follow-up	Reference
Netherlands	11	9 (85%)	20 years	[7]
Netherlands	12	2 (16%)	2 years	[8,37]
USA	48	12 (25%)	1-6 years	[6]
Finland	4	1 (25%)	4-5 years	[9]
Denmark	27	4 (15%)	1-3 years	[38]

infected children for 20 years [7]. Of the 9 individuals with lesions at 20 years, 5 first had lesions detected during infancy, 1 at 6 years, and in 3, lesions were first noted during adolescence but how often they were examined at younger ages is not clear. Studies based on case series of referred patients also rarely report late occurrence of lesions in previously unaffected children (no lesion in either eye). Mets et al followed children for a median of 5 years and [10] found that only 2 of 54 children with congenital toxoplasmosis followed beyond one year developed new lesions in previously uninvolved retina. Peyron et al [11] reported that, after a mean follow up of 12 years, only 2 of 37 patients with retinochoroiditis had lesions first noted after 10 years of age and in 28, lesions were diagnosed in the first year of life. Couvreur et al [12] found that of 49 children with retinochoroiditis due to congenital toxoplasmosis and followed for 2 to 11 years, only 2 developed lesions for the first time after 2 years of age.

Late appearance of first lesions is clearly affected by the thoroughness of early examinations and the length of follow-up. Data on follow-up beyond 10 years of age is limited, particularly of untreated children. However, all studies show evidence of a decline in the risk of first lesions with increasing age, and the majority of children who eventually develop lesions have their first lesion detected in the first 2 years of life.

In the cohort studies based on screening programmes, approximately half the patients had unilateral visual impairment or a lesion involving the macula. Some degree of visual impairment is therefore likely to have been detectable at least during school age. In the study by Guerina et al [6], all the children with a macula lesion had some degree of visual impairment, although even extensive macula lesions may be associated with reasonable visual acuity [10]. In preverbal children, visual impairment may be missed, but is likely to be picked up through vision screening and symptoms during the early school years. Therefore, if current teaching is correct and the majority of *Toxoplasma* retinochoroiditis seen by ophthalmologists is due to congenital infection, we would expect a history of visual symptoms during childhood in a substantial proportion of patients. This pattern is not observed in practice.

Acquired toxoplasmosis

In individuals known to have acquired toxoplasmosis, lesions can appear for the first time as early as 2 months after the onset of infection [13] or as late as 5 years [14]. New active lesions usually form a retinochoroidal scar after 6-8 weeks [15]. However, the age at onset of acquired *Toxoplasma* retinochoroiditis is difficult to determine from the literature. In case series of referred patients, the age distribution is determined by referral patterns. For example, a Dutch series of 8 patients, ranged from 42 to 75 years [16]. A Paris series of 49 patients ranged from 1 to 62 years over half of whom were under 16 years, probably reflecting the fact that the main author was a paediatrician [17]. Population-based studies avoid distortions due to referral bias but the age distribution may instead reflect atypical exposure. Thus, following an outbreak of toxoplasmosis linked to water-borne infection in Vancouver, 20 patients developed retinochoroiditis at a mean age of 56 years (range 15-83 years) [2]. Finally, in a population-based study in South Brazil of prevalent not first lesions, there was an increase in prevalence from 4% to 25% between 10 and 20 years of age after which prevalence remained steady [18]. Providing patterns do not change over time, these data suggest that, in South Brazil at least, most people developed retinochoroiditis for the first time during adolescence.

Recurrence of lesions

The risk of recurrence and the risk of bilateral lesions are both related to the length of follow-up and appear to be similar in congenital and acquired disease. Population-based studies of patients with acquired disease have not yet conducted long term follow-up but the Paris case series reported recurrences in 14/36 (39%) patients followed for a mean of 39 months [13]. This study may have been biased by referral of more severely affected patients. In population-based cohort studies of congenitally infected patients, lesions recurred at least once in 5/9 patients with retino-choroiditis followed for 20 years [7] and in 2/12 affected patients followed for 1-6 years [6]. In case series of congenitally infected patients, Peyron et al [11] reported recurrences in 5/37 (13%) followed for a mean of 12 years, Mets et al [10] in 13% of 54 children followed for more than 1 year, and Couvreur [12] in 3 of 38 (8%) children with lesions noted in the first year and followed 2-11 years.

Bilateral vs. unilateral lesions

The risk of bilateral lesions increases over time as lesions recur. Patients with congenital and acquired toxoplasmosis should therefore be compared at first presentation. Bilateral lesions were reported at presentation by Couvreur [13] in 2/45 patients with acquired infection and in 1 of 20 patients with infection acquired in the Vancouver outbreak [2]. In contrast, the proportion of congenitally infected children with bilateral lesions in the first year of life was higher in case series, which are likely to favour inclusion of more severely affected children, than in the population-based studies: 14-41% had bilateral lesions in the case series studies (4/28 [11], 13/38 [12], 31/76 [10]) but none in the population-based studies.

Clinical implications

The clinical implications of these findings are that most individuals with *Toxoplasma* retinochoroiditis due to congenital infection have lesions from early childhood, and approximately half of these would have some degree of visual impairment detectable during school years. Retinochoroiditis due to acquired infection can occur at any age but appears to occur mostly during adolescence and adulthood in western industrialised countries [2, 13, 18]. Both congenital and acquired infection are associated with a high rate of recurrence occurring in association with scars of old, healed retinochoroidal lesions. At first presentation, bilateral lesions are rare in both congenital and acquired infection, but become more common as lesions recur.

In a minority of individuals, other clinical characteristics help determine the aetiology as congenital or acquired. In individuals with retinochoroiditis, evidence of organ damage in utero or early infancy, such as microphthalmia or a history of intracranial calcification or hydrocephalus in early childhood, make the diagnosis of congenital toxoplasmosis almost certain. Evidence of retinitis in the absence of a scar in adolescence or adulthood makes acquired much more likely than congenital toxoplasmosis, particularly if associated with lymphadenopathy. Unfortunately, such findings are present in only a few patients with acquired [1] or congenital toxoplasmosis (ref 38) [6-9].

Serology

A further problem is that serological findings rarely provide evidence to date infection. Detection of *Toxoplasma* IgM and IgA antibodies in the first year of life or persistence of IgG beyond one year provides clear evidence of congenital toxoplasmosis, but IgM and IgA usually decline to undetectable levels in early infancy [4] and the presence of IgG in later childhood may be due to congenital or acquired infection. Similarly, production of IgM and IgA antibodies after acquired infection has usually subsided by 1 year post infection [4]. Therefore, most individuals with retinochoroidal lesions due to toxoplasmosis only have detectable IgG antibodies. Furthermore, detection of IgM antibodies in late child or adulthood does not necessarily date infection. Persistence or resurgence of IgM antibodies has rarely been reported in congenital infection [19] but occurs in about 5% of postnatally acquired infection [4]. Hence, presence of IgM in adults is more likely to reflect postnatally acquired infection but does not rule out congenital infection.

Risk of *Toxoplasma* retinochoroiditis due to congenital and acquired infection

Clinicians advice to patients should be based on the probability of disease due to acquired and congenital infection. Unfortunately, calculation of the expected risks of retinochoroiditis attributable to congenital or acquired infection, produces broad and uncertain estimates due to the paucity of published data. Recent cohort studies in northern Europe and North America give figures for the birth prevalence of congenital toxoplasmosis ranging from 0.8 to 5/10,000 live births (ref 38) [6, 8, 9, 20] (see Table 3). The birth prevalence for France is calculated from an incidence rate of 7.5/1000 susceptible pregnancies (based on 32/6442 "certain" diagnoses over an assumed 6 month mean time interval [21]), 46% of pregnancies are susceptible and the transmission rate is assumed to be 29% (ref 39). Based on these figures, the birth prevalence of congenital toxoplasmosis in France is estimated to be 1 per 1000 (7.5 x 0.46 x 0.29/1000). If we assume that 80% of congenitally infected children eventually develop retinochoroiditis, the estimated lifetime risk of retinochoroiditis due to congenital infection in the different centres studied is 6 to 80/100,000 (see Table 3).

Two pieces of information are required to determine the risk of acquired *Toxoplasma* retinochoroiditis. Firstly, the prevalence of previous infection by age 60, as retinochoroiditis is rare after this age [2, 13, 22]. As there is a lack of prevalence data for 60 year olds, the prevalence of *Toxoplasma* infection in pregnant women can be used. This slightly underestimates the risk of acquired infection (see Table 3). Secondly, the risk of retinochoroiditis in individuals who acquire toxoplasmosis is required. This can be derived from the lower estimate in the study in Vancouver by Burnett et al [2]. They calculated two estimates of the rate of infection, one based on the incidence in pregnant women and the other observed in control subjects. They estimated that between 2,894 and 7,718 individuals were infected in Greater Victoria of whom 20 developed *Toxoplasma* retinitis: a risk of 0.3% to 0.7%. More infected people may have developed lesions but not consulted the ophthalmologist, thereby underestimating the risk. However, the risk may have been overestimated if retinochoroiditis occurs more frequently following a water borne outbreak than following exposure experienced in the general population.

The risks of *Toxoplasma* retinochoroiditis following acquired infection estimated in other studies are higher than the estimates for Vancouver. Perkins [1] reported that 1.2% of 1,669 patients with acquired toxoplasmosis identified in case reports developed retinochoroidal lesions and provided some evidence that the risk may be higher (2.6%) in patients with neurologic or systemic signs and symptoms. A population-based study in South Brazil [18] showed that 21% of individuals aged 13 years or older had *Toxoplasma* retinochoroidal lesions when examined ophthalmologically. The prevalence of past infection was 77% in the age-matched population without lesions and 99.5% in those with lesions. Therefore, the risk of retinochoroiditis following *Toxoplasma* infection was approximately 25%. This extremely high rate of infection is almost all due to postnatal acquired infection as the authors' report that only 1% of cord blood samples tested in the same population were IgM positive.

Table 3. Estimated percentage of *Toxoplasma* retinochoroiditis due to congenital infection

Country	Risk due to Congenital Toxoplasmosis		Risk due to Acquired Toxoplasmosis		% Toxoplasma retinochoroiditis due to congenital infection
	Birth prevalence ** per 10,000 births	Risk of retinochoroiditis per 100,000	Risk of acquired infection*	Risk of retinochoroiditis *** per 100,000	
Switzerland [20]	1.7	13.6	29%	87	14%
USA [6]	0.8	6.4	10%	30	18%
France*	10	80	54%	162	33%
Netherlands [8]	4.3	34	45%	135	20%
Denmark [38]	3.0	23	28%	84	21%

* Prevalence of infection in pregnant women; ** risk of retinochoroiditis in congenitally infected individuals assumed to be 80%; *** risk of retinochoroiditis in individuals with acquired toxoplasmosis assumed to be 0.3% and based on incidence of certain diagnosis of 7.5/1,000 pregnant women (derived from Ancelle et al [21] and a transmission rate of 29% [39].

Finally, the risks of *Toxoplasma* retinochoroiditis due to congenital and acquired infection, and the proportion attributable to congenital infection are calculated (see Table 3). Until further research generates more robust estimates, these limited data suggest that two-thirds of retinochoroidal lesions seen by ophtalmologists due to acquired toxoplasmosis are at least as common as those due to congenital infection.

Patterns in practice

In a UK study of patients with suspected toxoplasmosis seen by ophthalmologists serving a population of 7 million, 83/84 patients presented with symptoms aged 10 to 54 years (Gilbert et al, In press. Epidemiology and Infection). Half reported never having had previous visual symptoms and presented at a mean age of 25 years. Of those with previous symptoms, only 2/84 had symptoms in early childhood and no others had symptoms before 10 years of age. In addition, 5/84 patients had detectable levels of *Toxoplasma*-specific IgM, suggesting that infection may have been acquired. Other studies similarly rarely report symptoms or serological evidence of congenital or acquired infection in patients with *Toxoplasma* retinochoroiditis [23].

The clinical implications of these findings for ophthalmologists seeing patients with *Toxoplasma* retinochoroiditis are that the cause is rarely known. Attribution to congenital infection can place an unnecessary emotional burden on the mother and is likely to be wrong. Lastly, there are major public health implications. Considerable expertise and expense is concentrated on screening and health information to reduce the risks of congenital toxoplasmosis. However, information about how to avoid infection is equally important for children and adults at risk of ocular disease due to postnatally acquired infection.

References

1. Perkins ES (1973) Ocular toxoplasmosis. Br J Ophthalmol 57:1-17
2. Burnett A, Shortt S, Isaac-Renton J, King A, Werker D, Bowie W (1998) Multiple cases of acquired toxoplasmosis retinitis presenting in an outbreak. Ophthalmology 105:1032-1037
3. Holland GN, Engstrom RE Jr (1988) Ocular toxoplasmosis in the United States. In: Belfort R, Petrilli A, Nussenblatt R (eds) World Uveitis Symposium. Roca, Sao Paulo, pp 315-322
4. Remington JS, McLeod R, Desmonts G (1995) Toxoplasmosis. In: Remington JS, Klein J (eds) Infectious Diseases of the Foetus and Newborn. WB Saunders, Philadelphia, 4th edn, pp 140-267
5. Rothova A (1993) Ocular involvement in toxoplasmosis. Br J Ophthalmol 77:371-377
6. Guerina NG, Hsu HW, Meissner HC, Maguire JH, Lynfield R, Stechenberg B, Abroms I, Pasternack MS, Hoff R, Eaton RB et al (1994) Neonatal serologic screening and early treatment for congenital *Toxoplasma gondii* infection. The New England Regional *Toxoplasma* Working Group. N Engl J Med 330:1858-1863
7. Koppe JG, Loewer Sieger DH, de Roever Bonnet H (1986) Results of 20-year follow-up of congenital toxoplasmosis. Lancet 1:254-256
8. Conyn van-Spaendonck MAE (1991) Prevention of congenital toxoplasmosis in the Netherlands. (Thesis). National Institute of Public Health and Environmental Protection (Netherlands) ISBN 90-9004179-6
9. Lappalainen M, Koskiniemi M, Hiilesmaa V, Ammala P, Teramo K, Koskela P, Lebech M, Raivio KO, Hedman K (1995) Outcome of children after maternal primary *Toxoplasma* infection during pregnancy with emphasis on avidity of specific IgG. Pediatr Infect Dis J 14:354-361

10. Mets MB, Holfels E, Boyer KM, Swisher CN, Roizen N, Stein L, Stein M, Hopkins J, Withers S, Mack D, Luciano R, Patel D, Remington JS, Meier P, McLeod R (1996) Eye manifestations of congenital toxoplasmosis. Am J Ophthalmol 122:309-324

11. Peyron F, Wallon M, Bernardoux C (1996) Long-term follow-up of patients with congenital ocular toxoplasmosis (letter). N Engl J Med 334:993-994

12. Couvreur J, Desmonts G, Aron-Rosa D (1984) Le prognostic oculaire de la toxoplasmose congénitale: role du traitement: communication préliminaire. Ann Pediatr Paris 31:855-858

13. Couvreur J, Thulliez P (1996) Acquired toxoplasmosis of ocular or neurologic site: 49 cases. Presse Med 25:438-442

14. Leblanc A, Bamberger J, Guillien F, Benoit A, Baufine Ducroq A, Quillet P (1985) Acquired toxoplasmic chorioretinitis with a late onset. Arch Fr Pediatr 42:37-39

15. Rothova A (1993) Ocular involvement in toxoplasmosis. Br J Ophthalmol 77:371-377

16. Ronday MJ, Luyendijk L, Baarsma GS, Bollemeijer JG, Van der Lelij A, Rothova A (1995) Presumed acquired ocular toxoplasmosis. Arch Ophthalmol 113:1524-1529

17. Couvreur J, Thulliez PH (1996) Toxoplasmose acquise a localisation oculaire ou neurologique. Presse Médicale 25:438-442

18. Glasner PD, Silveira C, Kruszon Moran D, Martins MC, Burnier M, Silveira S, Camargo ME, Nussenblatt RB, Kaslow RA, Belfort R (1992) An unusually high prevalence of ocular toxoplasmosis in southern Brazil. Am J Ophthalmol 114:136-144

19. Sibalic D, Djurkovic Djakovic O, Bobic B (1990) Onset of ocular complications in congenital toxoplasmosis associated with immunoglobulin M antibodies to *Toxoplasma gondii*. Eur J Clin Microbiol Infect Dis 9:671-674

20. Berger R, Merkel S, Rudin C (1995) Toxoplasmosis and pregnancy-findings from umbilical cord blood screening in 30,000 newborn infants. Schweiz Med Wochenschr 125:1168-1173

21. Ancelle T, Goulet V, Tirard-Fleury V, Baril L, du Mazaubrun C, Thulliez P, Wcislo M, Carme B (1996) La Toxoplasmose chez la femme enceinte en France en 1995. Résultats d'une enquête nationale périnatale. *Bulletin Épidémiologique Hebdomadaire* 51:227-229

22. Ronday MJH, Luyendijk L, Baarsma GS, Bollemeijer JG, Van der Lelij A, Rothova A (1995) Presumed acquired ocular toxoplasmosis. Arch Ophthalmol 113:1524-1529

23. Ronday MJ, Stilma JS, Barbe RF, McElroy WJ, Luyendijk L, Kolk AH, Bakker M, Kijlstra A, Rothova A (1996) Aetiology of uveitis in Sierra Leone, west Africa. Br J Ophthalmol 80:956-961

24. Darnell R, Wagener H, Kurland L (1962) Epidemiology of Uveitis. Arch Ophthalmol 62:100-112

25. Miettenen R (1977) Incidence of uveitis in Northern Finland. *Acta Ophthalmologica* 55:252-260

26. Mishima S, Masuda K, Igawa Y, Mochizuki M, Namba K (1979) Behçets disease in Japan: ophthalmological aspects. Trans Am Ophthalmol Soc 76:225-239

27. Perkins ES, Folk J (1984) Uveitis in London and Iowa. Ophthalmologica 189:36-40

28. Vadot E, Bartu E, Billet P (1984) Epidemiology of Uveitis-preliminary results of a prospective study in the Savoy. In: Saari K (ed) Uveitis update. Elsevier Science, Amsterdam, pp 13-17

29. Wakefield D, Dunlop I, McCluskey PJ, Penny R (1986) Uveitis: aetiology and disease associations in an Australian population. Aust New Zealand J Ophthalmol 14:181-187

30. Henderly DE, Genstler AJ, Smith RE, Rao NA (1987) Changing patterns of uveitis. Am J Ophthalmol 103:131-136

31. Palmares J, Coutinho MF, Castro Correia J (1990) Uveitis in northern Portugal. Curr Eye Res 9(Suppl):31-34

32. Baarsma GS (1992) The epidemiology and genetics of endogenous uveitis: a review. Curr Eye Res 11(Suppl):1-9

33. Paivonsalo Hietanen T, Tuominen J, Vaahtoranta Lehtonen H, Saari KM (1994) Incidence and prevalence of different uveitis entities in Finland. Acta Ophthalmol Scand 75:76-81

34. McCannel CA, Holland GN, Helm CJ, Cornell PJ, Winston JV, Rimmer TG (1996) Causes of uveitis in the general practice of ophthalmology. UCLA Community-Based Uveitis Study Group. Am J Ophthalmol 121:35-46

35. Lim VK, Ching N, Chee SP (1998) A review of uveitis cases seen at the Singapore National Eye Centre. In: Ohno S, Aoki K, Usui M, Uchio E (eds) Uveitis today. Elsevier Science BV, Amsterdam, pp 241-250

36. Secchi A, Tagnan S, Salmaso M, Cavaryeran F (1998) Uveitis in Italy: 10 years of experience in a referral centre. In: Ohno S, Aoki K, Usui M, Uchio E (eds) Uveitis today. Elsevier Science BV, Amsterdam, pp 232-238

37. Conyn van Spaendonck MA (1989) Prevention of congenital toxoplasmosis; experience in The Netherlands. Int Ophthalmol 13:403-406

38. Lebech M, Andersen O, Christensen N, Hertel J, Nielsen HE, Peitersen B, Rechnitzer C, Larsen SO, Norgaard-Pedersen B, Petersen E, and the Danish Congenital Toxoplasmosis Study Group. (1999) Feasibility of neonatal screening for toxoplasma infection in the absence of prenatal treatment. Lancet 353:1834-1837.

39. Dunn D, Wallon M, Peyron F, Petersen E, Peckham CS, Gilbert RE (1999) Mother to child transmission of toxoplasmosis: risk estimates for clinical counselling. Lancet 353:1829-1833.

4.3. Veterinary aspects of *Toxoplasma* infection

P. LIND, D. BUXTON

Toxoplasmosis and the cat

Cats (and other members of the cat family, Felidae) are the only final hosts for *Toxoplasma gondii*. The shedding of oocysts following the parasite's sexual reproduction in the cat's intestine is fundamental for the maintenance of the parasite in its natural reservoir populations. *Toxoplasma* may be transmitted as the tissue cyst (bradyzoite) stage between intermediate hosts, allowing it to move up the food chain to higher carnivores, and transplacental transmission of the parasite during acute infection has been demonstrated in many mammals. It is, however, unlikely that long-term reservoir populations are able to persist in wild or farming habitats without the presence of cats as shown by the virtual absence of *Toxoplasma* on some remote islands [1].

Reviews of the literature before 1990 on toxoplasmosis of cats have been published by Dubey [2], Dubey and Beattie [3] and Frenkel [4].

Transmission routes to cats

Small rodents and birds carrying the tissue cyst stage are the main source of infection for cats. Bradyzoites are liberated by gastric digestion of the cyst wall after which enterocyte invasion and initiation of the enteroepithelial cycles take place ultimately leading to oocyst formation. After a prepatency period of 3-10 days, shedding of oocysts in the feces continues for 1-2 weeks, with a total output of 0.3 – 100 millions of oocysts. Only bradyzoites may initiate the enteroepithelial cycles, a fact which has important implications for the duration of the prepatency periods after various types of transmission and for the development of intestinal immunity (resistance towards reshedding of oocysts).

Cats may acquire their infection directly from other cats by ingesting oocysts, although the importance of this transmission route is uncertain. A review and revision of the key parameters of infection of cats with *Toxoplasma* oocysts was recently given by Dubey [5]. A new inoculation study confirmed previous reports of a relatively high minimal infection dose for oocysts (size order of 100) to cats, compared with one or a few oocysts in the case of feeding oocysts to mice or pigs. The previously reported long prepatency period of 3 weeks or more was also confirmed. The new inoculation study, however, gave oocyst excretion in a significantly higher proportion (8/9) of infected cats (as assessed by seroconversion) than in most previous studies and also demonstrated that total oocyst outputs and patency periods are similar to those found after a primary infection of cats with tissue cysts. Suckling kittens appear less susceptible to infection with oocysts than weaned kittens.

Data on sporulation of oocysts and their resistance towards environmental conditions is given elsewhere in this volume (Chapter 4.3)

Clinical signs and pathology

A report of 100 fatal cases of toxoplasmosis in cats was given by Dubey and Carpenter [6].

Fever, dyspnea and abdominal discomfort were the most frequent signs of infection, but only 8 cases were conclusively diagnosed as toxoplasmosis antemortem. Generalized toxoplasmosis was the most frequent condition found postmortem followed by pulmonary, abdominal and neurological lesions. Ocular lesions were common.

Transplacental transmission of toxoplasmosis to cat litters is apparently of rare occurrence [6]. Congenital toxoplasmosis may or may not be associated with clinical manifestations. Important, however, is the fact that oocyst excretion may take place in these young kittens.

Immunity

Cats become immune to the clinical manifestations of toxoplasmosis after their first infection. Immunity towards the intestinal phase and oocyst excretion requires stimulation of local immune mechanisms with the enteroepithelial stages of *Toxoplasma*. The intestinal phase is initiated by bradyzoites, and infections with mutants or incomplete strains incapable of forming bradyzoites do not induce immunity towards reshedding of oocysts.

The duration of immunity after infection with tissue cysts was recently studied by Dubey [7], who challenged 9 cats with tissue cysts of a heterologous strain after 6 years. Two cats shed relatively few oocysts, while two cats shed oocysts in numbers (approx. 1 million) comparable to the challenge controls. All previously infected cats were seropositive at the time of challenge. Thus, immunity is not complete, even in healthy, seropositive cats.

Reactivation of intestinal infection with oocyst shedding may take place in severely immunocompromised cats (Dubey and Frenkel 1974) or during infection with the cat coccidian, *Isospora felis* (Chessum 1972).

Population aspects of transmission

The frequency of cats excreting oocysts at a given time (i.e. prevalence of oocysts in faecal samples) depends on geographical location, age group and nutritional habits. Faecal examinations by flotation techniques with proper microscopic identification or mouse inoculations are tedious and most surveys reported in the literature are based on sample sizes of some hundred specimens yielding none or small numbers of positive recordings (0-10) with resulting wide confidence limits for prevalence estimates. Surveys from Europe and North America generally yield prevalences in the size order of 1%. With the relatively short patency period of approx. 1 week, a straightforward calculation predicts that most cats will contract infection during their first 2 years of life. In a high-prevalence area (Costa Rica) [8], actually found high excretion frequencies in young cats (< 12 months) and low frequencies in adult cats.

Serological data is an alternative source for studies of the infection in cat populations. Seroprevalences reported range from zero to more than 80%, reflecting geographical area as well as age and hunting habits of the populations sampled. The sensitivity of the serological technique employed and the chosen cut-off value furthermore influence values reported. Seroprevalence increases with age and the proportion of seropositive cats may be modelled as an exponential function of a constant transmission pressure and cat age, assuming a persistent antibody response after infection [9]. According to the model, the incidence of newly acquired infections is highest in kittens and young cats and declines with age.

Examination of the avidity of specific anti-*Toxoplasma* antibodies also showed that the majority of seropositive cats aged less than 1 year had low-avidity antibodies, while most older cats had high-avidity antibodies [10], indicating that recent infection is more common among young cats.

Stray cats and farm cats, that hunt for food, have higher infection prevalences than cats kept as pets, particularly if these are mainly kept indoors and are fed processed food [11].

The diagnostic and prognostic value of serology on cats

Blood samples from cats for *Toxoplasma* serology are submitted to veterinary diagnostic laboratories for two main reasons: 1) verification of a diagnosis of toxoplasmosis in diseased cats or in the case of failed pregnancies, and 2) as an indicator of immunity in cats owned by a family with a pregnant woman.

False negative serology may occur in infected, but immunocompromised cats or during the early acute phase of infection. The latter problem may be resolved by taking a second blood sample after a few weeks. A positive serological test is of limited diagnostic value due to the long persistence of antibodies [12] and the high prevalence background. Specific IgG antibodies in young kittens (< 8 weeks) may be maternal antibodies transferred by colostrum [13, 14]. Various serological techniques exist for the determination of recent infection, such as the detection of specific IgM, the antibody avidity ELISA or the direct agglutination test employing acetone-fixed tachyzoites [12, 14]. IgA antibodies appear late in infection and tend to be associated with ocular disease [15].

Positive serology may be taken as an indication that the cat has passed the acute phase of infection and has developed immunity. However as noted above oocyst excretion may take place in some seropositive cats both because intestinal immunity tends to decline in the years after the initial infection [7] and because cats infected by ingesting oocysts have prepatency periods exceeding 3 weeks. The actual prognostic value of testing an individual cat by serology is thus limited, and pregnant women should adhere to the prescribed hygienic precautions irrespective of the serological status of the house cat.

Infection in sheep and goats

Toxoplasma gondii is a serious cause of abortion and neonatal mortality in sheep and goats, particularly in relatively temperate sheep-rearing areas such as may be found in the UK, France, Norway and New Zealand. Sporulated oocysts may contaminate pasture, feed, hay and water and when ingested by a susceptible pregnant sheep or goat they excyst in the small intestines, penetrate the intestinal wall and multiply in the mesenteric lymph nodes before initiating a parasitaemia. The cessation of the parasitaemia coincides with the onset of a protective immune response and infection then persists as bradyzoites within tissue cysts in muscle (Buxton 1998). Seroprevalence estimates of *Toxoplasma* infection in sheep in Northern Europe range from 20 to 70% depending on age group, geographic region and sampling year (Dubey and Beattie 1988). Sheep and lamb meat are therefore potentially important sources of infection for humans although meat that is frozen represents less of a risk.

In the pregnant ewe undergoing infection *Toxoplasma* may also establish in the gravid uterus with organisms initially parasitising the caruncular septa (the maternal tissues of the placentome) before invading the adjacent trophoblast cells of the fetal villi and from there the rest of the fetus (Buxton and Finlayson 1986). Typical clinical signs of *Toxoplasma* abortion usually result following infection in mid-gestation, with ewes producing stillborn and/or weakly lambs often accompanied by a small, mummified fetus. The outcome of infection early in gestation is often fetal death and resorption while infection in the latter part of gestation, when fetal immunity is relatively well developed, may have no clinical effect, the offspring being born normal but infected and immune. Abortion and neonatal mortality in goats is essentially similar to that seen in sheep (Munday and Mason 1979; Chhabra and Gautam 1984; Dubey 1981; Dubey et al 1981). During an acute infection in goats toxoplasms may be excreted in the milk and be a possible source of human infection if drunk unpasteurised (Dubey 1980; Skinner et al 1990).

Diagnosis of clinical disease in sheep and goats

The most obvious histopathological changes are the necrotic foci, visible macroscopically in the cotyledons. Microscopically they appear as large foci of coagulative necrosis, relatively free of inflammatory cells, which may become mineralised with time but only rarely are toxoplasms visible (Buxton and Finlayson 1986). In the fetal brain both primary and secondary lesions develop. Microglial foci, typically surrounding a necrotic and sometimes mineralised centre, often associated with a mild lymphoid meningitis, represent a fetal immune response following direct damage by local parasite multiplication. Again toxoplasms are only rarely found, usually at the periphery of the lesions. Focal leukomalacia, seen most commonly in the cerebral white matter cores, is also common and is probably due to fetal hypoxia in late gestation caused by advanced necrosis in the placentomes preventing sufficient oxygen transfer from mother to fetus (Buxton et al 1982).

Immunohistochemical techniques such as the ABC indirect immunoperoxidase method (Vector Laboratories, USA) and the peroxidase anti-peroxidase (PAP) technique (Uggla et al 1987) allow visualisation of both intact *T. gondii* and antigenic debris in tissue sections of aborted materials. Similarly the polymerase chain reaction (PCR) will detect viable and non viable toxoplasms in tissues. Amplification of the B1 gene rather than the P30 gene would seem to be more sensitive (Wastling et al 1993) and while the technique is not currently used in routine diagnosis its potential to identify specific DNA in paraffin sections cut from histopathological tissue blocks may broaden its applicability (Ellis 1997).

Serology is both an important epidemiological tool as well as a useful aid in the diagnosis of ovine and caprine *Toxoplasma* abortion (Uggla and Buxton 1990). The presence of specific antibodies in serum or tissue fluid from stillborn lambs or kids or in precolostral serum from live offspring indicates uterine infection. However, high *Toxoplasma* antibody titers in sera taken from ewes and nannys within a few weeks of abortion or production of stillborn lambs or kids can only suggest toxoplasmosis as titers remain relatively high for long periods after initial infection. Serology will also indicate the degree of exposure to infection in a group of animals.

Protective immunity to *T. gondii* is stimulated in both sheep and goats by natural infection (McColgan et al 1988). Currently a live *Toxoplasma* vaccine for the control of ovine toxoplasmosis is available in New Zealand (Toxovax, AgVax, New Zealand), the UK, Eire and France (Toxovax, Intervet, UK). The vaccine consists of live S48 tachyzoites which have lost their ability to develop bradyzoites in tissue cysts and unpublished data indicate that neither can the tachyzoites initiate the sexual life cycle of the parasite in cats (H. Bos, personal communication). While several instances of accidental injection of stockworkers have occurred the vaccine is supplied with clear instructions advising that medical attention is sought in such an instance. The authors are not aware of any cases of clinical illness occurring following such accidents. Goats also develop a protective immunity to the parasite so that they are protected against subsequent challenge during pregnancy (Obendorf et al 1990), although repeat abortions have been recorded (Dubey 1982). Toxovax is not licensed for use in goats.

Infection in pigs

Although severe clinical outbreaks of toxoplasmosis in swine herds have been reported, the course of infection under modern farming conditions is usually mild and inconspicuous. *Toxoplasma* infection in experimentally inoculated, pregnant sows has been demonstrated to give rise to transplacental transmission, resulting in mummified fetuses, stillbirths and congenital infections (Work et al 1970, Møller et al 1970, Dubey and Urban 1990) but the outcome of experimental inoculations can be variable. Mortality and serious pathology were seen in several cases with mouse-virulent isolates (Dubey et al 1991, 1997; Work et al 1970), but not consistently so (de Meuter et al 1978; Wingstrand et al, 1997). The dosage used, the route of inoculation and the life cycle stage of the inoculum as well as the age of pigs and the gestational stage of sows are all important parameters. The impact of swine toxoplasmosis on the farmers' economy is probably too small to act as a direct incentive for the introduction of control measures.

Serology applied to pigs is an alternative to direct demonstration of viable *T. gondii*, such as by mouse inoculation which requires the use of live animals and is a time consuming procedure (Work 1967, Dubey et al 1995c). Because infective tissue cysts as well as specific antibodies persist in pigs for several years after infection (as compared to the fattening period of less than 6 months) seroprevalence measurements correlate well with meat infectivity, provided the cut-off value is chosen so as to give optimal combined sensitivity and specificity (Dubey et al 1995c). Northern Europe and US prevalence estimates from the 1990s for *Toxoplasma* antibodies in slaughter pigs both show values at or below 5%. These values represent a distinct drop from corresponding estimates of 10-30% in previous decades (Dubey 1986b), a decline that is possibly associated with larger farm sizes and a shift in production management towards keeping slaughter pigs in confinement. However, high levels of *Toxoplasma* seroprevalence (> 20%) are found for the older age groups in some sow management systems, even where slaughter pig prevalences are low (Assadi-Rad et al 1995; Weigel et al 1995). Recent risk factor analyses performed on a large number of swine farms in Illinois, US, indicate that the presence of *Toxoplasma* infected cats (most notably the number of seropositive juvenile cats on the farm) is a strong parameter in determining seropositivity among sows and pigs (Weigel et al 1995) besides farm size and the access of swine to outdoor facilities (Assadi-Rad et al 1995; Davies et al,1998).

Toxoplasma gondii may be transmitted to man from meat-producing animals, such as swine and sheep, by way of unfrozen and lightly cooked meat (Work 1967, Dubey 1988, Smith 1991). Among meat-producing farm animals, cattle show an innate resistance to *T. gondii*. Acute disease or abortions are not seen, proliferation of parasites is terminated at an early stage and tissue cysts – although sometimes detectable by the most sensitive techniques, such as feeding raw tissue to cats – are very infrequently found by surveys of slaughter cattle (Dubey 1986 c; Dubey and Thulliez 1993). Thus meat from cattle is not considered significant in transmission of infection to humans. Tissue cysts have been found with variable frequency in the meat of chicken, after both natural and experimental infections. The public health consequences are probably very low, because broiler meat is usually well-heated before human consumption. No significant transmission from infected hen to egg is thought to occur.

The cat is the most significant factor in the transmission of toxoplasmosis to meat-producing animals – as a direct source of oocysts contaminating feed, bedding material and pastures and to some extent also by way of tissue cyst formation in farm rodents. Preventive measures may be directed towards preventing cats' access to feed and stables or preclusion of oocyst shedding by immunization.

A vaccine for cats based on the tissue cyst (bradyzoite) stage has recently been developed which is able to induce immunity against the intestinal coccidial cycle leading to oocyst production (Choromanski et al 1995). Its possible application on a broader scale will be facing the well-known problems in distributing live vaccines and the problems of motivating the swine producers without a direct economic incentive. Control and further reduction of the transmission pressure to humans from *Toxoplasma*-infected swine meat will probably rely on farmers' participation in integrated programmes that specifically address the production of human pathogen-free products so that the resulting added-value may make it cost-effective.

References

1. Dubey JP, Rollor EA, Smith K, Kwok OC, Thulliez P (1997) Low seroprevalence of *Toxoplasma gondii* in feral pigs from a remote island lacking cats. J Parasitol 83:839-841
2. Dubey JP (1986) Toxoplasmosis in cats. Feline Pract 16:12-26
   Dubey JP (1986) A review of toxoplasmosis in pigs. Vet Parasitol 19:181-223
   Dubey JP (1986) A review of toxoplasmosis in cattle. Vet Parasitol 22:177-202
3. Dubey, JP, Beattie CP (1988) Toxoplasmosis of animals and man, CRC Press, Boca Raton, FL
4. Frenkel JK (1990) Transmission of toxoplasmosis and the role of immunity in limiting transmission and illness. JAVMA 196:233-240
5. Dubey JP (1996) Infectivity and pathogenicity of *Toxoplasma gondii* oocysts for cats. J Parasitol 82:957-961
6. Dubey JP, Carpenter JL (1993) Histologically confirmed clinical toxoplasmosis in cats: 100 cases (1952-1990). JAVMA 203:1556-1566
7. Dubey JP (1995) Duration of immunity to shedding of *Toxoplasma gondii* oocysts by cats. J Parasitol 81:410-415
8. Ruiz A, Frenkel JK (1980) *Toxoplasma gondii* in Costa Rican cats. Am J Trop Med Hyg 29:1150-1160
9. Lind P, Skov I, Dietz HH, Olesen Larsen S (1997) A model for the transmission pressure of toxoplasmosis to Danish cats using age-related ELISA seropositivity. Bull Scand Soc Parasitol 7:44
10. Simon KGM (1995) Evaluierung diagnostischer Tests zur Untersuchung von Infektionen mit *Toxoplasma gondii* bei Katzen und Schafen. Thesis, Tierärztliche Hochschule Hannover
11. Tenter AM, Vietmeyer C, Johnson AM, Janitschke K, Rommel M, Lehmacher W (1994) ELISA based on recombinant antigens for sero-epidemiological studies on *Toxoplasma gondii* infections in cats. Parasitology 109:29-36
12. Dubey JP, Lappin MR, Thulliez P (1995b) Long-term antibody responses of cats fed *Toxoplasma gondii* tissue cysts. J Parasitol 81:887-893

13. Omata Y, Oikawa H, Kanda M, Mikazuki K, Dilorenzo C, Claveria FG, Takahashi M, Igarashi I, Saito A, Suzuki N (1994) Transfer of antibodies to kittens from mother cats chronically infected with *Toxoplasma gondii*. Vet Parasitol 52:211-218

14. Dubey JP, Lappin MR, Thulliez P (1995a) Diagnosis of induced toxoplasmosis in neonatal cats. JAVMA 207:179-185

15. Burney DP, Lappin MR, Cooper C, Spilker MM (1995) Detection of *Toxoplasma gondii*-specific IgA in the serum of cats. Am J Vet Res 56:769-773

Assadi-Rad AM, New JC, Patton S (1995) Risk factors associated with transmission of *Toxoplasma gondii* to sows kept in different management systems in Tennessee. Vet Parasitol 57:289-297

Buxton D (1998) Protozoan infections (*Toxoplasma gondii, Neospora caninum* and *Sarcocystis* spp.)in sheep and goats: recent advances. Vet Res 29:289-310

Buxton D, Finlayson J (1986) Experimental infection of pregnant sheep with *Toxoplasma gondii*: pathological and immunological observations on the placenta and foetus. J Comp Pathol 96: 319-333

Buxton D, Gilmour JS, Angus KW, Blewett DA, Miller JK (1982) Perinatal changes in *Toxoplasma* infected lambs. Res Vet Sci 32:170-176

Chessum BS (1972) Reactivation of *Toxoplasma* oocyst production in the cat by infection with *Isospora felis*. British Veterinary Journal 128:33-36

Chhabra MB, Gautam OP (1984) Caprine abortion and neonatal mortality associated with toxoplasmosis in India. In Les maladies de la chèvre, Niort (France) Les Colloques de l'INRA, No 28.719-726

Choromanski L, Freyre A, Popiel R, Brown K, Grieve R, Shibley G (1995) Safety anf efficacy of modified live feline *Toxoplasma gondii* vaccine. Dev Biol Stand 84:269-281

Davies PR, Morrow WEM, Deen J, Gamble HR, Patton S (1998) Seroprevalence of *Toxoplasma gondii* and *Trichinella spiralis* in finishing swine raised in different production systems in North Carolina, USA. Prev Vet Med 36:67-76

Dubey JP (1980) Persistence of encysted *Toxoplasma gondii* in caprine livers and public health significance of toxoplasmosis in goats. JAVMA 177:1203-1207

Dubey JP (1981) Epizootic toxoplasmosis associated with abortion in dairy goats in Montana. JAVMA 178:661-670

Dubey JP (1982) Repeat transplacental transfer of *Toxoplasma gondii* in goats. JAVMA 180:1220-1221

Dubey JP, Frenkel JK (1974) Immunity to feline toxoplasmosis: Modification by administration of corticosteroids. Vet Pathol 11:350-379

Dubey JP, Thulliez P (1993) Persistence of tissue cysts in edible tissues of cattle fed *Toxoplasma gondii* oocysts. Am J Vet Res 54:270-273

Dubey JP, Urban JF (1990) Diagnosis of transplacentally induced toxoplasmosis in pigs. Am J Vet Res 51:1295-1299

Dubey JP, Sundberg JP, Matiuck, SW (1981). Toxoplasmosis associated with abortion in goats and sheep in Connecticut. Am J Vet Res 42:1624-1626

Dubey JP, Urban JF, Davis SW (1991) Protective immunity to toxoplasmosis in pigs vaccinated with a nonpersistent strain of *Toxoplasma gondii*. Am J Vet Res 52: 1316-1319

Dubey JP, Baker DG, Davis SW, Urban JF, Shen SK (1994) Persistence of immunity to toxoplasmosis in pigs vaccinated with a nonpersistent strain of *Toxoplasma gondii*. Am J Vet Res 55:982-987

Dubey JP, Thulliez P, Weigel RM, Andrews CD, Lind P, Powell EC (1995c). Sensitivity and specificity of various serologic tests for detection of *Toxoplasma gondii* infection in naturally infected sows. Am J Vet Res 56:1030-1036

Ellis JT (1997) *Neospora caninum*: prospects for diagnosis and control using molecular methods. In Control of coccidiosis into the next millenium. Proceedings of the VII International Coccidiosis Conference and European Union COST 820 Workshop, 1-5 Sept., Oxford, pp 80-81

Janitschke K, Wormuth H-J (1970) Serologische, klinische und parasitologische Untersuchungen an spezifiziert-pathogenfreien Ferkeln vor und nach der Infektion mit *Toxoplasma gondii*. Zbl Bakt, I. Abt Orig 215:123-131

van Knapen F, Franchimont JH, van der Lugt G (1982) Prevalence of antibodies to *Toxoplasma* in farm animals in the Netherlands and its implication for meat inspection. Veterinary Quarterly 4:101-105

McColgan C, Buxton D, Blewett DA (1988) Titration of *Toxoplasma gondii* oocysts in non-pregnant sheep and the effects of subsequent challenge during pregnancy. Vet Rec 123:467-470

de Meuter F, Fameree L, Cotteleer C (1978) Influence de la virulence des souches toxoplasmiques pour la souris sur leur capacité de former des kystes chez le porc. Ann Soc Belge Méd Trop 58: 95-102

Møller T, Fennestad KL, Eriksen L, Work K, Siim JC (1970) Experimental toxoplasmosis in pregnant sows. II. Pathological findings. Acta Path Microbiol Scand Section B 78:241-255

Munday BL, Mason RW (1979) Toxoplasmosis as a cause of perinatal mortality in goats. Aust Vet J 55:485-487

Obendorf DL, Statham P, Munday BL (1990) Resistance to *Toxoplasma* abortion in female goats previously exposed to *Toxoplasma* infection. Aust Vet J 67:233-234.

Skinner LJ, Timperley AC, Wightman D, Chatterton JMW, Ho-Yen DO (1990) Simultaneous diagnosis of toxoplasmosis in goats and goat owner's family. Scand J Infect Dis 22:359-361

Smith JL (1991) Foodborne toxoplasmosis. J Food Safety 12:17-57

Uggla A, Buxton D (1990) Immune responses against *Toxoplasma* and *Sarcocystis* infections in ruminants: Diagnosis and prospects for vaccination. Rev sci tech Off int Epiz 9:441-462

Uggla A, Sjoland L, Dubey JP (1987) Immunohistochemical diagnosis of toxoplasmosis in fetuses and fetal membranes of sheep. Am J Vet Res 48:348-351

Wastling JM, Nicoll S, Buxton D (1993) Comparison of two gene amplification methods for the detection of *Toxoplasma gondii* in experimentally infected sheep. J Med Microbiol 38:360-365

Weigel RM, Dubey JP, Siegel AM, Kitron UD, Manelli A, Mitchell MA, Mateus-Pinilla NE, Thulliez P, Shen SK, Kwok OCH, Todd KS (1995) Risk factors for transmission of *Toxoplasma gondii* on swine farms in Illinois. J Parasitol 81:736-741

Wingstrand A, Lind P, Haugegaard J, Henriksen SA, Bille-Hansen V, Sørensen V (1997) Experimental infection of pigs with *Toxoplasma gondii*. II. Sensitivity of an indirect IgG-ELISA compared with clinical observations, pathology and bioassay in mice. Vet Parasitol 72:129-140.

Work K (1967) Isolation of *Toxoplasma gondii* from the flesh of sheep, swine and cattle. Acta Path Microbiol Scand 71:296-306

Work K, Eriksen L, Fennestad KL, Møller T, Siim, JC (1970). Experimental toxoplasmosis in pregnant sows. I. Clinical, parasitological and serological observations. Acta Path Microbiol Scand Section B 78:129-139

4.4. The scientific basis for prevention of *Toxoplasma gondii* infection: studies on tissue cyst survival, risk factors and hygiene measures

J.P. Dubey

Introduction

Ingestion of tissue cysts in uncooked, infected meat and oocysts in food or water contaminated with cat feces are the 2 major routes for transmission of *T. gondii* [1]. The survival of oocysts in the environment is covered by J.K. Frenkel in Chapter 1.2. This chapter covers formation, persistence, survival of tissue cysts in meat and the risk of acquiring *T. gondii* from ingesting infected meat.

Formation and persistence of tissue cysts

Tissue cysts are formed in many organs, including visceral, muscular and neural tissues, as early as 6-7 days after ingesting *T. gondii* oocysts or brady-zoites [2-4]. After ingestion of tissue cysts, bradyzoites survive digestive enzymes long enough to infect hosts [5]. Occasionally, also tachyzoites survive digestive enzymes [6]. Therefore, meat from both acutely and chronically infected animals would be a source of infection for humans. Tissue cysts probably survive for the life of the host. Among food animals, *T. gondii* is more prevalent in the tissues of sheep, goats, pigs, and feral chickens than in tissues of cattle, buffaloes, horses, and battery-raised chickens [1, 7-9]. Meat from wild animals is also a potential source of human infection [1]. For example, in the USA 80% of black bears are infected with *T. gondii* [10].

The risk of acquiring *T. gondii* may vary with the cultural habits of people and animal husbandry methods [1, 11, 12]. In the United States and probably in Europe, pigs are considered an important meat source of *T. gondii* infection for humans [13]. In pigs and lambs, *T. gondii* has been found in most edible parts [1, 14-17]. Therefore, any edible tissue from an infected animal should be considered a potential source of infection.

Survival of tissue cysts

The survival of tissue cysts in commercial cuts of meat and carcasses stored under different conditions has not been critically studied. Tissue cysts of *T. gondii* remained viable for at least 13 days in lamb carcasses chilled to 1 °C [16] and for 19 to 26 days in minced meat to 4 °C [18, 19]. Tissue cysts in mouse brains survived for 2 months at 4 °C [5, 20]. Thus, it is likely that tissue cysts survive in meat stored at 1 to 22 °C so long as the meat remains fit for human consumption.

Cooking meat in a conventional oven kills tissue cysts, provided the internal temperature reaches 66 °C (Fig. 1). Longer periods will be needed to inactivate *T. gondii* at lower temperatures [18]. A meat thermometer should be used to record the temperature while cooking and one should not depend on a color change. Microwave cooking cannot be relied upon to kill *T. gondii*.

Fortunately, *T. gondii* in meat is not resistant to freezing. Tissue cysts remained viable up to 22 days at -1 °C and -3.9 °C, and 11 days at -6.7 °C, but were rendered non-viable by freezing at -12 °C (Fig. 2). Thus, in a household freezer, maintained at a temperature of -10 °C or lower, tissue cysts will likely be killed. However, freezing alone cannot be relied upon to kill *T. gondii* because tissue cysts will occasionally survive freezing.

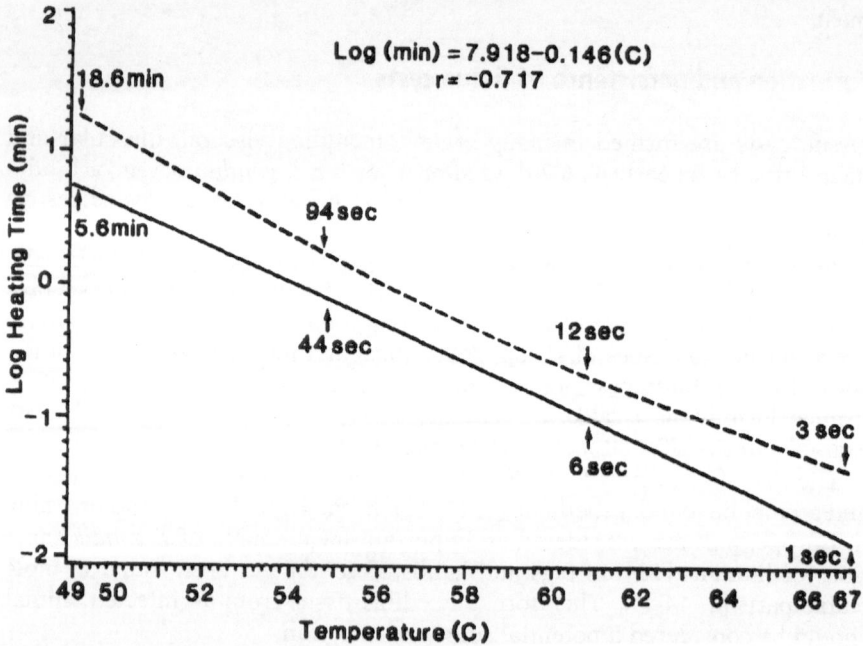

$$\text{Log (min)} = 7.918 - 0.146(C)$$
$$r = -0.717$$

Fig. 1. Linear regression (*solid line*) and the 99% upper confidence limits (*dotted line*) of the time required at each temperature for the inactivation of *Toxoplasma gondii*. Three and one-half minutes representing come-up and come-down times must be added to the times obtained from the equation on the curves. (From [18])

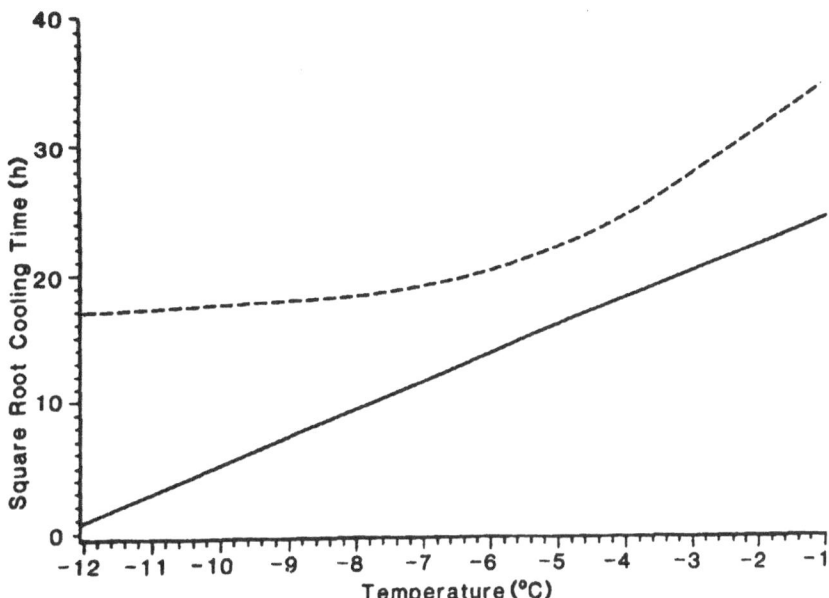

Fig. 2. The least squares linear regression of freezing times and temperatures for inactivation of *T. gondii* (*solid line*) expressed by the equation: Square root of time (h) = 26.72 + 16 (°C), with r = 0.77 and the 99% upper confidence interval for individual values (*broken line*). (From [19])

Tissue cysts are probably killed by commercial procedures of salting and curing [20, 22, 23]. Under laboratory conditions, the survival of tissue cysts in different concentrations of salt solutions (0.85% to 6.0% NaCl) varied with temperature of storage [20]. At 4 °C, tissue cysts survived for at least 56 days in 0.85% NaCl, for 49 days in 2.0% NaCl, and for 21 days in 3.3% NaCl solutions. At 10 °C, tissue cysts survived for at least 21 days in 0.85%, 2.0% and 3.3% NaCl solutions. At 15 °C, tissue cysts survived for at least 21 days in 0.85% NaCl, 14 days in 2% and 3.3% NaCl solutions. At 20 °C, tissue cysts survived for 14 days in 0.85% NaCl, 7 days in 2.0% NaCl and 3 days in 3.3% NaCl solutions. Tissue cysts can survive home-made procedures of salting [21, 24]. Tissue cysts were killed in 6.0% NaCl at all temperatures. Unless the salting procedures have been defined and tested for *T. gondii* infectivity, one should assume that salting is not enough to kill all tissue cysts.

Toxoplasma gondii tissue cysts are rendered non viable by gamma irradiation [12, 15, 25-28]. Most tissue cysts are killed by low dose irradiation (0.50 kGy cesium[137]) [25]. Although there may be some variability in the minimum dose needed to kill all tissue cysts in meat, depending on the irradiation source and temperature of irradiated meat [15, 25, 26], the 1.0 kGy already approved by the US Food and Drug Administration will kill tissue cysts in meat; at this dosages of irradiation, the quality of the meat is not affected.

Hygienic measures

To prevent human infection, hands should be washed thoroughly with soap and water after handling meat. All cutting boards, sink tops, knives, and other materials that come in contact with uncooked meat should be washed with soap and water because the stages of *T. gondii* that occur in meat are killed by water [5]. The meat of any animal should be cooked to 66°C before human or animal consumption, and tasting meat while cooking it or while seasoning home-made sausages should be avoided. Pregnant women definitely should avoid contact with cat feces or litter, soil, and raw meat.

Pet cats should be fed only dry, canned, or cooked food. Cat litter should be emptied every day, preferably not by a pregnant woman. Gloves should be worn while gardening. Vegetables should be washed thoroughly before eating because of the risk of contamination with cat feces. Because most cats become infected by eating infected tissues, cats should never be fed uncooked meat, viscera, or bones, and efforts should be made to keep cats indoors to prevent hunting. Trash cans should be covered to prevent scavenging. Cats should be spayed to control the feline population on farms and dead animals should be removed promptly to prevent scavenging by cats. Freezing meat overnight in a domestic freezer (-8 to -12 °C) can kill most *T. gondii* tissue cysts [29].

References

1. Dubey JP, Beattie CP (1988) Toxoplasmosis of animals and man. CRC Press, Boca Raton, Florida, pp 1-220
2. Dubey JP (1997) Bradyzoite-induced murine toxoplasmosis: stage conversion, pathogenesis, and tissue cyst formation in mice fed bradyzoites of different strains of *Toxoplasma gondii*. J Euk Microbiol 44:592-602
3. Dubey JP, Lindsay DS, Speer CA (1998) Structure of *Toxoplasma gondii* tachyzoites, bradyzoites and sporozoites, and biology and development of tissue cysts. Clin Microbiol Rev 11:267-299
4. Dubey JP, Speer CA, Shen SK, Kwok OCH, Blixt JA (1997) Oocyst-induced murine toxoplasmosis: life cycle, pathogenicity, and stage conversion in mice fed *Toxoplasma gondii* oocysts. J Parasitol 83:870-882
5. Jacobs L, Remington JS, Melton ML (1960) The resistance of the encysted form of *Toxoplasma gondii*. J Parasitol 46:11-21
6. Dubey JP (1998) Re-examination of resistance of *Toxoplasma gondii* tachyzoites and bradyzoites to pepsin and trypsin digestion. Parasitology 116:43-50
7. Dubey JP, Thulliez P, Powell EC (1995) *Toxoplasma gondii* in Iowa sows: comparison of antibody titers to isolation of *T. gondii* by bioassays in mice and cats. J Parasitol 81:48-53
8. Jacobs L, Moyle GG, Ris RR (1963) The prevalence of toxoplasmosis in New Zealand sheep and cattle. Am J Vet Res 24:673-675
9. Jacobs L. Remington JS, Melton ML (1960) A survey of meat samples from swine, cattle, and sheep for the presence of encysted *Toxoplasma*. J Parasitol 46:23-28
10. Dubey JP, Humphreys JG, Thulliez P (1995) Prevalence of viable *Toxoplasma gondii* tissue cysts and antibodies to *T. gondii* by various serologic tests in black bears (*Ursus americanus*) from Pennsylvania. J Parasitol 81:109-112
11. Buffolano W, Gilbert RE, Holland FJ, Fratta D, Palumbo F, Ades AE (1996) Risk factors for recent *Toxoplasma* infection in pregnant women in Naples. Epidemiol Infect 116:347-351
12. Weigel RM, Dubey JP, Dyer D, Siegel AM (1999) Risk factors for infection with *Toxoplasma gondii* for residents and workers on swine farms in Illinois, USA. Am J Trop Med Hyg (in press)
13. Dubey JP (1994) Toxoplasmosis. J Am Vet Med Assoc 205:1593-1598
14. Dubey JP (1988) Long term persistence of *Toxoplasma gondii* in tissues of pigs inoculated with *T. gondii* oocysts and effect of freezing on viability of tissue cysts in pork. Am J Vet Res 49:910-913
15. Dubey JP, Brake RJ, Murrell KD, Fayer R (1986) Effects of irradiation on the viability of *Toxoplasma gondii* cysts in tissues of mice and pigs. Am J Vet Res 47:518-522

16. Dubey JP, Kirkbride CA (1989) Economic and public health considerations of congenital toxoplasmosis in lambs. J Am Vet Med Assoc 195:1715-1716
17. Dubey JP, Murrell KD, Fayer R, Schad GA (1986) Distribution of *Toxoplasma gondii* tissue cysts in commercial cuts of pork. J Am Vet Med Assoc 188:1035-1037
18. Dubey JP, Kotula AW, Sharar A, Andrews CD, Lindsay DS (1990) Effect of high temperature on infectivity of *Toxoplasma gondii* tissue cysts in pork. J Parasitol 76:201-204
19. Kotula AW, Dubey JP, Sharar AK, Andrew CD, Shen SK, Lindsay DS (1991) Effect of freezing on infectivity of *Toxoplasma gondii* tissue cysts in pork. J Food Protection 54:687-690
20. Dubey JP (1997) Survival of *Toxoplasma gondii* tissue cysts in 0.85-6% NaCl solutions at 4-20 C. J Parasitol 83:946-949
21. Jamra LMF, Martins MC, Vieira MPL (1991) Açao do sal de cozinha sobre o *Toxoplasma gondii*. Rev Inst Med Trop Sao Paulo 33:359-363
22. Lundén A, Uggla A (1992) Infectivity of *Toxoplasma gondii* in mutton following curing, smoking, freezing or microwave cooking. Int J Food Microbiol 12:357-363
23. Work K (1968) Resistance of *Toxoplasma gondii* encysted in pork. Acta Pathol Microbiol Scand 73:85-92
24. Navarro IT, Vidotto O, Giraldi N, Mitsuka R (1992) Resistência do *Toxoplasma gondii* ao cloreto de sódio e aos condimentos em linguiça de suínos. Bol Of Sanit Panam 112:138-143
25. Dubey JP, Thayer DW (1994) Killing of different strains of *Toxoplasma gondii* tissue cysts by irradiation under defined conditions. J Parasitol 80:764-767
26. Song C-C, Yuan XZ, Shen LY, Gan XX, Ding JZ (1993) The effect of cobalt-60 irradiation on the infectivity of *Toxoplasma gondii*. Int J Parasitol 23:89-93
27. Wikerhauser T, Kuticic V, Marinculic A, Orsanic L (1988) Effect of gamma-irradiation on the infectivity of *Toxoplasma gondii* cysts in mouse brains. Veterinarski Arhiv 58:257-260
28. Wikerhauser T, Kuticic, V, Razem D, Besvir J (1992) A comparative study of the effect of gamma-irradiation on the infectivity of two isolates of *Toxoplasma gondii* cysts in porcine edible tissues. Veterinarski Arhiv 62:77-80
29. Dubey JP (1974) Effect of freezing on the infectivity of *Toxoplasma* cysts to cats. J Am Vet Med Assoc 165:534-536

4.5. Prevention of congenital toxoplasmosis in Austria: experience of 25 years

H. Aspöck

Introduction

During the fifties and sixties the Austrian paediatrician Otto Thalhammer carried out extensive studies on the prevalence and significance of *Toxoplasma* infections among pregnant women in Austria [1-15]. He confirmed earlier results that prenatal *Toxoplasma* infections need not necessarily be accompanied by clinical symptoms of the newborn, but that overt toxoplasmosis, mainly in the form of mental retardation (or, as it was shown later, of retinochoroiditis) may develop in childhood or even later. For this form of congenital toxoplasmosis Thalhammer [5] introduced the term "oligosymptomatic connatal toxoplasmosis". Moreover, he arrived at the conclusion that an infection of the unborn is usually only possible in the second half of the pregnancy after a primary infection of the woman and that an immediately initiated chemotherapy of the pregnant woman could prevent the parasite from infecting the unborn. Thalhammer was of the opinion that a prenatal infection during the first half of the pregnancy is a very rare event and, if it occurs, would always lead to an abortion. Finally he proposed to introduce regular serological tests of pregnant women in the 3rd and 8th month of pregnancy and to treat women in case of detection of a primary infection. His idea was to use a cheap skin test for the first examination, rule out the seropositive women and check only the seronegative women again. Today we know, of course, that Thalhammer's concept was correct in all main and basic aspects; he only underestimated the frequency of infections of the unborn in the first half of pregnancy which do not necessarily result in an abortion but may lead to the birth of infected children, and he may have underestimated the necessity of more than only two serological tests during pregnancy.

Thalhammer found that 6 to 8 out of 1.000 newborns suffer from congenital *Toxoplasma* infections and he therefore tried to convince the government authorities responsible for health affairs to establish a serological screening of pregnant women [8, 12, 16-21].

Establishment of the screening

In 1974, under the minister of health, Dr. Ingrid Leodolter, the so-called "Mutter-Kind-Pass" (mother-child-passport) was introduced in Austria (a number of medical examinations of the pregnant woman and, later, of the child, which were documented in a special "passport"), and it was soon considered to include also a serological screening of pregnant women for toxoplasmosis in order to detect primary infections and to treat them immediately, thus preventing an infection of the unborn. Finally, in July 1975, it was definitely decided to introduce a serological screening of pregnant women in Austria for prevention of toxoplasmosis following a certain procedure [22], and from autumn 1975 onwards almost 100% of all pregnant women were tested. Thus, Austria was the first country in the world with an overall toxoplasmosis screening of pregnant women. The basic concept was that of Thalhammer's first proposal [45]; it differed, however, in details of the procedure (see below).

The screening was called an "obligatory screening". In reality it was not obligatory as such, of course, but the women received – in four instalments, between the birth of the child and the end of the 4th year of age of the child – a total of 15.000,-- ATS (= at present about 1.200,-- US$) provided that all directed medical examinations included in the mother-child-passport had been carried out adequately and that the results had been recorded in the document. All tests and examinations were free of charge.

There is no doubt that a high percentage of all pregnant women would have had themselves tested for toxoplasmosis also, if only the tests had been free of charge, but with the reward of 15.000,-- ATS practically no woman in Austria renounced this relatively high sum. This is the simple explanation why the system worked through perfectly.

Procedure of the screening

When we introduced the screening in 1975, a procedure was established [22, 23] which we basically follow till now (Fig. 1).

The first serological test for specific antibodies to *Toxoplasma gondii* has to be carried out at the beginning of the pregnancy as soon as possible. In case of seronegativity the woman is tested again in the second and the third trimester. In case of seropositivity it has to be clarified whether this reflects an infection acquired before or during pregnancy. In case of a low antibody titer another sample is tested about three weeks later. If the titer remains more or less unchanged, this is regarded as a confirmation of an infection before pregnancy. If there is a significant rise, it is likely that the infection has been acquired recently, probably (or possibly) during pregnancy. In case that the first test already detects a high antibody titer, additional tests will be carried out with the same serum sample; moreover, a second serum sample will be taken from the woman immediately and checked in basic and supplementary tests. In case of suspicion of primary infection with *Toxoplasma gondii* acquired during pregnancy the woman is treated immediately. Primary infection during pregnancy is assumed in three situations:

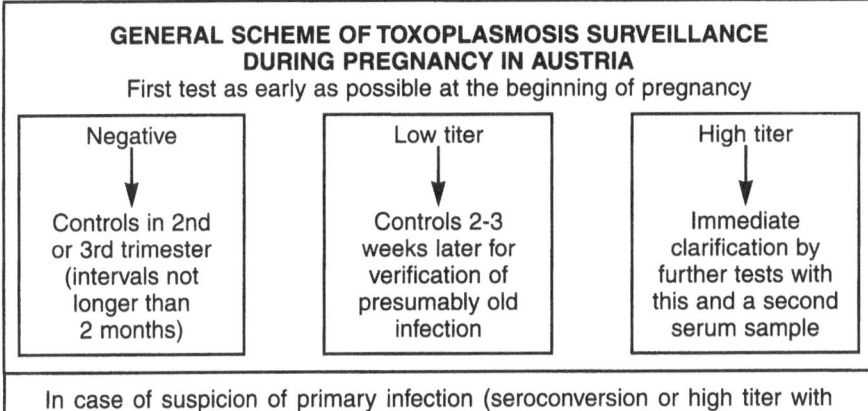

Fig. 1. Procedure of "obligatory" screening

1) seroconversion from seronegative to seropositive;
2) significant rise of titer in combination with detection of IgM antibodies;
3) high titer already in the first test, usually at the beginning of pregnancy, with detection of IgM antibodies.

It is of interest and should be mentioned that Thalhammer [24-26] was temporarily somewhat reluctant, when the screening basing upon his proposals given in 1957 and in many later publications was really introduced, particularly with respect to the necessity of a second test after three weeks in seropositive women with low titers. And even later, although apparently convinced of the benefit of the screening, and although he had found that the probability of the primary infection in a woman with a low titer may be 1:300, he questioned the necessity to test all seropositive women again [27, 28]. In his papers published in the eighties he recommended, however, the screening according to the official guidelines [29], but emphasized that the risk to overlook a relevant primary infection in a women with a low titer at the beginning of pregnancy is very low [30]. This can be understood as he was convinced that a primary infection at the beginning of the pregnancy would never result in the birth of a child with congenital toxoplasmosis.

At the introduction of the screening, it was regulated that alternatively the Indirect ImmunoFluorescence Test (IFAT) and the Sabin-Feldman Dye Test (SFT = DT) are acknowledged as basic tests and, in addition to these, any other test should be employed for clarification of a suspicion of a recent infection. In 1975 no other basic test was decidedly recommended, and among the supplementary tests, particularly a complement fixation test (CFT) and tests for detection of IgM antibodies (particularly the IgM-IFAT) were in use. Primarily IgM-tests were mainly used in newborns, while the CFT was employed in pregnant women [22, 31]; very soon, however, tests for detection of specific IgM were broadly applied in case of suspicion of primary infection of a pregnant woman [32]. IFAT (with conjugates against total Ig) and Dye-test were chosen because they detect IgM antibodies as well as IgG against membrane-bound antigens, thus warranting that also a very early stage of the infection can be revealed.

In the course of the following years the spectrum of tests has changed, of course (see below), but the basic tests are still IFAT and SFT (DT). Enzyme-linked immunosorbent assays were soon and repeatedly considered as basic tests [32-35], but were excluded as there were too many different products using different antigens which gave results not comparable to those obtained in IFAT and DT [23-36].

At the time of the introduction of the screening, re-examinations of women who were seronegative at the beginning of pregnancy were recommended to be performed in the 5th and 8th gestational month [22]. Soon it turned, out however, that this might lead to too long intervals, therefore we recommended not to exceed intervals of two months between each examination.

It was a great advantage for the effectiveness of the screening that only relatively few laboratories were involved into the testing which, moreover, sent all doubtful samples to one of the two national reference laboratories in Vienna (Dept. of Medical Parasitology, Institute of Hygiene, and Dept. of Neonatology, Clinics of Pediatry, both University of Vienna). Also this situation has remained more or less unchanged till today.

In some provinces (Upper Austria, Styria) almost 100% of all women were (and are) tested in one single laboratory each; for others a few other laboratories were (and are) involved besides one or two or three main laboratories.

Thus, the Austrian system of toxoplasmosis surveillance during pregnancy had some striking advantages from the beginning:

1) incorporation of practically 100% of all pregnant women of the whole country;

2) clear regulations on the procedure of the screening;

3) clear regulations on tests to be used, in particular with respect to the basic tests;

4) limited number of laboratories involved;

5) two co-operating reference laboratories acknowledged by all other laboratories in which any doubtful serological result is re-examined;

6) moreover, about 15 years ago a system of quality control has been established in which practically all laboratories involved in the toxoplasmosis screening take part. Twice per year they receive a number of coded serum samples to be tested for antibodies against Toxoplasma gondii.

There were, however, also some disadvantages which could not be removed:

1) The system did not (and does not) include any statutory measures for evaluation of the effectiveness of the screening.

2) In particular, there was and there is no duty of notification of a primary infection during pregnancy, of a prenatal infection or even of clinically symptomatic cases of toxoplasmosis.

3) There are no legal measures to warrant the long-term observation of children with congenital *Toxoplasma* infection.

The lack of a statutory system of evaluation of the effectiveness of the toxoplasmosis screening has not only been deplored by us, but also by others outside Austria [37].

Information on the course of detected primary infections during pregnancy always depended on voluntary activities and voluntarily given information of laboratories, gynaecologists, obstetricians, paediatricians, practitioners and mothers of infected children. Thousands of letters have been written to the concerning and concerned persons during these 25 years, the feed-back has, however, been moderate and often rather disappointing.

Repeated trials to encourage a prenatal screening on the basis of a cheap test (e.g. indirect hemagglutination) [38] failed entirely. We did not find any willingness or realistic basis, neither from the side of the health authorities nor of the physicians or of the non-pregnant young women, and we were soon convinced that this would not have any chance as the effectiveness depended highly on the premium in connection with the "Mutter-Kind-Pass".

Tests presently in use

The official basic tests for the screening are still IFAT and (alternatively) the Dye-test supplemented by any suitable test to reveal a primary infection as soon as possible. Some laboratories use enzyme-linked immunosorbent assays (ELISA) as basic tests, usually tests for detection of IgG in combination with tests for detection of IgM, sometimes also IgA. Unfortunately, sometimes ELISA extinction values are converted into IFAT (or DT) titers in order to express the result by means of an "official" test. Most of the present day ELISAs and ELFAs (Enzyme-Linked Fluorescent Assays) including competition tests offered by big companies are of high quality, and if two (or three) tests for detection of IgG and IgM (and IgA) are employed simultaneously, they certainly fulfil the requirements of a basic test. Also a modified ELISA using whole trophozoites has proved to yield results comparable to those in the standard basic tests [39]). Nevertheless, one should know that the Dye-test remains the golden standard and that – in case of any ambiguity of test results obtained with an ELISA – the serum sample must be tested in one of the standard basic tests and that, in particular, a possibility to perform a Dye-test must be available. This is the case in the two national laboratories. The complement fixation test has been in use as an important supplementary test throughout the first years of the screening up to the eighties but was left with the increasing quality of tests for detection of IgM. In the late eighties and throughout the first half of the nineties up to 1997 tests for detection of IgA (ELISA, ISAGA) gained growing interest and were frequently (usually in some laboratories) performed in all those cases in which – generally due to suspicion of primary infection – tests for IgM antibodies were done [40]. In retrospect we have to confess that the improvement of the assessment of the toxoplasmosis status by inclusion of tests for IgA was low and in a number of

cases the detection of (persisting) IgA antibodies may have led to false conclusions and to unnecessary treatment. It is important to emphasize that this sta-
tement pertains only pregnant women and not newborns, of course.
Detection of IgA in newborns, particularly in those cases where no IgM is
found, may have crucial importance to confirm a suspicion of a congenital
infection. One must be aware of the fact that in more than 30% (up to almost
50%) of infected newborns no specific *Toxoplasma* IgM antibodies are detectable, but in some of them IgA are, thus demonstrating a congenital infection.

One of the weak, or at least unsatisfactorily solved points of the screening
is the necessity to test women with low or moderate titers at first examination
again after 3 weeks. (This was also the main point critisized by Thalhammer,
see above.) There were many efforts to improve the situation and to find a
way to assess the toxoplasmosis status with one single serum sample [41, 42].
One way was the combination of the basic test (IFAT or DT) with a test for
detection of IgM at the first examination [43]. Due to the phenomenon of
long-persisting IgM antibodies and also possible false-negative tests (on the
other hand) this strategy proved to be unreliable. Another promising way
were tests for detection of circulating antigen [44-46], but the results were too
variable in various periods of the infection so that a general introduction as a
part of the screening was not justified. Also tests for specific IgA – although
useful in certain cases, and in particular in newborns – turned out not to ren-
der a second examination superfluous [47]. Moreover, application of PCR
with blood for detection of primary infections with *Toxoplasma gondii* in case
of suspicion due to serological tests was considered useful [48], but did not
really solve the problem either.

In recent years avidity tests have gained growing importance as supplementary tests in the toxoplasmosis screening of pregnant women in Austria.
Although a number of questions raised in an earlier study [49] must be thoroughly clarified, results obtained in another study using other reagents seem
to be very conclusive [41]. In particular, a high avidity apparently rules out a
recent infection (less than 3 months), while a low avidity gives an important
hint to a primary infection acquired within the past 3 months, but may also
be found occasionally in old infections. Thus, avidity tests may be suitable to
help to clarify the toxoplasmosis status of a pregnant woman with one serum
sample only, at least in a very high percentage. It appears that avidity tests
will gradually form a definite part of the serological procedures within the
Austrian system of prevention of congenital toxoplasmosis by screening pregnant women.

The present screening rests upon IFAT or Dye test or – inofficially – simultaneous IgG and IgM ELISA or competition tests (ELFA) as basic tests supplemented by IgM tests and avidity tests in case of suspicion.

Since 1990 polymerase chain reaction has gained growing importance
within the screening of pregnant women to prevent congenital toxoplasmosis
[50, 51]. Both national reference laboratories are regularly performing PCR
for *Toxoplasma gondii*. In case of serologically verified suspicion of a primary infection, the pregnant woman is advised to have an amniocentesis performed, if possible, shortly before the beginning of treatment with pyrime-

thamine in order to clarify whether the unborn has already been infected or not. A positive PCR results in a treatment with pyrimethamine plus sulfadiazine alternating with courses of spiramycin throughout the whole pregnancy. In case of a negative PCR it is supposed that the unborn has not yet been infected, which results in a different treatment for the remaining time of the pregnancy (Fig. 2).

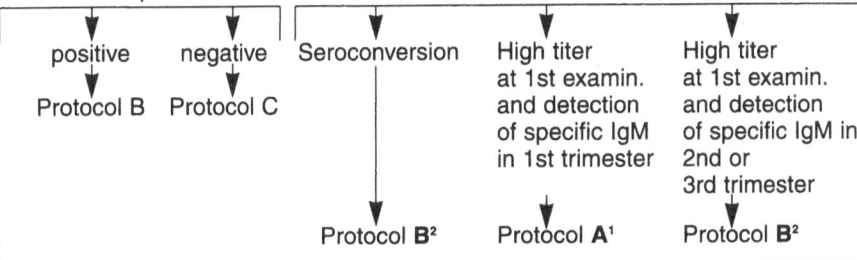

Procedure

Suspicion of primary infection ➤ immediate therapy according to protocol **A** and recommendation of amniocentesis for PCR with amniotic fluid before starting **A₂**

PCR performed		No PCR performed		
positive	negative	Seroconversion	High titer at 1st examin. and detection of specific IgM in 1st trimester	High titer at 1st examin. and detection of specific IgM in 2nd or 3rd trimester
Protocol B	Protocol C	Protocol **B²**	Protocol **A¹**	Protocol **B²**

1) Low risk for fetus supposed
2) High risk for fetus supposed

Regimens of chemotherapy of *Toxoplasma* infections in Austria

Protocol A:

A₁: From diagnosis until the last day of the 15th week of gestation: 4 weeks **Spiramycin (Rovamycin®)**: 3g/day (1-2-2-1)

A₂: Subsequently from the 1st day of 16th week of gestation (also for pregnant women who have not completed a 4 weeks therapy with **Spiramycin** till the end of 15th week of gestation) throughout 4 weeks

Pyrimethamine (Daraprim®)
1st day: twice 25mg;
afterwards: 25mg/day, **plus**

Sulfadiazine
1st day: 1.5g;
afterwards: 0.75g/day, **plus**

Folinic acid (Leucovorin®)
15mg (1tbl) every 3rd day

Protocol B: **A₂** alternating with Rovamycin (3g/day, for four weeks) **A₁**, throughout the whole pregnancy until delivery

Protocol C: Spiramycin (3g/day) only, for the whole pregnancy until delivery

Fig. 2. During therapy weekly blood count

Epidemiological data

In the period before the introduction of the toxoplasmosis screening several studies on the prevalence of *Toxoplasma* infections among the normal population and on the incidence of prenatal infections were carried out by Thalhammer [summarized in 8 and 15]. He found a prevalence of about 30% in the age group of 15-20 years, about 58% in the age group 21-30 years and about 60% in the age group 31-40 years. On the basis of his studies he arrived at the conclusion that in the region of Vienna about 7 per 1.000 newborns are infected with *Toxoplasma gondii*.

At the time of the introduction of the toxoplasmosis screening of pregnant women in 1975 and throughout the subsequent years the percentage of seropositive women in the child-bearing age was around 50% [28, 32, 53], in cohorts of younger women somewhat lower [54].

The percentage of primary infections during pregnancy varied from (at least) 0.2 [32, 36, 55] to 0.86% [28], but the incidence of congenital *Toxoplasma* infections and of congenital toxoplasmosis dropped significantly. After the introduction of the screening the disease was only very rarely diagnosed in newborns.

Thalhammer and Szöllösy [28] found among 4.310 pregnant women 37 suspected primary infections during the gestational period, which means 8.6‰. All these 37 women were treated and none gave birth to a child with a congenital *Toxoplasma* infection.

Flamm and Aspöck [35] found among 48.832 pregnant women tested between 1976 and 1980 52.61% seronegative and 47.32% seropositive persons. Suspicion of primary infection was found in 205 (= 0.42%), but could be confirmed only in 102 cases. This means a minimum incidence of 0.2%. (The real rate was certainly higher as many women were tested only once at the beginning of their pregnancies and had then changed the laboratory – a well-known problem today as well as 25 years ago.) At any rate none of the children from these pregnancies had a congenital toxoplasmosis. We must, however, emphasize that the follow-up of many of these pregnancies and, moreover, of the children has not been possible. A similar situation was found in 1982 among 70.000 women; 47% of them were seropositive already at the beginning of pregnancy, in 0.2% a primary infection was found, but again it was demonstrated that this figure was below the real rate of seroconversions [56]. In 1985 the overall seropositivity rate was still 48%, the frequency of suspicion of primary infections during pregnancy 0.5% (the incidence of verified infections somewhat lower) and the incidence of congenital *Toxoplasma* infections about 1 per 10.000 newborns [53].

In a study comprising about 167.000 pregnant women tested in Vienna in the period between 1981 to 1991 57% proved to be seronegative, in 0.68% a primary infection was suspected (in 0.32% already at the first test). The overall seropositivity was 43%; when split in several subsequent periods, it came out that the seropositivity rates had decreased constantly from almost 50% at the end of the seventies to 36.7% in the period 1989 to 1991. Interestingly, the percentage of pregnant women with suspected primary infection tested in

Vienna had constantly increased from less than 0.4% to 0.83% in the same period [57]. Among 2.413 pregnant women tested between VIII 1994 and VIII 1995 in Vienna, 37.7% proved to be seropositive and among them 1% with suspicion and 0.66% with verified primary infection [58].

A similar course, although at a different level was observed in Styria [59]. During the period 1978 to 1997 altogether 70.366 pregnant women were examined. In 1978/79 the seronegativity was 32.2%; in 1983/84 45.5%; in 1993/94 49.6%; in 1995/96 56.6%, and in 1997 58.2%. Primary infection rates with *Toxoplasma gondii* were 0.3% in 1978/79, 0.42% in 1983/84, 0.39% in 1993/94, 0.73% in 1995/96 and 0.7% in 1997.

Thus, the rates of incidence of suspected and/or verified primary *Toxoplasma* infections in various studies in different parts of Austria, carried out within the past 25 years, varied from > 0.2% to < 0.9%. Critically reflected, it is quite possible that higher rates in certain periods were due to the increased use of certain tests (e.g. IgA) which may have resulted sometimes in a unjustified suspicion of primary infection. Probably, at present, on an average about 0.5% of all pregnant women in Austria acquire a primary infection. The incidence of congenital toxoplasmosis (including oligosymptomatic cases) is > 1 < 2 per 10.000 births.

The significant decrease of seropositivity in all parts of Austria has most probably several reasons, possibly the most important one being the decrease of *Toxoplasma* infections among pigs during the past two decade, e.g. from 13.7% in 1982 to 0.9% in 1992 [60]. The decrease of *Toxoplasma* infections in the human population would be possibly even higher, if the consumption of mutton had not increased in recent years. In a study on Austrian sheep and goats infection rates of 66.4% (n = 4079) and 68.7% (n = 687), respectively were found [60].

It is also likely that the increased use of tinned cat food may play a role. Certainly also factors of generally improved hygiene may be of some influence. It is, however, interesting that the percentage of primary infections has increased which can partly and easily be explained by the higher number of seronegative and therefore susceptible women.

We suspect that the importance of infections by oocysts has been generally underestimated in the past and that – at least presently – the largest part of infections is due to ingested oocysts. Seroepidemiological studies on *Toxoplasma* infections among cats in Austria have shown that the seroprevalence is 48.2% (n = 456); out of 1.386 cats tested for oocysts, 2% were positive [60].

Therapeutical concepts within the Austrian system of prevention of congenital toxoplasmosis

The basic concept throughout the 25 years since the introduction of the toxoplasmosis screening in Austria has always been to initiate a chemotherapy as soon as possible after the diagnosis of a primary infection during pregnancy.

During the first years spiramycin was usually administered during the first trimester, afterwards pyrimethamine plus sulfadiazine was given. Very soon, however, for reasons of safety due to a possible teratogenity of pyrimethamine, this drug was given (together with sulfadiazine) only after the 20th week of gestation, and spiramycin was given up to the 20th week [36]. In the seventies and early eighties usually only one 3-4 weeks course of pyrimethamine plus sulfadiazine was given [21]. Later – after various WHO-conferences on toxoplasmosis – spiramycin was given only during the first 15 weeks of gestation, but pyrimethamine was administered from the 1st day of the 16th week onwards, and later on – in case of strongly suspected or verified infection of the unborn – it became usual to treat with pyrimethamine plus sulfadiazine in several courses alternating with spiramycin.

After all, a consensus paper of Austrian gynaecologists, paediatricians, parasitologists and serologists was published [52], in which the procedure of chemotherapy in various situations of an infection with *Toxoplasma gondii* was explained (Fig. 2). The regimen depends on the PCR result with amniotic fluid. Detection of *Toxoplasma* DNA in the amniotic fluid requires the administration of pyrimethamine plus sulfadiazine alternating with spiramycin throughout the whole pregnancy.

This regimen has proved very successful. We have never observed any irreversible side-effects.

Children with a confirmed congenital *Toxoplasma* infection, revealed in prenatal diagnosis by a positive PCR with amniotic fluid or by detection of IgM or IgA in the newborn, regardless whether there are clinical symptoms or not, will receive a chemotherapy throughout one year [50-52] (Fig. 3). In case of negative IgM or IgA and absence of any clinical symptoms, but serologically diagnosed primary infection of the mother during pregnancy, the child is serologically checked at birth and usually after 1, 3, 6, (9) and 12 months in order to follow the course of antibody titer. If the child is seronegative after one year, a congenital *Toxoplasma* infection is ruled out. In case of suspicion of congenital infection, chemotherapy is initiated immediately.

Benefit of the toxoplasmosis screening in Austria

In the fifties and sixties, Thalhammer [8, 61] found that 17% of all congenital cerebral damages in children in Vienna, not explainable otherwise, are due to congenital *Toxoplasma* infections, which means an incidence of about 6 per 1.000 newborns, and he estimated that the incidence of congenital *Toxoplasma* infections in Vienna and other European regions may even reach 1% of all born children. This is certainly a surprisingly high figure, and today it is difficult to clarify whether congenital *Toxoplasma* infections were really so frequent throughout the whole period before the introduction of the screening. Seitz [37] has questioned whether the incidence of congenital *Toxoplasma* infections has really been so high 40 years ago. Also in later publications, soon after the introduction of the screening, Thalhammer presented, however, similar figures, e.g. 0.86% primary infections during pregnancy [28]. Hayde et al [51] estimate the incidence of symptomatic congenital toxoplasmosis with hydrocephalus, intracranial calcifications and chorioretinitis in Austria for the period before the introduction of the toxoplasmosis screening as 1.5-2.5 per 1.000 living newborns. At any rate, the infection rates were high as can be derived from the conversion rates even to be found today (see above). It is a matter of fact, on the other side, that congenital *Toxoplasma* infections and, in particular, congenital toxoplasmosis have become very rare in Austria. Today the incidence of congenital toxoplasmosis (including late clinical manifestations) is 1 to 2 per 10.000 living newborns [51, 57, 58]. We have no doubt that this is mainly due to a rigorous and immediate chemotherapy in case of suspicion. It is a dangerous strategy to have additional tests performed, if valuable time for the beginning of the chemotherapy is lost. We are aware of the fact that during the past years sometimes women were treated in whom the suspicion of a primary infection could not be confirmed or had been unjustified [62]. Nevertheless, we believe that this strategy to treat as soon as possible is not only important with respect to prevention of transplacental infection but – after the 15th week of gestation when pyrimethamine plus sulfadiazine is given – also if the unborn has already been infected. Probably this is one of the main reasons for the success of the Austrian screening. In some pregnant women the treatment was stopped after further tests which revealed an "old" infection. It is again important to emphasize that we do not know any case, presenting any irreversible side-effect of the treatment. Since the introduction of PCR with amniotic fluid during pregnancy on one hand, and later on of avidity tests, the diagnostic basis for an optimal treatment has been considerably improved so that unnecessary chemotherapy, in particular with pyrimethamine plus sulfadiazine, can largely be avoided.

Gratzl et al [63] could convincingly demonstrate the validity and reliability of PCR with amniotic fluid for detecting a fetal *Toxoplasma* infection. Out of 49 specimens of amniotic fluid of women with suspected or proven primary infection, 38 gave a negative PCR. All women were treated, the children remained uninfected also after one year follow-up. Eleven samples gave a positive PCR. Fetal death occurred in one case, abortion was done in another case. The 9 children (2 with clinical symptoms) were treated throughout the first year of life and experienced normal development. In the cases with fetal death and abortion respectively and in those with clinical symptoms at birth the screening recommendations had not been followed properly.

In Austria about 85.000 children are born per year (1975: 93.757; 1980: 90.872; 1985: 87.440; 1990: 90.454; 1995: 88.669; 1997: 84.045). Based upon an (average) incidence of primary infections with *Toxoplasma gondii* during pregnancy of 0.4% - 0.6%, we may conclude that at least 200 (possibly up to 300) cases of congenital toxoplasmosis per year can be avoided in Austria due to early detection of this infection and thus early treatment [64].

Cases of congenital *Toxoplasma* infections and also of overt congenital toxoplasmosis do also occur in Austria, of course. In each single case, however, the regulations of the screening were not followed adequately. In the majority of these cases the intervals between the examinations were too long or the first examination was performed too late [51, 57, 59, 63, 65, 66]. According to the legal regulations, the screening comprises at least three exa-

minations, one in each of the three trimesters of the pregnancy. This is usually done in this way in seronegative women. In case of suspicion any test
which appears to be necessary may be performed, of course. However, we
have been emphasizing the importance not to exceed an interval of two
months between two examinations in seronegative women. Thus, in certain
cases (if the first test is performed very early in pregnancy) four (and, very
exceptionally, five) examinations may be performed.

In some cases of congenital toxoplasmosis the infection of the unborn was
due to delayed or even failed treatment, or to the use of inadequate drugs.

On the other hand it is a great satisfaction to be able to state that we do not
know of any case of congenital toxoplasmosis in a child born from a mother
who had undergone the examinations (and, in case of suspicion of primary
infection, the chemotherapy) in accordance with the regulations and recommendations within the framework of the toxoplasmosis screening system.

Moreover, it is another great satisfaction that we have never recommended
an induced abortion due to results of serological examinations. Sometimes it
is claimed that a toxoplasmosis screening may be associated with an increased number of induced abortions and – in case of unjustified suspicion – even
of abortions of healthy, uninfected fetuses. This is an absolutely wrong impu-
tation. Those who are familiar with the infection, with laboratory diagnosis
and with the interpretation of results will never (or, at most, in very exceptional, carefully proven cases) give such a recommendation. This is another reason why in case of suspicion of primary infection one of the reference laboratories should always be contacted.

The impact of education

From the very beginning of the toxoplasmosis screening in Austria the information of pregnant women, but also of physicians, in particular practitioners
and gynaecologists, was regarded as an important part of the overall strategy to
prevent congenital toxoplasmosis. Seronegative women are warned of eating
raw or undercooked meat, of having close contact with cats (in particular of
cleaning a cat's box) and of getting infected via contaminated hands (e.g. when
gardening). Moreover, all media (newspapers, popular journals, radio, televi-
sion) have been brought into action to inform the population on toxoplasmosis
and how to prevent the infection and the disease. In addition, we have organized various courses for biology teachers in gymnasia to transport the information on *Toxoplasma* and toxoplasmosis to the youth, particularly to young girls.

On the other hand, lectures on toxoplasmosis are a permanent topic of
postgraduate medical education. It is out of question that the present-day-
community of medical doctors is much better informed on toxoplasmosis
than the older generations. Nevertheless, often unnecessary, surprising lacu-
nae in the knowledge of physicians can be observed.

The main problem, however, is the severe ignorance of the problem in the
population. There are, of course, some women who have a good knowledge
of the problem and who know a lot about all important measures to prevent

Medication (per os):

1) **Pyrimethamine (Daraprim®):** 1mg/kg/day (1 dose at meal); blood count twice per week
2) **Sulfadiazine:** 85mg/kg/day in 4 doses
3) **Spiramycin:** 100mg/kg/day in 2 doses
4) **Corticosteroids (Prednisolon®):** 1,5mg/kg/day in 2 doses until ease off of retinochoroiditis and decrease of elevated proteins in liquor cerebrospinalis
5) **Folinic acid (Leucovorin®):** 5mg twice per week during chemotherapy with pyrimethamine

Indications

A: Congenital toxoplasmosis with clinical manifestation
   Duration of therapy 1 year (two periods)
   • Period A (6 months): medications 1+2+5
   • Period B (6 months): medications 1+2+5 (4 wks) alternating with 3 (4 wks)

B: Congenital toxoplasmosis with inflammation
   Scheme A, in addition medication 4

C: Subclinical congenital Toxoplasma infection
   Duration of therapy 1 year: medication 1+2+5 for 6 weeks, followed by medication 3 for 6 weeks, afterwards medications 1+2+5 (4 wks) alternating with medication 3 (6 wks)

Fig. 3. Recommendations for treatment of congenital *Toxoplasma* infections in Austria [52]

an infection, but the vast majority does not know anything on toxoplasmosis and certainly not enough to decrease infection rates. Two decades ago we were convinced that education may be another important tool to prevent congenital toxoplasmosis. Today we must accept that even many pregnant women are not willing to invest time into collecting information which may be important for them but which does not concern them at the moment – at least as regards toxoplasmosis. On the other hand, in case of a primary infection, however, when women are told that they have to be treated, they try to get any information on *Toxoplasma* and toxoplasmosis and sometimes become almost "toxoplasmatologists". It is therefore our deep conviction that education is of very little influence on the epidemiology of *Toxoplasma* infections in Austria. In particular, it can by no means replace a serological screening of pregnant women.

Due to economic measures of the government the reward of 15.000, -- ATS for every woman who had all medical examinations performed according to the "Mutter-Kind-Pass" was drastically reduced from January 1997 onwards. Only those women whose family (i.e. a woman and her husband or mate) has an annual income of less than 462.000,-- ATS (= ca. 38.000 US $) will receive 2.000 ATS (= ca. 170,-- US $) one year after the birth of the child. Women with a higher income do not receive any premium. All medical examinations have remained free of charge. Nevertheless, this has resulted in a significant decline of participation. At present reliable data are not yet available, but it is estimated that now only 90% of the women have the tests for toxoplasmosis performed. The ministry has received many telephone calls in which women have expressed sharpest protest against the cut of the reward and some of them have menaced that they would not participate in any examination. The arguments of the ministry that all tests are free of charge and that they are primarily in the interest of the pregnant woman and of the child were repelled.

Outlook

The introduction of the toxoplasmosis screening of pregnant women almost 25 years ago as a part of the "Mutter-Kind-Pass" in Austria was a far-sighted measure which has most probably prevented at least 4.000, possibly more than 7.000 children from congenital *Toxoplasma* infections and/or congenital toxoplasmosis. Due to the generous linking with a high premium, practically 100% of the Austrian pregnant women were screened until 1997. After the reduction of the reward the compliance of the women has decreased; it is, however, hoped that it will get consolidated at a high level. It would be also highly desirable to include statutory measures for a follow-up at least of confirmed cases of congenital *Toxoplasma* infections and for an evaluation of the effectiveness of the system. Due to considerable advances in the laboratory diagnosis of *Toxoplasma* infections, the reliability of a rapid assessment of the toxoplasmosis status of a woman and (by performing PCR with amniotic fluid) also of the unborn has been largely improved so that optimal chemotherapy can be initiated rapidly and unnecessary treatment can largely be ruled out. Toxoplasmosis screening of pregnant women will therefore be continued under improved cost-benefit conditions, thus preventing grievous misery in many families.

References

1. Thalhammer O (1951) Die Teste auf Toxoplasmose. Vorläufig eigene Ergebnisse. Österr Z f. Kinderheilk 6:53-66
2. Thalhammer O (1951) Zur Therapie der Toxoplasmose. Interruptio nach vorangegangener Geburt eines toxoplasmotischen Kindes. Österr Z f Kinderheilk 6:99-108
3. Thalhammer O (1951) Erfahrungen mit Toxoplasmose in Wien vom November 1949 bis November 1950. Klin Med 6:204-209
4. Thalhammer O (1951) Der Stand der Toxoplasmoseforschung in Wien. Wien Klin Wschr 63:565-569
5. Thalhammer O (1954) Oligosymptomatische Toxoplasmose. Helv Paediat Acta 9:50-58
6. Thalhammer O (1954) Zwei bemerkenswerte Fälle frischer Toxoplasmainfektion. Österr Z f Kinderheilk 10:316-321
7. Thalhammer O (1955) Über die Diskrepanz zwischen der Häufigkeit von mütterlichen Toxoplasmainfektionen und der Zahl angeborener Toxoplasmoseerkrankungen. Statistisches und kasuistisches zur oligosymptomatischen connatalen Toxoplasmose. Wien Klin Wschr 67:697-700
8. Thalhammer O (1957) Die Toxoplasmose bei Mensch und Tier. Maudrich Verlag Wien, p 307
9. Thalhammer O (1957) Place de la toxoplasmose oligosymptomatique dans la genese des encéphalopathies congénitales. Médecine et Hygiène 17:97-103
10. Thalhammer O (1960) Heutige Anschauungen über die angeborene Toxoplasmose und die Infektion der Graviden. Arch f Kinderheilk 162:105-114

11. Thalhammer O (1960): La Toxoplasmose congénitale. – Bol Soc Val Ped 2:231-233
12. Thalhammer O (1961) Pränatal verursachte Schädigungen, die vermieden werden könnten. Mittl.d österr Sanitätserw 62:332-337
13. Thalhammer O (1961) Die oligosymptomatische, angeborene Toxoplasmose. Untersuchung an 1332 angeborenen hirngeschädigten Kindern. Wien Klin Wschr 73:885-889
14. Thalhammer O (1966) Die angeborene Toxoplasmose. In: Kirchhoff H, Kräubig H (eds) Toxoplasmose. Georg Thieme Verlag, Stuttgart, pp 151-173
15. Thalhammer O (1967) Pränatale Erkrankungen des Menschen. Georg Thieme Verlag Stuttgart, p 442
16. Thalhammer O (1961) La prévention de la toxoplasmose congénitale. La méthode et l'indication régionale. Aktuelle Probleme der Paediatrie 8:95-104
17. Thalhammer O (1962) Probleme auf dem Gebiet der angeborenen Toxoplasmose. Göttinger Symposium 18-19 November 1960. In: Kirchhoff H, Kräubig H (eds) Toxoplasmose. Georg thieme Verlag, Suttgart, pp 59-74
18. Thalhammer O (1963) Toxoplasmose. In: Opitz H, Schmid F (eds) Handbuch der Kinderheilkunde. Springer-Verlag, Berlin, Göttingen, Heidelberg Vol 5, pp 957-979
19. Thalhammer O (1970) Congenital Toxoplasmosis in Vienna. Summing up findings and opinions. In: Colloque sur la toxoplasmose de la femme enceinte. "Monographie du – Lyon Medical", pp 109-118
20. Thalhammer O (1973) Prevention of Congenital Toxoplasmosis. Neuropädiatrie 4:233-237
21. Thalhammer O, Coradello H (1974) Toxoplasmose in der Schwangerschaft. Mittlg Österr San Verw 75:345-348
22. Flamm H, Aspöck H, Picher O, Werner H (1975) Die Toxoplasmose-Untersuchung von Schwangeren und Neugeborenen. Öst Ärzteztg 30 (1): 15-17
23. Aspöck H (1986) Prevention of Congenital Toxoplasmosis by Serological Surveillance during Pregnancy: Current Strategies and Future Perspectives. In: Marget L, Lang W, Gabler-Sandberger (eds) Proc. IXth Int Congr Infectious and Parasitic Diseases. MMV Medizin Verlag München, Munich, Vol. III, pp 69-72
24. Thalhammer O (1975) Toxoplasmose und Schwangerschaft. Verhütung angeb. Toxoplasma-Infektion. Der praktische Arzt 19:2800-2811
25. Thalhammer O (1975) Die Toxoplasmose als angeborene Krankheit und ihre Verhütung. Österr Ärztezeitung 3:381-383
26. Thalhammer O (1975) Die Toxoplasmose-Untersuchung von Schwangeren und Neugeborenen. Wien Klin Wschr 87:676-681
27. Thalhammer O (1980) Toxoplasmose in der Schwangerschaft. Mittlg Österr San Verw 81. Nr 7/8 1-4
28. Thalhammer O, Heller-Szöllösy E (1979) Erfahrungen mit routinemässigem Toxoplasmose-Screening bei Schwangeren zwecks Verhütung angeborener Toxoplasmose. Eine prospektive Untersuchung. Wien Klin Wschr 91:10-25
29. Thalhammer O (1984) Toxoplasmose-Screening bei Schwangeren. Speculum 2:13-16
30. Thalhammer O (1988) Toxoplasmose und Schwangerschaft. In: Spiess H (ed) Prophylaxe in der Schwangerschaft. Deutsches Grünes Kreuz EV, pp 189-198
31. Aspöck H (1976) Diagnostik pränataler Infektionen II: Toxoplasmose. Laboratoriumsblätter (Behring) 26:12-15
32. Aspöck H (1980) Die Diagnostik der Toxoplasma-Infektionen. Med Laboratorium 33:240-247
33. Aspöck H, Flamm H (1984) Die Toxoplasmose-Überwachung während der Schwangerschaft. ApibioMerieux-Monographien I:10-26
34. Auer H, Picher O, Aspöck H (1980) Der Peroxidase-Test (ELISA) zum Nachweis von Antikörpern gegen *Toxoplasma gondii*. Vortr XII Tg Österr Ges Tropenmed. Hoffmann-La Roche, Wien, pp 46-51
35. Flamm H, Aspöck H (1981) Die Toxoplasmose-Überwachung der Schwangerschaft in Österreich – Ergebnisse und Probleme. Pädiatr Grenzgeb 20:27-34
36. Aspöck H (1982) Toxoplasmose. Hoffmann-La Roche, Wien, p 43
37. Seitz HM (1997) Toxoplasmose-Screening: tu felix Austria? Wien Klin Wschr 109:621-622
38. Picher O, Aspöck H (1980) Die Bedeutung des Indirekten Hämagglutinationstests für die Diagnostik von *Toxoplasma*-Infektionen. Vortr XII Tg Österr Ges Tropenmed. Hoffmann-La Roche, Wien, pp 41-45
39. Obwaller A, Hassl A, Picher O, Aspöck H (1995) An enzyme-linked immunosorbent assay with whole trophozoites of *Toxoplasma gondii* from serum-free tissue culture for detection of specific antibodies. Parasitol Res 81:361-364
40. Aspöck H (1994) Protozoen als Erreger von Krankheiten des Menschen: Übersicht und aktuelle Probleme in Mitteleuropa. In: Die Urtiere. Eine verborgene Welt. Katalog OÖ. Landesmuseum N F, Linz 71:219-266
41. Auer H, Vander-Möse A, Walochnik J, Picher O, Aspöck H (1999) Ermittlung des Toxoplasmose-Status mittels einer Serumprobe? Mitt Österr Ges Tropenmed Parasitol 20 (in press)

42. Hassl A, Aspöck H (1996) Neue Verfahren in der Laboratoriumsdiagnostik der *Toxoplasma*-Infektionen. Mitt Österr Ges Tropenmed Parasitol 18:121-124
43. Aspöck H, Picher O, Flamm H, Auer H (1981) Aktuelle Probleme der Serodiagnostik im Rahmen der Toxoplasmose-Überwachung während der Schwangerschaft. Mitt Österr Ges Tropenmed 3:20-25
44. Hassl A, Auer H, Hermentin K, Picher O, Aspöck H (1987) Experimental studies on circulating antigen of *Toxoplasma gondii* in intermediate hosts: critera for detection and structural properties. Zbl Bakt Hyg A 263:625-634
45. Hassl A, Picher O, Aspöck H (1987) Untersuchungen über die Bedeutung des Nachweises von zirkulierendem Antigen für die Aufdeckung einer Erstinfektion mit *Toxoplasma gondii* während der Schwangerschaft. Mitt Österr Ges Tropenmed Parasitol 9:91-94
46. Hermentin K, Hassl A, Picher O,& Aspöck H (1989) Comparison of different serotests for specific *Toxoplasma* IgM-antibodies (ISAGA, SPIHA, IFAT) and detection of circulating antigen in two cases of laboratory acquired *Toxoplasma* infection. Zbl Bakt Hyg A 270:534-541
47. Obwaller A, Hassl A, Picher O, Aspöck H (1994) Vergleich und Bewertung des quantitativen Nachweises spezifischer IgM-und IgA-Antikörper gegen *Toxoplasma gondii* in Serumproben von Schwangeren. Mitt Österr Ges Tropenmed Parasitol 16:127-132
48. Hassl A, Tuma W, Bünger G, Weber, E. Niebecker A, Giesing M, Maass G, Aspöck H (1995) Möglichkeiten des Einsatzes der PCR zur Aufdeckung von frischen Infektionen mit *Toxoplasma gondii*. Mitt Österr Ges Tropenmed Parasitol 17:39-44
49. Hassl A, Aspöck H (1997) Der Aviditätstest zum Nachweis von *Toxoplasma*-Frischinfektionen. Mitt Österr Ges Tropenmed Parasitol 19:125-128
50. Hayde M, Pollak A, Aspöck H (1998) Toxoplasmose-Screening: tu felix Austria. – Eine Entgegnung. Wien Klin Wochenschr 110:63-65
51. Hayde M, Pollak A, Gratzl R, Hermon M, Trittenwein G, Häusler M, Arzt W, Bernaschek G (1996) Die Bedeutung der Nachsorge von Kindern mit pränataler *Toxoplasma*-Infektion. Mitt Österr Ges Tropenmed Parasitol 18:125-130
52. Aspöck H, Husslein P, Janisch H, Möse JR, Pollak A, Vander-Möse A, Winter R (1994) Toxoplasmose. Empfehlungen zur Behandlung der Toxoplasma-Erstinfektion in der Schwangerschaft und der konnatalen Toxoplasmose. Gynäkol Geburtshilfl Rundsch 34:50-51
53. Aspöck H, Flamm H, Picher O (1986) Die Toxoplasmose-Überwachung während der Schwangerschaft – 10 Jahre Erfahrungen in Österreich. Mitt Österr Ges Tropenmed Parasitol 8:105-113
54. Aspöck H, Korbei V, Picher O (1983) Versuche zum Nachweis von *Toxoplasma gondii* in menschlichen Embryonen von Müttern mit latenter Toxoplasma-Infektion. Mitt Österr Ges Tropenmed Parasitol 5:93-97
55. Aspöck H (1981) Toxoplasmose-Diagnostik. Behring-Sympos. Diagnostik und Therapie pränataler Infektionen. Aktuelles aus Diagnostik und Therapie, 1979 (1981):81-90
56. Aspöck H (1983) Überwachung von Toxoplasmose während der Schwangerschaft. Gynäk Rdsch 23:57-65
57. Aspöck H, Pollak A (1992) Prevention of prenatal toxoplasmosis by serological screening of pregnant women in Austria. Scand J Infect Dis 84:32-38
58. Aspöck H (1996) Österreichs Beitrag zur Toxoplasmose-Forschung und 20 Jahre Toxoplasmose-Überwachung der Schwangeren in Österreich. Mitt Österr Ges Tropenmed Parasitol 18:1-18
59. Moese JR, Vander-Moese A (1998) Mother-child pass in Austria and primary toxoplasmosis infections in pregnant women. Centr Eur J Publ Hlth 6 (4):261-264
60. Edelhofer R, Aspöck H (1996) Infektionsquellen und Infektionswege aus der Sicht des Toxoplasmose-Screenings der Schwangeren in Österreich. Mitt Österr Ges Tropenmed Parasitol 18:59-70
61. Thalhammer O (1963) Klinik, serologische Diagnostik und Therapie der Toxoplasmose. Wien Klin Wschr 17/18:375-381
62. Picher O, Auer H, Aspöck H (1996) Toxoplasmose-Screening in Österreich - Problemfälle der Serodiagnostik. Mitt Österr Ges Tropenmed Parasitol 18:115-120
63. Gratzl R, Hayde M, Kohlhauser Ch, Hermon M, Burda G, Strobl W, Pollak A (1999) Follow up of Infants with Congenital Toxoplasmosis Identified by Amniotic Fluid Polymerase Chain Reaction Eur J Clin Microbiol (in press)
64. Flamm H, Aspöck H (1990) 15 Jahre Toxoplasmose-Überwachung der Schwangeren: Jährlich 200 bis 300 Fälle verhindert. Österr Ärzteztg 45 (9): 8-11
65. Fast ChM, Rosegger H, Mayer HO, Aspöck H, Schuhmann G (1984) Ausgebrannte intrauterine Toxoplasmose trotz Screening. Pädiatrie und Pädologie 19:93-97
66. Kuchar A, Hayde M, Steinkogler FJ (1996) Konnatale Toxoplasmose Retinochoroiditis nach Primärinfektion der Mutter in der Schwangerschaft. Ophthalmologe 93:190-193

4.6. Prenatal screening and prevention of congenital toxoplasmosis in France

P. Thulliez, S. Romand

After the first case of congenital toxoplasmosis in France was diagnosed in 1947, surveys carried out in the fifties demonstrated both a high frequency of congenital *Toxoplasma gondii* infection and its occurrence as a consequence of a maternal infection acquired during pregnancy. The high seroprevalence rate, i.e. 80%, in women of childbearing age [1] proved suitable for the setting up of a programme for the prevention of congenital toxoplasmosis since only about 20% of women required repeated testing throughout pregnancy.

A systematic surveillance of seronegative pregnant women was first proposed in 1959 [2] and a serological screening on a voluntary basis was widespread in the sixties and the seventies. When the mode of transmission of *Toxoplasma gondii* was elucidated, health education of seronegative women was introduced [3]. Serological screening became compulsory in 1978.

Serological surveillance

An antibody test for *Toxoplasma* is required at the premarital medical visit which is compulsory for any woman under 50 years of age willing to get married (Decree n° 78-396, March 17, 1978). During pregnancy the serological screening is achieved together with other tests at the time of compulsory antenatal examinations (Table 1). The first one must be performed before the end of the third month of pregnancy and includes a test for toxoplasmosis if no positive previous results are available. Then, this test must be repeated every month throughout pregnancy in seronegative women (Decree n° 92-144, February 14, 1992).

Defects of the serological screening programme

Ideally, thanks to the premarital examination, every woman should know her serological status before pregnancy. In fact, it is often unknown why the number of women being pregnant for the first time without being married has been continuously increasing during the last decades. Consequently, the initial serological test is performed at the first antenatal visit, usually at the end of the second month but sometimes later in pregnancy, which may lead to interpretation difficulties for timing the infection when both specific IgG and IgM antibodies are detected. In spite of the use of complementary tests for IgG [4, 5] to rule out a recent infection, a doubt can remain in certain cases and be a source of unnecessary anxiety and unwarranted treatment, ultrasound monitoring and amniocentesis. Efforts should be made by physicians to obtain a blood test from all women who intend to be pregnant with or without a compulsory premarital examination. In a given pregnancy with no previous positive result available, the test should be performed as early as possible, the best being before the first prenatal visit.

Besides, it is not clearly specified in the programme whether the last test of the follow-up of seronegative women must be done at the time of delivery or within the following three weeks, otherwise there is a risk of misdiagnosing infection acquired in the very late pregnancy.

Table 1. Compulsory medical examinations before and during pregnancy

Medical examinations	Serological tests for infections	Other tests
Premarital visit	Toxoplasmosis*, rubella*	ABO, Rh, typing**. Irregular antibodies if necessary
First antenatal visit	Toxoplasmosis*, rubella*, syphilis	• ABO, Rh, Kell typing** • Irregular antibodies • Albumin, glucose in urine
Six subsequent antenatal visits	Toxoplasmosis* every month HBs antigen at 6 months	• ABO typing and irregular • antibodies if necessary • Albumin, glucose in urine RBC-WBC counts at 6 months

* if no previous positive results available; ** if no previous results available

Laboratory obligations

Almost 3800 private and public laboratories can perform serological tests. They are free to choose kits among some forty for IgG and some forty for IgM which are commercially available. All these reagents are registered by the Agence du Medicament after having been evaluated by experts. Twice a year the laboratories receive serum specimens for a quality control from the Agence du Medicament.

Every serum sample must be examined by two methods at least, one for specific IgG antibodies and another one for IgM.

The price is defined by law. The first serological test costs from 16 Euros for a single specimen to 22 Euros if a second sample, tested in parallel, is necessary for definite conclusion. No extra charge can be applied if more than two methods are used. The price of the monthly follow-up of a non immune patient is 11 Euros per serological test.

Every specimen sampled for the diagnosis of parasitic or viral infections must be kept frozen at least for one year in order to make a retrospective study possible.

The laboratory report must specify the methods used, the name of the reagents and of the manufacturing companies, and the cut-off values. Lastly, a conclusion must be given according to clinical data when available.

Health education

Physicians are responsible for educating seronegative women with preven-tive measures and all pregnant women are given a general guide to pregnancy containing advices to avoid sources of infection. Additionally, laboratories were instructed in 1983 to give seronegative women a letter describing hygienic measures together with the laboratory report; they are reported in Table 2.

Table 2. Measures for prevention of toxoplasmosis in pregnancy

– Do not eat any raw or undercooked meat. Cook it to well done
– Wash hands after handling raw meat
– Wash fruits and vegetables before consumption
– Wash cooking utensils and preparation surfaces that come into contact with raw meat, fruits and vegetables
– Wash hands before eating
– Avoid raw vegetables when not eating at home
– Wear gloves when gardening and wash hands afterwards
– Do not feed cats with raw meat. Wash hands after contact with them. Arrange for someone else to clean litter and to sanitize the pan with boiling water, or wear disposable gloves

The routine serological screening implemented for twenty years has given the opportunity to French centers to greatly improve the diagnostic tools and the management of infection in the mother, the fetus and the infant. However, primary prevention seems to have been neglected so far as shown by some studies which underlined a poor compliance to preventive measures likely due to a deficient information [6, 7]. It is obvious that a comprehensive health education of seronegative women has to be reinforced. It should be achieved by national or local health authorities involving physicians, midwives and family planning services by means of materials printed in an appropriate language and short teaching sessions.

Additionally, since consumption of meat is one of the chief modes of transmission it would be relevant to control the extent of infection in meat animals, particularly in sheep and cattle [8, 9].

Objectives of the screening and management during pregnancy

The objective of the first screening test at the premarital visit is to distinguish immune women, who will no longer be tested, from the seronegative ones who will have to take precautions during pregnancy to reduce the risk of infection. The identification before or early in pregnancy of non immune women allows to give health education only to them which may be more effective than if directed towards all pregnant women. The monthly repeated testing of seronegative women leads infection to be prospectively recognized and dealt with at any stage of pregnancy.

The short interval time between blood tests enables an early diagnosis of seroconversion and a prompt beginning of therapy. Among drugs which have proved effective *in vitro* and in animal models, spiramycin is the most widely used. It concentrates markedly in placenta and reduces both duration of placental infection and parasite burden. However, this drug does not significantly modify the pattern of infection in an already infected foetus, and most probably it does not enter the foetal brain, so it should be considered to prevent mother to child transmission rather than to treat congenital infection. Spiramycin, 3 g (i.e. 9 MIU) is given continuously throughout pregnancy unless fetal infection is demonstrated which leads to modify therapy.

Once maternal infection is diagnosed, clinical monitoring of the foetus is achieved by a monthly ultrasound examination in order to detect possible effects of the transmission of parasites. Since demonstration of ultrasound abnormalities can be delayed regarding the date of fetal infection and above all, since most infected fetuses are not severely damaged, a biological prenatal diagnosis should be attempted.

It has been proved that cordocentesis is no longer necessary thanks to the reliability of the PCR testing on amniotic fluid; thus, prenatal diagnosis with amniocentesis alone can be offered to women infected during pregnancy. Amniocentesis is usually performed from the 18th week onwards and at least four weeks after the suspected date of maternal infection, not to increase the risk of negative result due to the delay transmission of *Toxoplasma* from the placenta to the foetus [10].

When foetal infection is proved by the amniotic fluid testing, the treatment with spiramycin is replaced by the combination of pyrimethamine and sulfonamides for the rest of pregnancy, to reduce the severity of infection and the incidence of late sequelae [11]. Additionally, folinic acid (50 mg weekly) is administered to prevent bone marrow suppression and haematological monitoring is required. Besides, it is recommended to repeat ultrasound examination fortnightly considering the rapidity of evolution of cerebral ventricular dilatation [10]. Given the high risk of congenital infection when maternal occurs in late pregnancy, i.e. after the 34th week, some authors institute the regimen with pyrimethamine and sulfonamides right away without attempting a prenatal diagnosis [12].

There is a general agreement on using the ultrasonographic demonstration of ventricular dilatation as indication for the consideration of therapeutic abortion. The prognosis of intracranial densities without evidence of ventricular enlargment is not known so far but from the comparison of ultrasound and autopsy findings, it is obvious that both number and size of lesions are underestimated by ultrasonography. Finally, the documentation of an early maternal infection combined with an early demonstration of foetal infection without ultrasound abnormalities poses a difficult dilemma since despite prolonged treatment of the mother with pyrimethamine and sulfonamides, offsprings may be severely damaged [12].

Management at birth

The treatment with pyrimethamine and sulfonamide initiated during pregnancy for mothers whose foetus was identified as infected, should be continued in the infant from birth until one year of life [13]. Clinical evaluation includes complete general and neurological examinations as well as ophthalmological and ultrasonographic examinations.

The same evaluation should be performed in newborns for which the prenatal diagnosis was not attempted, and also when negative, since some cases of congenital infection are not prenatally identified because of a delayed transplacental transmission. Furthermore, isolation of *Toxoplasma* from the placenta or the blood and detection of a specific humoral response should be tried. In case of negative results at birth, a serological follow-up must be continued until *Toxoplasma* IgG antibodies turn to negative, which constitutes the definitive proof of the absence of congenital infection.

Missing data

Information from French paediatric departments concur to assess that both the incidence and the severity of congenital toxoplasmosis has been markedly reduced during the last twenty years probably as a consequence of the implementation of the comprehensive programme. As a matter of fact, no general statistics are available because the disease is not officially notifiable and there is no centralization of data from regional centres for epidemiological purposes.

On the basis of a national study on seroprevalence carried out in 1995 [14], the rough estimate of infected pregnant women per year would be 4900, which may result in 980 to 1470 infections among the offsprings, according to a vertical transmission rate from 20 to 30%. The assessment of a decrease in the number of *Toxoplasma* infections would necessarily require both maternal and congenital cases to be registered.

The costs of medical examinations as well as those of laboratory testing are taken over by the Social Security system. In 1992, the annual cost of all serological tests performed for toxoplasmosis was estimated at 41 million Euros. No evaluation of the total cost of the whole public health intervention for toxoplasmosis has been made since the screening programme has been introduced. It could be expected that it has increased for two reasons at least.

First, the number of seronegative women to be followed-up during pregnancy is higher since the seroprevalence which was up to 80% in the sixties in certain regions [1] has decreased to a national rate of 54.3% in 1995 [14]. Secondly, the management of infection during pregnancy has been reinforced by the use of prenatal diagnosis and ultrasound monitoring [11].

References

1. Desmonts G, Couvreur J, Ben Rachid MS (1965) Le toxoplasme, la mère et l'enfant. Arch Fr Pediatr 22:1183-1200
2. Lelong M (1959) Prophylaxie des toxoplasmoses du nouveau-né et de la femme enceinte. Rev Hyg Méd Soc 7:71
3. Roux C, Desmonts G, Muliez N, Gaulier M, Tufferaud G, Marmor D, Herbillon A (1976) Bilan de deux ans de prophylaxie de la toxoplasmose congénitale à la maternité de l'hôpital Saint-Antoine. J Gynecol Obstet Biol Reprod 5:249-264
4. Dannemann BR, Vaughan WC, Thulliez Ph, Remington JS (1990) Differential agglutination test for diagnosis of recently acquired infection with *Toxoplasma gondii*. J Clin Microbiol 28:1928-1933
5. Pelloux H, Brun E, Vernet G, Marcillat S, Jolivet M, Guergour D, Fricker-Hidalgo H, Goullier-Fleuret A, Ambroise-Thomas P (1998) Determination of *anti-toxoplasma gondii* immunoglobulin G avidity: adaptation to the Vidas system (bioMérieux). Diagn Microbiol Infect Dis 32:69-73
6. Goulet V, Le Magny F, Iborra M (1990). Enquête sur la connaissance des mesures préventives contre la toxoplasmose auprès de femmes venant d'accoucher. BEH 4:14-15
7. Wallon M, Mallaret MR, Mojon M, Peyron F (1994) Toxoplasmose congénitale, évaluation de la politique de prévention. Presse Med 23:1467-1470
8. Baril L, Ancelle T, Thulliez Ph, Goulet V, Tirard-Fleury V, Carme B (1999) Risk factors for *toxoplasma* infection in pregnant women: a case-control study in France. Scand J Infect Dis (in press)
9. Desmonts G, Couvreur J, Alison F, Baudelot J, Gerbeaux J, Lelong M (1965) Étude épidémiologique sur la toxoplasmose : de l'influence de la cuisson des viandes de boucherie sur la fréquence de l'infection humaine. Rev Fran Etudes Clin Biol 10:952-958
10. Hohlfeld P, Daffos F, Costa JM, Thulliez Ph, Forestier F, Vidaud M (1994) Prenatal diagnosis of congenital toxoplasmosis with a polymerase chain reaction test on amniotic fluid. N Engl J Med 331:695-699
11. Daffos F, Forestier F, Capella-Pavlovsky M, Thulliez Ph, Aufrant C, Valenti D, Cox WL (1988) Prenatal management of 746 pregnancies at risk for congenital toxoplasmosis. N Engl J Med 318:271-275
12. Pratlong F, Boulot P, Villena I, Issert I, Tamby I, Cazenave J, Dedet JP (1996) Antenatal diagnosis of congenital toxoplasmosis: evaluation of the biological parameters in a cohort of 286 patients. Br J Obst Gyn 103:552-557
13. Remington JS, McLeod R, Desmonts G (1995) Toxoplasmosis. In: Klein JO, Remington JS (eds) Infectious diseases of the fetus and newborn infant. WB Saunders, Philadelphia, pp 140-268
14. Ancelle T, Goulet V, Tirard-Fleury V, Baril L, du Mazaubrun C, Thulliez Ph, Wcislo M, Carme B (1996) La toxoplasmose chez la femme enceinte en France en 1995. Résultats d'une enquête nationale périnatale. BEH 51:227-229

4.7. What informations should be extracted from the national programs for the prevention of congenital toxoplasmosis in Austria and in France?

P. Ambroise-Thomas

Toxoplasmosis is one of the most frequent congenital diseases. In several European countries many practitioners, and particularly gynaecologists and paediatricians in their everyday practice, regularly prescribe patients systematic tests and prevention measures. Two European countries, Austria and France, have implemented nation-wide prevention programmes. These programmes were set more than 20 years ago. It is interesting to put them side by side and extract their successes, restraints, failures and uncertainties before specifying to what extent it may be possible to transpose them to other countries.

The first nation-wide prevention programme was decided in Austria in 1975. It was followed by the French programme in 1978. Originally, the decision was taken in Austria because of the high prevalence of congenital toxoplasmosis found in the fifties. There was also a strong prevalence of toxoplasmic seropositivity in young adult women: more than 58% in Austria, from 60 to 80% in France, depending on the regions.

The preventive or therapeutic methods and schemes

Serological screening

In both countries, the programmes are based on the systematic serological screening of all young women, before pregnancy as in France or at the beginning as in Austria. For pregnant women who are seronegative at the first examination, regular serological screening is performed every month in France and every two months in Austria in order to detect and treat toxoplasmosis as early as possible, if the mother becomes infected during pregnancy.

Many serological tests are used and they are slightly different in the two countries. This is mainly due to the local experience which can be derived from each method. Detailing the choice of these serological procedures has no practical value. But it is essential, in order to detect a seropositivity corresponding to a long-acquired immunity, to use a technique whose results remain positive for life – as it is the case with immunofluorescence (IFAT), dye-test or ELISA tests with certain antigens. Weakly positive serological results, i.e. at the threshold of specificity, give rise to difficult interpretation problems, even when the tests are performed simultaneously using two methods for the detection of IgG and IgM antibodies – as is compulsory in France. With such weakly positive results, another test is required two or three weeks later, using different complementary procedures. The most difficult problems however are, for recently acquired toxoplasmosis, to determine the time of maternal seroconversion in relation to the time of conception. Several procedures are concurrently used in order to evaluate the time of infection, such as avidity test for IgG and differential agglutination assay (France), or a second control test, three weeks after the first one, to determine the evolution of specific IgG antibodes titers (Austria).

In Austria, the serological tests are carried out in a relatively small number of laboratories and the results may be confirmed in two reference centres, while in France these tests are performed in more than 3,800 laboratories (university-hospitals, general hospitals, or private-practice laboratories). Thus, it is easy to meet the demand (several millions of serological tests each year) but it is also essential to control the results, as only a few laboratories are specialised in this field. This has been possible since a nation-wide quality control has been implemented by the French Agency for the safety of health products (Agence Française de Sécurité Sanitaire des Produits de Santé). This has also been ensured thanks to stringent regulations (such as requiring that serum samples be kept deep-frozen for one year) and the evaluation and registration with an official visa for the corresponding biological reagents. The last measure has recently been the subject of a European directive, but it has not yet been applied in all the European countries. This control is needed and its necessity is more and more urgent because of the commercial significance of the "market" represented by serological tests for toxoplasmosis, which leads to the proliferation of a variety of reagents, sometimes produced by non-specialised companies and whose quality is not always satisfactory.

Prevention measures. Therapeutic protocols, drugs and regimens

Prevention measures and treatment regimens, based on serological screening, are more or less the same in France and in Austria.

Seronegative pregnant women are given recommendations about food hygiene, which reduces the risk of toxoplasmic infection. This is a simple prevention measure which could be improved if the pregnant women were better informed and with a higher circulation of the text presenting these prophylactic recommendations.

In both countries the treatment of infected mothers, or rather the chemoprophylaxis of mother-to-child transmission, and the treatment of infected foetuses are conducted using the same drugs and similar protocols. The rule is that polytherapy, combining pyrimethamine and sulfadoxine or pyrimethamine and sulfadiazine, which are the most effective but also with adverse side-effects, should be reserved for proven cases of foetus infection and administered only after twelve or fifteen weeks of pregnancy, over a period of limited duration. During the first trimester of pregnancy or when maternal infection acquired during pregnancy is only suspected and not certainly proven, only spiramycin is prescribed in France at a dose of 3 grams daily until the delivery. Spiramycin is clearly less active than the other drugs given in combinations, but it is devoid of unwanted side-effects and has the advantage of concentrating in placenta.

Results, advantages, costs, limits and drawbacks

It is always very difficult to assess the results of prophylactic measures. This is particularly true for a congenital disease like toxoplasmosis. Transmission from mother to foetus is very inconstant and varies according to gestational age at the time of maternal infection, so that even in the absence of preventive measure, no *in utero* infection may be occured.

Furthermore, a large part of the national programs of prevention, in Austria and France, is based on the treatment of pregnant women. Some of these treatments are prescribed when maternal infection acquired during pregnancy is only strongly suspected and not proven. When infection is proven, treatments are initiated more or less immediately after maternal infection, depending on how early the diagnosis could be established. Infection itself may also occur at different periods of pregnancy. In such conditions, clinical observations cannot easily be compared to one another and it is very difficult to accurately assess the efficacy of the treatment.

In spite of such reserves, it may reasonably be concluded however that the therapeutic protocols that have been proposed lead to a decrease of both the frequency of transplacental infection and the severity of foetus lesions if transmission had occurred.

Regarding its action on the risk of *in utero* transmission, surveys conducted in France quite a long time ago revealed that the risk decreased from about 55% to less than 25% when spiramycin was prescribed. However, more recent studies in France and in other countries have not confirmed such a significant drop in the transmission rate, although these have confirmed the overall preventive action of the treatment. This should be expressed, in Austria as in France, by a decrease in the number of cases of congenital toxoplasmosis, starting when the national prevention programmes were implemented. This seems to be true although difficult to assert, congenital toxoplasmosis being most often poorly symptomatic or asymptomatic in neonates. Besides, leaving aside these prevention programmes, the prevalence of acquired toxoplasmosis among adults has fallen quite markedly, more particularly in Austria, during the last two or three decades. This is likely due to factors such as changes in food habits, mainly since people eat deep-frozen meat more often, general improvement of food hygiene, and to a greater proportion of cats fed with tinned food, thus keeping away from infection risks and, subsequently, from contagiousness.

The curative efficacy of the different therapeutic protocols are also very difficult to assess than their efficacy on mother-to-child transmission. It is noteworthy, however, that in Austria as well as in France, only on rare occasions are severe cases of congenital toxoplasmosis now observed, combining encephalitic and ocular lesions (hydrocephalus, intracerebral calcifications, retinochoroiditis etc.) with the corresponding functional disorders. In the past, these forms of the disease were more frequent. Their decline is probably due, at least in part, to the fact that treatments of infected foetuses are initiated as early as possible.

In compensation for their advantages, the two national prevention programmes have various drawbacks and may be improved in various ways.

The first drawback is the cost which, only for the serologic tests, has been estimated at 41 million Euros in France every year. The total expenses (including medical examinations, ultrasonographies, treatments etc.) are certainly three times as high, around 90 million Euros. Such expenses may seem excessive; they should be compared, however, to the psychological, social and emotional cost of the handicaps caused by congenital toxoplasmosis. A purely financial approach to this question should also take into account the considerable amounts of money involved in the hospitalisation, treatment and nursing of severely handicapped children. Besides, these expenses related to congenital toxoplasmosis should be put back in the more general context of the measures taken for the prevention of other various congenital diseases, such as blood-group incompatibility, rubella, etc.). It will surely be possible to reduce some of the expenses due to congenital toxoplasmosis mainly by avoiding repeated useless serological tests, for instance in young women who are seropositive before pregnancy. This is now possible thanks to a correct computerised follow-up of patients.

Finally, the results of the prevention programmes should take into account not only the consequences immediately detectable at birth but also (and perhaps mainly) the long-term effects and the risk of late reactivations causing mainly retinochoroiditis. In France, about 25% of cases of retinochoroiditis in young adults are considered to have a toxoplasmic origin. Some of them may result from acquired toxoplasmosis, although most of the cases seem to be secondary to an undetected congenital infection. If their number may be decreased thanks to the prevention programmes, although this evaluation is still impossible with the current system, this would correspond to great savings, which would partly compensate for the cost of such programmes.

The necessary improvements obviously concern the screening procedures, more particularly the timing of infection in relation to the beginning of pregnancy. Other major improvements should focus on our drugs and regimens. The drugs which are used are not all available in all countries (for example, spiramycin). These have been prescribed for many years and could be probably replaced by more recent and more active drugs. But a major improvement to prevention schemes should concern the duration of treatment of asymptomatic infected newborns to prevent late onset of toxoplasmosis. Above all, no programme exists to follow these babies over several years, which would allow the detection and, maybe, the prevention of late reactivations, and would have an effect on the frequency of toxoplasmic retinochoroiditis.

Conclusion

When considering the details they currently contain, the national programmes for the prevention of toxoplasmosis are clearly not perfect, not more in France than in Austria. These programmes are costly, and can be improved in several ways. They have however proved to be effective, even though it is difficult, for many reasons, to demonstrate their efficacy from a statistically indisputable standpoint.

Can such preventive measures be directly applied to other countries, mainly in Europe? Very probably not, but they can be most likely transposed and adapted. Indeed, it is clearly impossible to formulate a univocal answer to all the difficult problems of the prevention of toxoplamosis. Both the prevalence and epidemiology of toxoplasmosis vary from one country to another. It is therefore logical that the prophylactic measures should also vary to be adapted to the local conditions. The main part of the debate deals with the type of prevention that should be carried out: either screening before or during pregnancy to avoid maternal infection and transplacental transmission, or screening at birth with treatment given to infected newborns. Until more effective prevention tools, such as vaccination, become available, no miracle solution exists that could be applied in all countries. Therefore, for moral as well as medical reasons, the only rule is to ensure maximum protection.

4.8. Neonatal screening for congenital infection with *Toxoplasma gondii*

E. Petersen, R. B. Eaton

Background

Toxoplasma gondii is a zoonotic infection, i.e. an infection transmitted from animals to man, and it is therefore in theory possible to prevent infection by prevention of transmission. The reservoirs are known (see chapters 1.2. and 4.3.), but the relative contribution to human infections from cats and meat are not known in detail. Based on the knowledge of the transmission routes and the reservoirs, simple advice on preventive measures (see chapter 4.4.) can be given.

However, the effect of health education on prevention of infection with *Toxoplasma gondii* during pregnancy has never been proven [1], although one study found a reduction of 63% in the seroconversion rate during a seven-year period where primary systematic health education was given. Unfortunately, the study used historical controls, and during the same period the risk of infection with *Toxoplasma* declined throughout Europe [2].

Because infection with *Toxoplasma gondii* is asymptomatic or passes unrecognized in more than 80% of cases, and since more than 80% of newborns with congenital toxoplasmosis are asymptomatic at birth [3], systematic screening programs is the only possible way to detect the infection at an early stage.

Some countries have chosen to perform screening for primary infection with *Toxoplasma gondii* during pregnancy (see chapters 4.5. and 4.6.), but the concept of prenatal screening has not been adopted nationwide by other countries, although extensive screening during pregnancy is performed in Germany, Switzerland, Italy and Belgium. In many countries or areas, the majority of pregnant women have not been previously infected, but the risk of new infection during pregnancy is low. At the same time the possibilities for pre- and neonatal diagnosis are under rapid development, and neonatal screening is now performed for diseases as rare as less than 1 per 100,000 (Maple Syrup Urine Disease, homocysteinuria), so it is becoming common practice to diagnose rare diseases by screening programs in the continued effort to lower infant mortality and morbidity.

In such a situation neonatal screening is an alternative to prenatal screening, and in the following we will discuss the advantages and disadvantages of neonatal screening for congenital Toxoplasma infection based on experience from two on-going programs in New England (United States) and Denmark.

Epidemiological background

The decision to perform screening in France and Austria was taken based on data where up to 85% of the pregnant women were immune and the remaining 15% had a very high risk, estimated to be 60 infected women per 1,000 seronegative pregnant women in 1960 [4]. However, the epidemiology of the infection has changed during the past 25 years with decreasing risk to the population including pregnant women (chapter 4.1.) [5, 6].

The seroprevalence in pregnant women in New England was 17% when newborn screening was initiated in 1986, and has decreased slightly to 13% since that time. The seroprevalence in Denmark was approximately 28% in pregnant women when the neonatal screening programme was first planned [7].

The New England newborn screening programme for congenital toxoplasmosis

The decision to perform neonatal screening in New England

Population-based universal newborn screening began in the state of Massachusetts, USA, in 1962, using a bacterial inhibition assay for phenylketonuria (PKU) developed by Robert Guthrie of New York. Some additional metabolic disorders were soon added. A significant expansion of the scope of newborn screening occurred in 1976 with the addition of a relatively common endocrine disease (congenital hypothyroidism) to the traditional list of metabolic diseases screened for in all Massachusetts newborns. In the 1980s, the newborn screening program came under the leadership of George F. Grady. Dr. Grady explored whether the strong background of the Massachusetts State Laboratories in the areas of infectious diseases and epidemiology might be applicable to another expansion of the newborn screening program, to include infectious diseases. After serious considerations of other candidates such as hepatitis and HIV, Dr. Grady enlisted the assistance of Rod Hoff to implement a congenital toxoplasmosis program in 1986 [8]. Because no organized screening for congenital toxoplasmosis was being performed in any part of the US, and the impetus for the program came from within the newborn screening program, attention was focused on comparing the advantages of adding congenital toxoplasmosis to the existing newborn screening program, rather than on a comparison of the virtues of prenatal vs. newborn screening.

Detection of Toxoplasma-*specific IgM-antibodies from PKU-cards*

The New England Program makes use of a single 6mm disk from the dried filter paper blood spot already obtained from every baby born in Massachusetts for routine newborn screening for PKU and eight other disorders (samples from New Hampshire are also tested for congenital toxoplasmosis by this Program). This sample is analyzed for Toxoplasma-specific IgM by an IgM capture enzyme immunoassay produced in-house, which is an adaptation for filter papers of an assay previously described [9]. Briefly, the filter paper disks are eluted overnight with 0.2 ml of a PBS-TWEEN-milk buffer, then 0.1 ml of eluate is removed and added to wells pre-coated with goat anti-human IgM. A source of Toxoplasma antigen is added (soluble saline extract from sonicated parasites grown in mouse cell cultures), followed by alkaline phosphatase-conjugated rabbit anti-*Toxoplasma* antibodies, and substrate. Each microtiter plate contains standards and controls to allow identification of newborn samples with elevated reactions. The sensitivity is purposefully set high at some expense to specificity, so that elevated results may be examined carefully with appropriate follow-up testing on the original sample (for Toxoplasma-IgM in wells with and without antigen to study specificity, and also for Toxoplasma-IgG).

The current program

When screening identifies a suspected baby with congenital toxoplasmosis, the baby's pediatrician is notified. Follow-up liquid serum samples from the baby and mother are obtained to establish the diagnosis. Occasionally the serology is unclear, and diagnosis requires special clinical evaluation, longer term follow-up serology, or both. Overall, more than 99.9% of all babies are screened as negative on initial testing. The remaining are enriched for a group of babies in which more than 1 out of ten are determined to be infected after all analysis is complete. Overall detection rate of congenital toxoplasmosis in New England is 1:10,000. We are aware of three babies during the 12 years of screening, who showed severe clinical manifestations of Toxoplasma infection but did not show elevated IgM antibody in the newborn filter paper specimen (one of the three had low levels of detectable Toxoplasma-IgM in the follow-up serum). Presumably these babies were infected early in gestation, and either never developed antibody or lost IgM antibody by birth. We are not aware of any babies with congenital toxoplasmosis who were missed by both clinical and screening analysis, but we assume that some subclinical infections will not be detected. Babies who are identified as infected are referred to a network of pediatric infectious disease specialists in Massachusetts, who also serve as a clinical advisory committee for this toxoplasma program.

Infected babies are evaluated with extensive blood analysis, a retinal eye examination, cranial CT scan, neurological exam, and lumbar puncture (for protein, cells, glucose, and antibody). Infected babies are treated regardless of the presence of clinical signs.

Treatment consists of a one-year regimen of pyrimethamine, sulfadiazine, and folinic acid. During the early stages of the study (40 cases), pyrimethamine was administered for the first six months, then every other month for the rest of the first year. Sulfadiazine was administered for one year. Folinic acid was administered during pyrimethamine administration, and adjusted as needed. The clinical advisory committee reconsidered the treatment regimen, noting that compliance with therapy was generally good and well tolerated, and that several infants had retinal scars that had not been noted at birth. The advisory committee agreed to increase the treatment so that pyrimethamine, sulfadiazine, and folinic acid are now all administered for one year. Long term follow-up includes monitoring for drug toxicity, Toxoplasma-specific antibodies, audiologic and neurologic evaluation, and further retinal exams. Not surprisingly, the cohort of babies identified through newborn screening appeared to show better clinical outcome (five year) than cohorts identified clinically [10]. Evaluation of long term efficacy of early identification and treatment of newborns with subclinical infections at birth are complicated by the paucity of data regarding the natural course of infection of such newborns, and the wide range of results reported by those studies [11, 12]. At short (less than five year) follow-up, four of 39 babies may have developed new retinal lesions (only one macular, and some minor lesions which may not have been detected at birth), and only one of 46 had a neurologic deficit (mild hemiplegia attributable to a cerebral lesion present at birth) [10]. Evaluation of a ten year follow-up of the New England cohort is in preparation.

The Danish neonatal screening programme for congenital toxoplasmosis

The decision to perform neonatal screening in Denmark

During 1990 we were assessing the problem of congenital toxoplasmosis in Denmark, and we performed a pilot study of the prevalence of IgM-antibodies in first trimester samples from 5,402 pregnant Danish women [7]. We found an annual increase in IgG-seroprevalence rate of 1.16% equivalent to about 1 per 160 pregnant women infected during pregnancy. Based on these results it was decided to perform a larger, prospective study to confirm the results, and during 1992-1996 we performed a study including 89,873 pregnant women with follow up of all children born to infected mothers.

The results showed considerably lower numbers of infected women and infected children compared to the pilot study [13], but it also showed that neonatal screening for Toxoplasma-specific IgM-antibodies would reliably identify 75%-80% of infected newborns. The study further showed that clinical symptoms were not more frequent compared to children born to mothers treated during pregnancy [14]. Based on the results from the study we found that a neonatal screening program would be a cheap and reliable method which would identify at least 75% of infected children who would otherwise be missed, and these children could be offered early treatment [15].

It is clear, however, that the rationale for a neonatal screening program is that early treatment should prevent later disease, which for congenital toxoplasmosis is retinochoroiditis and probably minor psychomotor developmental problems.

When screening for a rare disease, the performance of the screening test is most important to ensure that healthy children are not wrongly told that they are infected, and to make sure that no infected child is missed, which would severely decrease the value of the program.

The pilot program in Denmark evaluated the value of neonatal IgM-screening based on the PKU-filter paper (Guthrie-card) on 21,163 newborns by following IgG-seroconversions in their mothers at the same time [15], which would reveal any false negative IgM-results.

It is well known that some children are born with no specific IgM-antibodies at birth and these can not be regarded as diagnostic "false-negatives" but merely emphasize that the biology of the infection is so, that a few children will have ended the IgM-response before being born. For these children an additional analysis for specific IgA would pick up the child in about 5% of the cases [14]. Assays of Toxoplasma-specific IgA eluted from the PKU-card is currently under development.

Based on the results of the pilot study, the National Health Board decided in June 1998 to offer newborn screening for congenital toxoplasmosis to all newborns based on the analysis of Toxoplasma-specific IgM-antibodies eluted from the PKU-card. The screening started 1 January 1999.

Detection of Toxoplasma-specific IgM-antibodies from PKU-cards

From all incoming PKU-cards a 3 mm disk is punched into a microtiter well precoated with an anti-IgM antibody (DAKO, Denmark, Cat. no. A0425). The spots are eluted at 28 °C temperature for 1 hours and a *Toxoplasma gondii* antigen added from lysed RH-strain parasites cultured *in vitro*. The assays are performed on a single 3 mm disk from each card and whenever the OD value is above the defined cut-off two new spots are analyzed.

In the pilot study 21,163 PKU-cards were analysed for Toxoplasma-specific IgM- and IgG antibodies. If IgG or IgM antibodies were detected, the maternal first trimester sample was analyzed to identify women who had seroconverted between the two samples. Thirty women seroconverted and 11 PKU-cards were found positive in the screening test of which 7 had Toxoplasma-specific IgM-antibodies in a serum sample obtained a few weeks after birth. One child was diagnosed with congenital toxoplasmosis due to persistent IgG-antibodies at one year. The sensitivity of the assay was thus 100% and the positive predictive value 50% (4/7).

The current programme

When the results of the IgM-analysis persistently show a value above the cut-off, the local department of paediatrics is informed and a serum sample for confirmatory testing is requested from the mother and the newborn. The samples are analyzed for Toxoplasma-specific IgM using an ISAGA test (bioMerieux), IgA antibodies using an EIA test (Pasteur), and the Sabin-Feldman dye test. If the presence of Toxoplasma-specific IgM-antibodies are confirmed, the child is investigated by ultrasound of the skull for intracranial calcifications and dilated ventricles, an ophthalmoscopy is performed for retinitis or scars in the retina, and a physical examination is performed including a neurological assessment. Treatment is started with sulfadiazine, pyrimethamine and folinic acid according to the standard guidelines by the WHO [16]. The WHO recommend 4 courses of sulfadiazine combined with pyrimethamine interspersed with 4 weeks of spiramycin. There is very little if any evidence that spiramycin is effective [17], and so with the American recommendations in mind (where the child is treated with sulfadiazine and pyrimethamine continuously for a year without spiramycin), we chose for our treatment regimen sulfadiazine and pyrimethamine combined with folinic acid as a single, 3 months course.

Advantages and disadvantages of neonatal screening

The advantages of neonatal screening should be considered on the background of the disadvantages of performing prenatal screening in low risk areas like New England and Denmark.

In prenatal screening a series of samples are collected from the pregnant women during pregnancy and analyzed for Toxoplasma-IgM and IgG-antibodies. It is normally recognized that about 3% of all samples obtained in a diagnostic laboratory will show a positive test for Toxoplasma-IgM antibodies. In IgM-positive patients a new blood sample is required and further testing is usually done in attempts to decide whether the infection occurred at a time that indicates risk for fetal infection.

In the Danish situation this would mean that for every 10,000 seronegative women, 300 would be further investigated, but only 16 found infected giving birth to 3 infected children. In New England, again, 300 women would be further investigated with perhaps 5 found infected and one child ending up with proven congenital Toxoplasma-infection.

Furthermore, in a certain number of cases it will not be possible to determine the precise date of infection and it can not be ruled out that infection occurred after conception, in which case it may be decided to perform an amniocentesis. If in the above scenario one half of the IgM-positive women undergo an amniocentesis, approximately one fetus will be lost due to the procedure, and the fetus will very probably not be infected.

In neonatal screening the problems of prenatal diagnosis naturally do not exist, but the infected fetuses are not treated, and some fetuses will end up as late abortions or intrauterine deaths, and it can be argued that a neonatal screening programme deprived these fetuses of treatment.

The argument that neonatal screening deprives the unborn infected child from treatment is certainly correct, but it has been very difficult to document a clear effect of prenatal treatment.

In the study from Denmark, only 5 out of 27 children had symptoms at birth, which is comparable with data reported from prenatal screening programmes. A recent review from the Cochrane initiative could not find any evidence of effect of spiramycin treatment in delaying materno-fetal transmission or on the outcome of the child [17].

It is therefore questionable if early treatment with spiramycin influences the outcome in the majority of children.

Congenital toxoplasmosis results in significant morbidity in all populations. Some regions have chosen to implement wide scale prenatal screening to detect congenital infection. This approach is not well suited to regions with a low seroprevalence. An alternative approach is to conduct newborn screening. There are theoretical advantages and disadvantages to each approach. Comparative analyses of these approaches in regions with differing epidemiological pictures are difficult, but will be important as countries develop the most effective strategies for the public health of their populations.

References

1. Jeanel D, Cosatgliola D, Niel G, Hubert B, Danis M (1990) What is known about the prevention of congenital toxoplasmosis? Lancet 336:359-361
2. Foulon W, Naessens A, Derde MP (1994) Evaluation of the possibilities for preventing congenital toxoplasmosis. Am J Perinatol 11:57-62
3. Hohlfeld P, Daffos F, Thulliez P, Aufrant C, Couvreur J, MacAleese J, Descombey D, Forestier F (1989) Fetal toxoplasmosis: Outcome of pregnancy and infant follow-up after in utero treatment. J Paediatrics 115:765-769
4. Desmonts G (1985) Prevention of Toxoplasmosis: Observations on follow-up experience in France. Prog Clin Biol Res 163B:333-337
5. Forsgren M, Gille E, Ljungström I, Nokes DJ (1991) *Toxoplasma gondii* antibodies in pregnant women in Stockholm in 1969, 1979 and 1989. Lancet 337:1413-1414
6. Edelhofer R (1994) Prevalence of antibodies against *Toxoplasma gondii* in pigs in Austria - An evaluation of data from 1982 and 1992. Parasitol Res 80:642-644
7. Lebech M, Larsen SO, Petersen E (1993) Prevalence, incidence and geographical distribution of *Toxoplasma gondii* antibodies in pregnant women in Denmark. Scand J Infect Dis 25:751-756
8. Grady G (1990) Newborn screening and surveillance for infectious diseases: anticipation of treatment options and impact on minority groups. In: Knoppers BM, Laberge CM (eds) Genetic screening from newborns to DNA typing. Excerpta Medica, New York
9. Naot Y, Desmonts G, Remington JS (1981) IgM enzyme-linked immunosorbent assay test for the diagnosis of congenital *Toxoplasma* infection. J Pediatrics 98:32-36
10. Guerina NG, Hsu HW, Meissner HC, Maguire JH, Lynfield R, Stechenberg B, Abroms I, Pasternack MS, Hoff R, Eaton RB, Grady GF, Cheeseman SH, Mcintosh K, Medearis DN, Robb R, Weiblen BJ (1994) Neonatal serologic screening and early treatment for congenital *Toxoplasma gondii* infection. N Engl J Med 330:1858-1863
11. Wilson CB, Remington JS, Stagno S, Reynolds DW (1980) Development of adverse sequelae in children born with subclinical congenital *Toxoplasma* infection. Pediatrics 66:767-774
12. Koppe JG, Loewer-Sieger DH, Roever-Bonnet H (1986) Results of 20-year follow-up of congenital toxoplasmosis. Lancet 1:254-256
13. Larsen SO, Lebech M (1994) Models for prediction of the frequency of toxoplasmosis in pregnancy in situations of changing infection rates. Intl J Epidemiol 23:1309-1314
14. Pratlong F, Boulot P, Issert E, Msika M, Dupont F, Bachelard B, Sarda P, Viala JL, Jarry D (1994) Fetal diagnosis of toxoplasmosis in 190 women infected during pregnancy. Prenatal Diag 14:191-198
15. Lebech M, Andersen O, Christensen NC, Herlel J, Nielsen HE, Peitersen B, Rehnitzer C, Larsen SO, Nørgaard-Pedersen B, Petersen E and the Danish Congenital Toxoplasmosis Study Group (1999) Feasilibity of neonatal screening for toxoplasma infection in the absence of prenatal treatment. Lancet 353:1834-1837.
16. WHO ((1988) Report of the WHO consultation on Public Health Aspects of Toxoplasmosis. WHO/CDS/VPH/88.74
17. Wallon M, Liou C, Garner P, Peyron F (1999) Congenital toxoplasmosis: systematic reviews of evidence of efficacy of treatment in pregnancy. Br Med J 318:1511-1514

4.9. Strategies for development of vaccines against *Toxoplasma gondii*

H.V. NIELSEN, E.A. INNES, E. PETERSEN, D. BUXTON

Toxoplasma gondii can infect a wide range of intermediate hosts and, as outlined elsewhere (chapter 4.1.), transmission from the meat of pigs and lambs is an important route of infection for humans. Another source is oocysts shed by cats into the environment, thereby contaminating soil, vegetables and childrens' sand pits. In humans, more than 90% of primary infections pass either unnoticed or with only mild clinical symptoms. However, if a primary infection occurs during pregnancy, the child may be born congenitally infected with varying degrees of damage (chapter 2.1.). Infection with *T. gondii* is therefore theoretically a preventable disease and it is important that advice on hygiene, aimed at breaking the two main routes of transmission, is heeded by those most at risk such as pregnant women. However, if education could be supported by an effective vaccine the incidence of disease could be further reduced.

Immunization has proven one of the most cost effective strategies for preventing many infectious diseases, but to date a vaccine against *Toxoplasma* suitable for human use has not been developed. In addition, vaccination to prevent tissue cyst formation in food animals or targeted at cats to prevent the parasite's sexual life cycle in the intestine, and so prevent oocyst shedding would be valuable public health measures. The livestock industry would also benefit both in terms of reduced losses and the ability to sell meat of "proven safety" and therefore added value. In summary, the main targets for a vaccination strategy would be to: a) control the acute parasitaemia during a primary infection in a pregnant woman to protect the vulnerable fetus; b) protect sheep (and goats) against *Toxoplasma* abortion and also reduce the numbers of tissue cysts in food animals; c) reduce environmental contamination of oocysts by vaccinating cats.

In most immunocompetent animals, a primary infection with *T. gondii* results in the development of a life-long protective immune response. This immune response will not always protect against reinfection but will protect against disease [1]. As *T. gondii* is a very potent inducer of protective immunity, control of the disease by vaccination is a real possibility. In order to develop an effective vaccine against *Toxoplasma gondii*, it is necessary to identify the critical immune responses that a vaccine would be required to induce.

Mechanisms of protective immunity

Pregnant women infected with *T. gondii* only transmit infection to the fetus during a primary infection. A primary infection in a pregnant or non-pregnant woman results in complete clinical immunity against reinfection in a subsequent pregnancy and so also protects the fetus. Thus, infection results in protective immunity even though bradyzoites in tissue cysts remain viable in the host probably for the rest of life (chapter 1.4.). As *T. gondii* is an obligate intracellular parasite, cell-mediated immune mechanisms are thought to be important in the development of protective immunity. Much of the work elucidating immune mechanisms has been done using experimentally infected mice, although there have been several studies looking at immune responses in humans and in experimentally infected sheep.

Some recent work has shown the importance of the innate immune system during the very early stages of *T. gondii* infection. Parasites have been shown to directly stimulate macrophages to produce the cytokines IL12 and TNF-α and these cytokines in turn will induce interferon-γ (IFN-γ) synthesis from NK cells [2]. Interferon-γ is a key cytokine in development of protective immunity to *T. gondii*. The presence of IFN-γ at this early stage of infection will provide the appropriate cytokine environment to "bias" the CD4+ T-cell response to a Th1 type during the subsequent priming of the adaptive immune response [3]. Clearly for vaccine development the adaptive immune response needs to be understood, as this is what will need to be induced by a given vaccine preparation.

In mice, infection with *T. gondii* stimulates the development of a Th1 type of immune response including the development of high titres of IgG_{2a} antibody against *T. gondii* antigens [4]. Specific T lymphocytes secrete the Th1-cytokines IL-2 and IFN-γ in response to specific stimulation [5, 6], and it has been clearly demonstrated that infection in mice also induces a cytotoxic T lymphocyte (CTL) response (mainly CD8+ T cells) against *T. gondii* infected target cells [7]. Evidence is accumulating to show that both CD4+ T lymphocytes together with CD8+ T cells are required for protective immunity [8, 9]. Protective immunity has also been transferred from mice orally dosed with live *Toxoplasma gondii* to naïve mice, by isolating gut derived intraepithelial lymphocytes from the former and injecting them into the latter [10]. The protection induced may be longlasting [11], emphasising the potential importance of mucosal immunity.

In experiments using the technique of lymphatic cannulation it was possible to study the kinetics of development of a primary immune response to *T. gondii* in sheep [12]. This study showed that the lymphoblasts were initially mainly comprised of CD4+ T-cells. However, during the peak lymphoblast response the predominant T-cell population had changed to CD8+ cells and this coincided with the disappearance of parasite from the efferent lymph [13]. The activated CD4+ cells produced IFN-γ which is thought to be important in the induction and maturation of CD8+ T-cells [14, 15]. Adoptive transfer experiments are also a powerful tool in determining the critical immune responses to *T. gondii*.

Adoptive transfer of splenocytes depleted of CD4+ T lymphocytes promotes protection against a challenge with *T. gondii* tissue cysts as do to a lesser extent, splenocytes depleted of CD8+ T lymphocytes [16]. Adoptive transfer of CD8+ T cells has also been shown to confer protection in mice [17]. In human infection with *T. gondii* both CD4+ and CD8+ T lymphocytes have been shown to be cytolytic against specific target cells [18, 19], and it now seems clear that CD8+ T lymphocytes play a key role in control of both the acute and the long term infection with *T. gondii*. CD8+ T lymphocytes are generally considered to be cytotoxic killer cells capable of causing cytolysis of specific target-cells, and this is also the case in *T. gondii* infected mice where specific CTL have been shown to be cytolytic to both *T. gondii* infected and antigen loaded target cells [20, 21]. A well described mode of action by which CTL effect their lytic activities are mediated by perforin. However, perforin knockout mice infected with the attenuated *Toxoplasma* mutant strain ts-4 were as fully protected against challenge with the lethal RH strain as were wild-type mice, even though their cytolytic capacity was greatly impaired [22]. This suggests that these mice are able to control infection by other CTL cytolytic pathways, such as by granzyme mediated target cell lysis or by the induction of apoptosis [23, 24]. While these latter mechanisms cannot be excluded, it seems likely that another key factor provided by *T. gondii* specific CD8+ T lymphocytes is IFN-γ [25-27], perhaps the primary molecule in controlling the acute *T. gondii* infection. This was clearly shown by Scharton-Kersten and colleagues [28] using IFN-γ knockout mice which were unable to control an acute *T. gondii* infection, succumbing to the parasite at day eight to nine, even when challenged with the attenuated mutant ts-4 strain. As well as CD8+ cells, CD4+ and NK-cells contribute to the early production of IFN-γ but it appears that the secretion of IFN-γ from activated CD8+ T lymphocytes is pivotal in promoting resistance against the acute infection. This is shown when *T. gondii* infected mice are depleted of NK cells on day 1 of infection by anti-asialo GM1 antibody. In this case, even though the IFN-γ level in these mice is decreased, mortality is not significantly altered [7]. *In vivo* adoptive transfer experiments have reported that the protective effect of the transferred CD8+ cells is ablated if the recipient mice are treated with antibody to IFN-γ [29]. As is the case with many other intracellular pathogens including viruses, *T. gondii* multiplies within the cells of the host. The endogenously generated antigen is processed within the infected cell and presented along with MHC Class I on the cell surface. CD8+ T cells recognise parasite antigen in association with MHC Class I and, following further secondary signals from co-stimulating molecules such as CD8, CD3, CD80 and CD86, are activated to deal with the antigen presenting cell [30].

The major challenge is to induce an effective CD8+ T-cell response by vaccination. This is comparatively easy if a live vaccine preparation such as the S48 strain vaccine is used, as the parasite undergoes limited multiplication within the host [31]. As a result of this intracellular multiplication, the parasite antigens are presented in the appropriate way to the immune system to stimulate the required CD8+ T-cell response. However, major hurdles have to be overcome if one wishes to try and use recombinant antigens or other non-replicating antigen preparations to stimulate a protective cell-mediated immune response. Various strategies are being examined to "deliver" antigens in an appropriate form for processing within the cell in order to stimulate the necessary CD8+ T-cell response. Some of these are discussed further below.

Although T. gondii induces a very strong antibody response following infection, this response is generally not considered to be as important in terms of protection of the host as a cell-mediated immune response. In a primary infection in sheep antibody responses are not detected until eight to nine days after challenge [32]. Data from lymph node cannulation studies in sheep showed that this response did not occur until after the cell-mediated immune response and after the parasite was no longer detectable within the efferent lymph [12]. Clearly, during a secondary challenge antibody responses will play a more significant role. It is known that specific antibody will lyse extracellular tachyzoites [33] and passive transfer of immune serum [34] or monoclonal antibodies [35] can confer partial protection against challenge infection. But unfortunately, it appears that an antibody response is insufficient on its own to protect against T. gondii. It is certainly an easier prospect to induce an antibody and Th2 type response using a killed antigen preparation than to induce a Th1/CD8+ cell mediated immune response.

Vaccine models

Live attenuated vaccines

Live, attenuated strains of T. gondii, which have incomplete life cycles and do not produce tissue cysts, have been used to induce protective immunity in animals against subsequent infections [36-40]. The S48 strain is commercially available for the immunisation of sheep (Toxovax, Intervet, Cambridge, UK and AgVax, Upper Hutt, New Zealand) to prevent abortion caused by T. gondii infection. Live, attenuated vaccines are relatively expensive but have a short shelf-life and require care in their use to prevent accidental infection of those administering the vaccine. The protective immunity is longlasting [41] and there are no significant side effects. The vaccine produces significant economic benefits and possibly even reduces the weight of muscle infection by subsequently acquired natural T. gondii infection, thus making the meat safer for human consumption. Sheep also provide a very valuable model of the human infection which in many respects is more appropriate than the infection in mice [1].

The RH strain of T. gondii has also been reported to induce a degree of protective immunity in pigs against an oral challenge with T. gondii oocysts [42, 43]. Although this research suffered from small animal groups, evidence was presented that fewer tissue cysts were present in pigs vaccinated with the RH strain compared to the uninoculated control pigs, after challenge with a complete strain of the parasite. Therefore, both the S48 and the RH strains of T. gondii, which undergo a limited replication and do not persist in the animal, may provide a means of reducing the number of *T. gondii* tissue cysts that develop in muscle following natural challenge with a complete strain of the parasite. This could significantly affect transmission of the parasite to humans and animals through the ingestion of raw or lightly cooked infected meat.

Attenuation of *T. gondii* oocysts using γ-irradiation has also been attempted. The oral dosing of mice with γ-irradiated, sporulated, *Toxoplasma* oocysts induced partial protection against subsequent lethal challenge. However, the results favoured the conclusion that the treatment had killed a proportion of the initial oocyst dose rather than cause attenuation of the inoculum [44, 45].

Another approach to the control of toxoplasmosis by vaccination has been described by Frenkel and colleagues [46]. The target for their vaccine was to prevent cats from shedding oocysts, so contaminating the environment. A mutant strain of *T. gondii*, known as T-263, was selected on the basis that it would only undergo partial enteric development within the gut of the cat and therefore would not result in the production of oocysts. This strain was tested on naïve kittens and was found to protect 84% of the animals from shedding oocysts [46]. Further studies reinforced its efficacy and safety [47], but as this is a live vaccine and the only source of the bradyzoites is from harvesting infected mouse brains, large scale production of this vaccine is problematic.

Inactivated and subunit vaccines

Toxoplasma gondii tachyzoites, inactivated following harvest from either mice or *in vitro* culture, have been used in several studies both in mice and sheep but have not been successful in inducing protective immunity [34, 37, 48, 49]. Use of immunostimulating complexes (ISCOMS) as an adjuvant capable of stimulating both antibody and cell-mediated responses, combined with surface antigens of the parasite (including the SAG1 antigen) provided protection in studies in mice [50], but in a follow-up study in pregnant sheep the immunity induced was insufficient to prevent abortion [51], although this preparation can induce significant immune responses in sheep [52]. The SAG1 (or P30) molecule, is an abundant surface protein of the tachyzoite stage and has been intensively studied as it is probably the most immunogenic *Toxoplasma* antigen, capable of inducing strong T and B cell responses [53, 54]. While the antigen(s) selected is of great importance, the choice of adjuvant and the route of administration are also crucial, as shown by Bülow and Boothroyd [55], who showed strong protection to *Toxoplasma* challenge in mice immunised with purified SAG1 formulated with liposomes. This was further demonstrated by Bourguin and colleagues [56] when they showed protection in mice dosed orally with *T. gondii* sonicate using cholera toxin as an adjuvant. In further studies, Debard and colleagues [57] combined SAG1 with cholera toxin and gave it intranasally to mice. They were able to show that both cellular and humoral immune mechanisms were induced. Furthermore, following oral infection with a tissue cyst producing strain of the parasite, significantly fewer tissue cysts developed in the brains of treated mice when compared with control mice. This approach has a lot of advantages and may be the most feasible route for vaccination of people. On the other hand, in one particular study mice immunised with purified, native SAG1 combined with Freund's Complete Adjuvant (FCA) showed a significant increase in mortality and brain cyst numbers [58], but another study using recombinant SAG1 with alum as adjuvant found a significant protection in mice challenged with the RH-strain [4]. These contradictory results show the importance of the selection of adjuvant as well as the specific antigen and the route of administration, as all may profoundly influence the resultant protective immune response. While cholera toxin and ISCOMs are potentially suitable adjuvants, with the latter also effective by the oral route [59], so are liposomes.

As well as SAG1, other major surface antigens on the tachyzoite have been identified (SAG2, 3) [60, 61] and are potential targets for a subunit vaccine. Antigens expressed exclusively in the bradyzoite stage have also been identified [62, 63], and may prove of interest as potential candidates for vaccines designed to prevent tissue cyst formation and persistence. Various recombinant antigens have been identified for *T. gondii*. The major challenge is probably not to identify specific antigens but to examine different methods of delivering these antigens to the immune system by targetting appropriate antigen presenting cells or creating the necessary cytokine environment for optimal induction of the immune response.

Vaccination of mice with a soluble tachyzoite antigen preparation was found to reduce *T. gondii* induced abortion in mice if the antigen was delivered within lipid vesicles [64]. One property of liposomes in vaccines, is their capacity to induce a pronounced CD8+ T lymphocyte immune response including CTL [65], emphasising that the method of antigen presentation to the immune system is pivotal in the eventual outcome. As discussed above, it is very difficult to induce CD8+ T-cell responses using exogenous antigen. It is thought that introducing the antigen to the immune system within a lipid vesicle may allow appropriate processing and presentation of antigen to activate the required CD8+ T-cell response [6].

Another approach is to use cytokines as adjuvants to stimulate the required cell-mediated immune response by providing the appropriate cytokine microenvironment during the critical induction phase of the immune response. A potential candidate would be IL12 as it is a potent inducer of IFN-γ and has been used successfully in vaccination studies of *Leishmania major* [67]. Experiments with SCID mice have shown that the administration of IL12 has significantly prolonged time to death following infection with *T. gondii* [2].

Genetic immunisation

Genetic immunisation is a rapidly developing technique making use of the great oportunities provided by the recent significant advances in the field of molecular biology. The most frequently used construction vehicle for genetic vaccination is based on the use of a plasmid of prokaryotic origin. A strong promotor, such as the CMV promotor, drives the transcription and a poly-adenylation site is included. Genetic immunisation or gene vaccination is highly effective at inducing a strong MHC I restricted CTL response [68, 69]. This is probably because gene vaccination provides a mechanism by which the antigen is synthesized within antigen-presenting cells allowing MHC I presentation of CTL epitopes by the classical pathway. In this manner gene vaccination mimicks the *in vivo* situation that occurs in a viral or intracellular parasite infection, such as with toxoplasmosis. So far gene vaccination has successfully induced antibody and CTL responses in several parasite models [70, 71]. The DNA constructs used have included both whole genes and subunits of genes, some so small that they encode only a single CTL epitope of 8-10 amino acids [72]. The intracellular malaria parasite, against which it has proved so difficult to vaccinate, has been a target for studies with gene vaccination and some promising results have been obtained, including CTL and antibody responses and protection in mice [73-75]. Our own recent data shows that the SAG1 gene provided as a DNA vaccine, raise a strong antibody response, and protects mice from an otherwise lethal challenge with the RH strain. The level of protection is between 80-100% in two different mice trains used, and excess the protection obtained with recombinant SAG1 formulated in either alum or freunds adjuvants (Petersen et al., unplished).

Concluding remarks

We are clearly at a very exciting stage in the development of vaccines against *T. gondii*. It is likely that several different vaccines may become available which may target the different life-cycle stages of the parasite. Currently, the only commercially available vaccines use live S48 strain tachyzoites to prevent abortion in sheep and the T-263 mutant to prevent oocyst excretion by cats. A vaccine for use in people must be both safe and effective and this is likely to involve using a non-replicating antigen formula, with all the inherent difficulties in delivering such a preparation, to induce an appropriate immune response. It is also very important to consider who would benefit from a vaccine against *T. gondii*. The major risk group is clearly pregnant women but those who are immunocompromised are also at risk from the parasite but it is unlikely that vaccination would be effective in such individuals. It is also important to focus attention on reducing the environmental contamination by *T. gondii* which would include the wider use of a vaccine to prevent oocyst excretion by cats and a vaccine for food animals to reduce the numbers of tissue cysts in muscle destined for human consumption. Success with these measures would significantly decrease the incidence of human *T. gondii* infection and so reduce the incidence of disease.

References

1. Innes EA (1997) Toxoplasmosis: comparative species susceptibilty and host immune response. Comp Immun Microbiol Infect Dis 20:131-138
2. Gazzinelli RT, Hieny S, Wynn TA, Wolf S, Sher A (1993) Interleukin 12 is required for the T-lymphocyte-independent induction of interferon γ by an intracellular parasite and induces resistance in T-cell deficient hosts. Proc Natl Acad Sci USA 90:6115-6119

3. Gazzinelli RT, Denkers EY, Sher A (1993) Host resistance to *Toxoplasma gondii*: model for studying the selective induction of cell-mediated immunity by intracellular parasites. Infect Agents Dis 2:139-149

4. Petersen E, Nielsen HV, Christiansen L, Spenter J (1998) Immunization with E-coli produced recombinant T. gondii SAG1 with alum as adjuvant protect mice against lethal infection with *Toxoplasma gondii*. Vaccine 16:1283-1289

5. Gazzinelli RT, Hayashi S, Wysocka M, Carrera L, Kuhn R, Muller W, Roberge F, Trinchieri G, Sher A (1994) Role of IL-12 in the initiation of cell mediated immunity by *Toxoplasma gondii* and its regulation by IL-10 and nitric oxide. J Eukar Microbiol 41 (Suppl)5:9

6. Denkers EY, Gazzinelli RT (1998) Regulation and function of T-cell-mediated immunity during *Toxoplasma gondii* infection. Clin Microbiol Rev 11:569-580

7. Shirahata T, Yamashita T, Ohta C, Goto H, Nakane A (1994) CD8[+] T lymphocytes are the major cell population involved in the early gamma interferon response and resistance to acute primary *Toxoplasma gondii* infection in mice. Microbiol Immunol 38:789-796

8. Suzuki Y, Remington JS (1988) Dual regulation of resistance against *Toxoplasma gondii* infection by Lyt-2[+] and Lyt-1[-], L3T4[+] T cells in mice. J Immunol 140:3943-3946

9. Curiel TJ, Krug EC, Purner MB, Poignard P, Berens RL (1993) Cloned human CD4[+] cytotoxic T lymphocytes specific for *Toxoplasma gondii* lyse tachyzoite-infected target cells. J Immunol 151:2024-2031

10. Buzoni-Gatel D, Lepage AC, Dimier-Poisson IH, Bout DT, Kasper LH (1997) Adoptive transfer of gut intraepithelial lymphocytes protects against murine infection with *Toxoplasma gondii*. J Immunol 158:5883-5889

11. Lepage AC, Buzoni-Gatel D, Bout DT, Kasper LH (1998) Gut-derived intraepithelial lymphocytes induce long term immunity against *Toxoplasma gondii*. J Immunol 161:4902-4908

12. Innes EA, Wastling JM (1995) Analysis of in vivo immune responses during *Toxoplasma gondii* infection using the technique of lymphatic cannulation. Parasitol Today 11:268-271

13. Innes EA, Panton WRM, Sanderson A, Thomson K, Wastling JM, Maley S, Buxton D (1995) Induction of CD4[+] and CD8[+] T-cell responses in efferent lymph responding to *Toxoplasma gondii* infection: analysis of phenotype and function. Parasit Immunol 17:151-160

14. Zanovello P, Vallerani E, Biasi G, Landolfo S, Collavo D (1988) Monoclonal antibody against IFN-γ inhibits Maloney murine sarcoma virus-specific cytotoxic T-lymphocyte differentiation. J Immunol 140:1341-1344

15. Innes EA, Panton WRM, Thomson KM, Maley S, Buxton D (1995) Kinetics of interferon gamma production in vivo during infection with the S48 vaccine strain of *Toxoplasma gondii*. J Comp Pathol 113:89-94

16. Parker SJ, Roberts CW, Alexander J (1991) CD8[+] T cells are the major lymphocyte subpopulation involved in the protective immune response to *Toxoplasma gondii* in mice. Clin Exp Immunol 84:207-212

17. Khan IA, Ely KH, Kasper LH (1994) Antigen-Specific CD8[+] T Cell Clone Protects Against Acute *Toxoplasma gondii* Infection in Mice. J Immunol 152:1856-1860

18. Montoya JG, Lowe KE, Clayberger C, Moody D, Do D, Remington JS, Talib S, Subauste CS (1996) Human CD4[+] and CD8[-] T lymphocytes are both cytotoxic to *Toxoplasma gondii*-infected cells. Infect Immun 64:176-181

19. Purner MB, Berens RL, Nash PB, Vanlinden A, Ross E, Kruse C, Krug EC, Curiel TJ (1996) CD4-mediated and CD8-mediated cytotoxic and proliferative immune responses to *Toxoplasma gondii* in seropositive humans. Infect Immun 64:4330-4338

20. Hakim FT, Gazzinelli RT, Denkers E, Hieny S, Shearer GM, Sher A (1991) CD8+ T cells from mice vaccinated against *Toxoplasma gondii* are cytotoxic for parasite-infected or antigen-pulsed host cells. J Immunol 147:2310-2316

21. Subauste CS, Koniaris AH, Remington JS (1991) Murine CD8[+] cytotoxic T lymphocytes lyse *Toxoplasma gondii* infected cells. J Immunol 147:3955-3959

22. Denkers EY, Yap G, Scharton-Kersten T, Charest H, Butcher BA, Caspar P, Heiny S, Sher A (1997) Perforin-mediated cytolysis plays a limited role in host resistance to *Toxoplasma gondii*. J Immunol 159:1903-1908

23. Kägl D, Ledermann B, Bürkl K, Seller P, Odermatt B, Olsen KJ, Podac ER, Zinkernagel RM, Hengartner H (1994) Cytotoxicity mediated by T cells and natural killer cells is greatly impaired in perforin-deficient mice. Nature 369:31-37

24. Shresta S, Pham CTN, Thomas DA, Graubert TA, Ley TJ (1998) How do cytotoxic lymphocytes kill their targets? Curr Opin Immunol 10:581-587

25. Gazzinelli RT, Hakim FT, Hieny S, Shearer GM, Sher A (1991) Synergistic role of CD4[+] and CD8[+] T lymphocytes in IFN-gamma production and protective immunity induced by an attenuated *Toxoplasma gondii* vaccine. J Immunol 146:286-292

26. Johnson L, Vander Vegt FP, Havell EA (1993) Gamma interferon-dependent temporary resistance to acute *Toxoplasma gondii* infection independent of CD4[+] or CD8[+] lymphocytes. Infect Immun 61:5174-5180

27. Beaman MH, Hunter CA, Remington JS (1994) Enhancement of intracellular replication of *Toxoplasma gondii* by IL-6 - Interactions with IFN-gamma and TNF-alpha. J Immunol 153: 4583-4587

28. Scharton-Kersten TM, Wynn TA, Denkers EY, Bala S, Grunvald E, Hieny S, Gazzinelli RT, Sher A (1996) In the absence of endogenous IFN-gamma, mice develop unimpaired IL-12 responses to *Toxoplasma gondii* while failing to control acute infection. J Immunol 157:4045-4054

29. Suzuki Y, Remington JS (1990) The effect of anti-IFN-γ antibody on the protective effect of Lyt 2+ immune T-cells against Toxoplasmosis in mice. J Immunol 144:1954-1956

30. Horspool JH, Perrin PJ, Woodcock JB, Cox JH, King CL, June CH, Harlan DM, St. Louise DC, Lee KP (1998) Nucleic acid vaccination-induced immune responses require CD28 costimulation and are regulated by CTLA4. J Immunol 160:2706-2714

31. Buxton D, Innes EA (1995) A commercial vaccine for ovine toxoplasmosis. Parasitol 110(Suppl.):11-16

32. Wastling JM, Harkins D, Maley S, Innes EA, Panton WRM, Thomson K, Buxton D (1995) Kinetics of the local and systemic antibody response to primary and secondary infection with S48 *Toxoplasma gondii* in sheep. J Comp Path 112:53-62

33. Schreiber RD, Feldman HA (1980) Identification of the activator system for antibody to *Toxoplasma* as the classical complement pathway. J Inf Dis 141:366-369

34. Krahenbuhl JL, Ruskin J, Remington JS (1972) The use of killed vaccines in immunization against an intracellular parasite: *Toxoplasma gondii*. J Immunol 108:425-431

35. Johnson AM, McDonald PJ, Neoh SH (1983) Monoclonal antibodies to Toxoplasma cell membrane surface antigens protect mice from toxoplasmosis. J Protozool 30:351-356

36. Pfefferkorn ER, Pfefferkorn LC (1976) *Toxoplasma gondii*: isolation and preliminary characterisation of temperature-sensitive mutants. Exp Parasitol 39:365-376

37. Waldeland H, Frenkel JK (1983) Temperature sensitive mutants of *Toxoplasma gondii*: pathogenicity and persistence in mice. J Parasitol 69:171-175

38. O'Connell E, Wilkins MF, TePunga WA (1988) Toxoplasmosis in sheep. II. The ability of a live vaccine to prevent lambing losses after an intravenous challenge with *Toxoplasma gondii*. N Z Vet J 36:1-4

39. Wilkins MF, O'Connell E, TePunga WA (1988) Toxoplasmosis in sheep. III. Further evaluation of the ability of a live *Toxoplasma gondii* vaccine to prevent lamb losses and reduce congenital infection following experimental oral challenge. N Z Vet J 36:86-89

40. Buxton D, Thomson K, Maley S, Wright S, Bos HJ (1991) Vaccination of sheep with a live incomplete strain (S48) of *Toxoplasma gondii* and their immunity to challenge when pregnant. Vet Rec 129:89-93

41. Buxton D, Thomson K, Maley S, Wright S, Bos HJ (1993) Experimental challenge of sheep 18 months after vaccination with a live (S48) *Toxoplasma gondii* vaccine. Vet Rec 133:310-312

42. Dubey JP, Urban JF, Davis SW (1991) Protective immunity to toxoplasmosis in pigs vaccinated with a nonpersistent strain of *Toxoplasma gondii*. Am J Vet Res 52:1316-1319

43. Dubey JP, Baker DG, Davis SW, Urban JF, Sken SK (1994) Persistence of immunity to toxoplasmosis in pigs vaccinated with a nonpersistent strain of *Toxoplasma gondii*. Am J Vet Res 55:982-987

44. Dubey JP, Jenkins MC, Thayer DW, Kwok OCH, Shen SK (1996) Killing of *Toxoplasma gondii* oocysts by irradiation and protective immunity induced by vaccination with irradiated oocysts. J Parasit 82:724-727

45. Dubey JP, Lunney JK, Shen SK, Kwok OCH (1998) Immunity to toxoplasmosis in pigs fed irradiated *Toxoplasma gondii* oocysts. J Parasit 84:749-752

46. Frenkel JK, Pfefferkorn ER, Smith DD, Fishback JL (1991) Prospective vaccine prepared from a new mutant of *Toxoplasma gondii* for use in cats. Am J Vet Res 52:759-763

47. Choromanski L, Freyre A, Popiel R, Brown K, Grieve R, Shibley G (1995) Safety and efficacy of modified feline *Toxoplasma gondii* vaccine. Dev Biol Stand 84:269-281

48. Beverley JKA, Archer JF, Watson WA, Fawcett AR (1971) Trial of a killed vaccine in the prevention of ovine abortion due to toxoplasmosis. Br Vet J 127:529-534

49. Wilkins MF, O'Connell E, TePunga WA (1987) Toxoplasmosis in sheep. I. Effect of a killed vaccine on lambing losses caused by experimental challenge with *Toxoplasma gondii*. N Z Vet J 35:31-34

50. Uggla A, Araujo FG, Lundén A, Lövgren K, Remington JS, Morein B (1988) Immunizing effects in mice of two *Toxoplasma gondii* Iscom preparations. J Vet Med B 35:311-314

51. Buxton D, Uggla A, Lövgren K, Thomson K, Lundén A, Morein B, Blewett DA (1989) Trial of a novel ISCOM vaccine in pregnant sheep. Br Vet J 145:451-457

52. Lundén A (1995) Immune responses in sheep after immunization with *Toxoplasma gondii* antigens incorporated into iscoms. Vet Parasit 56:23-35

53. Khan IA, Smith KA, Kasper LH (1988) Induction of antigen-specific parasiticidal cytotoxic T cell splenocytes by a major membrane protein (P30) of *Toxoplasma gondii*. J Immunol 141:3600-3605

54. Mineo JR, McLeod R, Mack D, Smith J, Khan IA, Ely KH, Kasper LH (1993) Antibodies to *Toxoplasma gondii* major surface protein (SAG-1, P30) inhibit infection of host cells and are produced in murine intestine after peroral infection. J Immunol 150:3951-3964
55. Bülow R, Boothroyd JC (1991) Protection of mice from fatal *Toxoplasma gondii* infection by immunization with p30 antigen in liposomes. J Immunol 147:3496-3500
56. Bourguin I, Chardes T, Bout D (1993) Oral immunization with *Toxoplasma gondii* antigens in association with cholera toxin induces enhanced protective and cell-mediated immunity in C57BL/6 mice. Infect Immun 61:2082-2088
57. Debard N, Buzoni-Gatel D, Bout D (1996) Intranasal immunization with SAG1 protein of *Toxoplasma gondii* in association with cholera toxin dramatically reduces development of cerebral cysts after oral infection. Infect Immun 64:2158-2166
58. Kasper LH, Currie KM, Bradley S (1985) An unexpected response to vaccination with a purified major membrane tachyzoite antigen (P30) of *Toxoplasma gondii*. J Immunol 134:3426-3431
59. Mowat A Mcl, Donachie AM, Reid G, Jarret O (1991) Immune stimulating complexes containing Quil A and protein antigen prime class I MHC-restricted T lymphocytes in vivo and are immunogenic by the oral route. Immunol 72:317-322
60. Cesbron-Delauw MF, Tomavo S, Beauchamps P, Fourmaux MP, Camus D, Capron A, Dubremetz JF (1994) Similarities between the primary structures of two distinct major surface proteins of *Toxoplasma gondii*. J Biol Chem 269:16217-16222
61. Lundén A, Parmley SF, Bengtsson KL, Araujo FG (1997) Use of a recombinant antigen, SAG2, expressed as a glutathione-S-transferase fusion protein to immunize mice against *Toxoplasma gondii*. Parasitol Res 83:6-9
62. Bohne W, Gross U, Ferguson DJ, Heesemann J (1995) Cloning and characterization of a bradyzoite-specifically expressed gene (hsp30/bag1) of *Toxoplasma gondii*, related to genes encoding small heat-shock proteins of plants. Mol Microbiol 16:1221-1230
63. Odberg Ferragut C, Soete M, Engels A, Samyn B, Loyens A, Van Beeumen J, Camus D, Dubremetz JF (1996) Molecular cloning of the *Toxoplasma gondii* SAG4 gene encoding an 18 kDa bradyzoite specific surface protein. Mol Biochem Parasitol 82:237-244
64. Roberts CW, Brewer JM, Alexander J (1994) Congenital toxoplasmosis in the Balb/c mouse: Prevention of vertical disease transmission and fetal death by vaccination. Vaccine 12:1389-1394
65. Powers DC, Manning MC, Hanscome PJ, Pietrobon PJ (1995) Cytotoxic T lymphocyte responses to a liposome-adjuvanted influenza A virus vaccine in the elderly. J Infect Dis 172:1103-1107
66. Zhou F, Rouze B, Huang L (1992) Induction of cytotoxic T lymphocytes in vivo with protein antigen entrapped in membranous vesicles. J Immunol 149:1599-1604
67. Scott P (1993) IL-12: initiation cytokine for cell-mediated immunity. Science 260:496-497
68. Tighe H, Corr M, Roman M, Raz E (1998) Gene vaccination: plasmid DNA is more than just a blueprint. Parasitol Today 19:89-97
69. Fomsgaard A, Vedel Nielsen H, Johansson K, Nielsen, Machuca R, Bruun L, Hansen J, Buus Søren (1998) Improved humoral and cellular immune responses against the gp 120 V3 loop of HIV-1 folowing genetic immunization with a chimeric DNA vaccine encoding the V3 inserted into the Hepatitis B Surface antigen. Scand J Immunol 47:289-95
70. Alarcon JB, Waine GW, McManus DP (1999) DNA vaccines: technology and application as anti-parasite and anti-microbial agents. Adv Parasitol 42:343-410
71. Burns JM Jr, Adeeku EK, Dunn PD (1999) Protective immunization with a novel membrane protein of *Plasmodium yoelii*-infected erythrocytes. Infect Immun 67:675-680
72. Rodriguez F, An LL, Harkins S, Zhang J, Yokoyama M, Widera G, Fuller JT, Kincaid C, Campbell IL, Whitton JL (1998) DNA immunization with minigenes: low frequency of memory cytotoxic T lymphocytes and inefficient antiviral protection are rectified by ubiquitination. J Virol 72:5174-5181
73. Leitner WW, Seguin MC, Ballou WR, Seitz JP, Schultz AM, Sheehy MJ, Lyon JA (1997) Immune responses induced by intramuscular or gene gun injection of protective deoxyribonucleic acid vaccines that express the circumsporozoite protein from *Plasmodium berghei* malaria parasites. J Immunol 159:6112-6119
74. Becker SI, Wang R, Hedstrom RC, Aguiar JC, Jones TR, Hoffman SL, Gardner MJ (1998) Protection of mice against *Plasmodium yoelii* sporozoite challenge with *P. yoelii* merozoite surface protein 1 DNA vaccines. Infect Immun 66:3457-3461
75. Hanke T, Schneider J, Gilbert SC, Hill AV, McMichael A (1998) DNA multi-CTL epitope vaccines for HIV and *Plasmodium falciparum*: immunogenicity in mice. Vaccine 16:426-435

Conclusion

P. AMBROISE-THOMAS, E. PETERSEN

Thanks to the collaboration of many colleagues who are among the most experienced specialists in this field, we hope that this book will contribute to a better knowledge of the latest data of several biological, clinical and therapeutic aspects of congenital toxoplasmosis, as well as of the prospects for the diagnosis, treatment and prevention of this disease.

This book cannot provide all the answers to all questions. As a matter of fact, toxoplasmosis is a complex protozoan disease, just like the biology of its causative agent, *Toxoplasma gondii*.

Concerning some important aspects, particularly screening and prevention measures, we have deliberately decided to present different solutions adopted in different countries, or groups of countries, rather than a mere general overview of all the European countries. This presentation will perhaps give the impression that discrepancies exist, although these are more apparent than real since the solutions that have been adopted in each case depend on the local epidemiological situation and experience. The decision to perform routine screening or not, before or after birth, and the choice of the appropriate therapeutic protocol give rise to questions to which univocal answers do not – and probably cannot – exist. It is indeed always very difficult to validate a prophylactic protocol, and this is true in particular for a congenital disease. For congenital toxoplasmosis, the experience of only one country cannot serve as a universal model as it corresponds to a given epidemiological situation. Conversely, the idea to group together widely different observations, from different countries, in order to draft a general overview may lead to erroneous conclusions.

It is important to avoid dogmatic positions and until our diagnostic and therapeutic tools are improved or until new prophylactic tools are available (vaccination), a state of relative uncertainty will undoubtedly prevail as to the best course of action.

The efficacy of prophylactic measures is particularly difficult to evaluate in a congenital disease as congenital toxoplasmosis, whose consequences, mainly ocular, sometimes appear several years later. From a very pragmatic medical, but also ethical, point of view, a parallel can be drawn between therapeutic rules and prophylactic measures during pregnancy. The rule is indeed that a pregnant woman should never be prescribed a drug which could be only suspected of being potentially teratogenic or embryotoxic. In a similar way, it is logical to accept that if an infected pregnant woman may transmit a disease to her fetus, prevention methods will be used even if they are only partly effective, provided they cause no harm. The different policies in different countries on treatment and prevention clearly demonstrate that we need more knowledge which can only obtained by clinical studies with careful collection and registration of data.

CET OUVRAGE A ÉTÉ ACHEVÉ D'IMPRIMER EN OCTOBRE 1999
SUR LES PRESSES DE L'IMPRIMERIE DE L'INDÉPENDANT
53200 CHÂTEAU-GONTIER - FRANCE
DÉPÔT LÉGAL : 4ᵉ TRIMESTRE 1999